W9-BAC-382

Hospital Economics

Hospital Economics

Sylvester E. Berki
University of Michigan

Lexington Books
D.C. Heath and Company
Lexington, Massachusetts
Toronto London

Fifth printing December 1977

Published simultaneously in Canada.

Printed in the United States of America.

International Standard Book Number: 0-669-75366-1

Library of Congress Catalog Card Number: 72-165462

Contents

List of Figures

List of Tables

Preface

My purpose in this book is to address the issue of how the central part of the American medical care system, the hospital, can be understood. For the understanding of its objectives, functions, and contributions, the understanding of its economic bases of operations, is prerequisite to the formulation of policies to assure that all Americans, regardless of race, color, religion, economic status, sex, national origin, and cultural values, can best benefit from the medical services our technology and resources can provide.

While I have made the attempt, I claim no success. My hope is that hospital administrators, medical care specialists, economists, planners, and policy analysts will find this book sufficiently stimulating and irritating to make them consider the unresolved issues, to engage in the requisite research, to rethink the unanswered questions which are required to enable us to construct a system of medical care within which our resources are most efficiently used in the betterment of life.

I have many debts. But I shall not name all those from whom I have learned, for I do not wish them to share in the blame my errors will elicit. Nonetheless, and with the usual proviso that they have attempted, without success, to correct my errant ways, I must acknowledge my indebtedness to my colleagues Professors S.J. Axelrod, A. Donabedian, W.L. Dowling, and C.A. Metzner, and to Uwe Reinhardt.

My wife Minnie and my Mother sustained me as much as the memory of my Father. Indulgence though it may be, I must thank my children Lisa and Matthew for trying to live with the nervous wreck of an absent father. To my son Andrew's question, "Daddy, why did you have to write a book?" I could only answer, "Because it was there." I hope the reader will have a better one.

Introduction

> The hospital is to modern America what the cathedral was to Europe in the Middle Ages: a complex social institution serving simultaneously a variety of purposes—welfare center, object of civic pride, major source of employment, market for artists, artisans, and architects, inspirer of saintly deeds and beneficiary of repentant sinners, occasional "cover-up" for hypocrites and exploiters, source of power, and object of political conflict.
>
> —A. Somers, *Hospital Regulation*, p. ix.

With the essential elimination or control, at least in our society, of the major contagious and parasitic diseases, the current function of the medical care sector is restorative and ameliorative. It is sickness care. Medical services are provided to retard the progression and to alleviate the implications of chronic diseases, to terminate successfully episodes of acute illness, and to attempt to ease the process of dying. Medical care is designed to cure when it can, to manage when it cannot cure, and to dignify when it can do neither. There is a consensus that the medical care sector, while ever costing more, is not performing any of its functions well for all those who could benefit by them, a nearly ubiquitous view that there is a "health care crisis." The multiplicity of proposals for the cure in terms of delivery, organization, financing, and control is evidence that dissatisfaction with the performance of the medical care sector has reached the status of a politicized social problem. As in other complex diseases, while there is agreement that something is drastically wrong, there is no consensus on either the diagnosis or the therapy. And the prognosis is pessimistic.

Of the large set of proximate causes of the malfunctioning of the medical care sector—which in a more detailed analysis are seen as symptoms—we may identify the four salient ones:

1. Shortages in the availability of providers and resources—particularly in the inner cities of large metropolitan areas and in the low population density sectors of the country—as well as barriers to access to the available resources. This is demonstrated in long waiting times in doctors' offices and in hospital outpatient clinics, difficulties in getting appointments and admissions for elective procedures where service capabilities are present, and the high incidence of remediable conditions together with low rates of utilization for the poor, the black, and the other socially disadvantaged population groups.
2. High and still rapidly rising costs with no dampening mechanism in sight. Increases in the prices of medical care services exceed those of the general inflation or price increases in all other services, with hospital prices rising at the rate of 15 percent per year. Yet there is no obvious equilibrating tendency that might eventually retard or eliminate these price and cost increases.

3. With multiple and uncoordinated entry points to an increasingly mass production system of fragmented care, the patient is lost in the maze.
4. The rapidly rising cost of services together with shifts in the age distribution of the population and selected increases in utilization rates by certain cohorts have resulted in a significant relative enlargement of the medical care sector. In fiscal year 1971 the medical care sector of the American economy absorbed 7.4 percent of the Gross National Product, or $75 billion, representing a per capita expenditure of $358. The largest single component of this expenditure, 39 percent, or almost $30 billion, was for hospital services.

That part of the hospital industry which provides the bulk of general clinical services, and which is the focus of our analysis, is comprised of voluntary, proprietary, and state and local governmental short-term general and special hospitals, generally known as community hospitals. While employing more than 76 percent of the sector's personnel, they provide 74 percent of outpatient visits, more than 92 percent of all admissions, and absorb 77 percent of the cost of hospital care. More than 241 million patient days of care and almost 134 million outpatient visits were produced by community hospitals at a cost exceeding $22 billion (see table I-1). And these costs are expected to more than double by 1980.

The hospital can be conceived to be a flexible set of departments within an institutional setting which produce a mix of multidimensional services. The services can be categorized as: (a) consumption and investment, (b) medical and hotel type services, (c) inpatient and ambulatory, (d) personal and community, depending on the purposes of analysis. If our focus of interest is the assessment of the hospital's role in satisfying patient preferences by producing those services which the patient considers desirable and which, therefore, enter his preference

Table I-1
Some Selected Characteristics of Community Hospitals

	Total	Nonprofit	For-profit	State and Local Government
		Number		
Hospitals	5,859	3,386	769	1,704
Beds	848,232	591,937	52,739	203,556
Admissions	29,251,655	20,948,080	2,030,669	6,272,906
Patient days	241,458,815	173,154,540	13,903,215	54,401,060
Outpatient visits	133,544,672	90,922,193	4,698,200	37,854,279

Source: *Medical Care Costs and Prices: Background Book.* Department of Health, Education and Welfare, Social Security Administration, Office of Research and Statistics Document 72-11908.

function, its output is correctly seen as a bundle of consumption goods. From the perspective of social resource allocation, the same set of goods and services may be seen as investment in human capital, designed to maintain or to improve the quantity and quality of the economy's pool of potential labor inputs. There are two factors, however, which we must note in any analysis: the interconnectedness of the medical care sector and the hospital's pervasive centrality within it.

The medical care sector provides a wide variety of services which have but one common denominator: the expectation that either in the short or the long run they will lead to the maintenance or improvement of human health, or, failing that, will minimize the effects of disease and injury. Even though the implicit definition of health here, in terms of functional abilities, is rather narrow, disregarding as it does the social and political dimensions, the set of services produced on the assumption that medical intervention will yield beneficial results is complex.

Classificatory schemes of services may be based on morphological principles, giving rise to their categorization by the organ systems at which they are directed. In such a scheme services are seen as medical, dental, optometric, etc., or, at a higher level of specificity, as internal, neurological, orthopedic, thoracic, orthodontic, ophthalmic, etc. Yet other methods of classification envisage services as direct patient and auxiliary, with functions performed on the fluids, tissues, and cells in the laboratory, such as pathology and microbiology, falling in the latter category. Note that, with the exception of the laboratory, we have not considered so far any method of classification that relies on the site at which the services are provided. In such a system one differentiates home, office, and clinic visits, inpatient care in short-term and long-term hospitals, and domiciliary care in extended care facilities such as nursing homes.

It is useful to classify services according to their primary purpose. In this taxonomy by function we can identify seven basic categories of services:

1. *Preventive*, designed to minimize the likelihood of events or conditions resulting in the diminution of attainable health levels;
2. *Diagnostic*, designed to identify such conditions in individual humans, usually termed disease;
3. *Therapeutic*, services which are expected to terminate successfully episodes of acute illness or to minimize the severity and impact of chronic conditions;
4. *Maintenance*, services designed to maintain attained health levels;
5. *Ameliorative*, processes whose purpose is to reduce the physiological and psychological discomforts of incurable conditions and to ease the process of dying for terminal patients;
6. *Research*, activities whose fundamental long-term objectives are improvement in the processes of prevention, diagnosis, and therapy; and
7. *Medical education*, activities designed to disseminate accepted medical knowl-

edge and the techniques required for the production of the first five categories, the preventive and curative processes.

While medical research and education can be identified with a relatively narrow spectrum of providers such as the medical schools, teaching hospitals, governmental, foundation, and private laboratories, all of the other services are provided by a multiplicity of individual practitioners in a variety of institutional settings.

The community hospital is not only the most resource intensive source of care, not only the primary and often sole source of care for large urban populations, it is unique in that while there are some services in the medical care sector of which the hospital is the unique producer, there exist no services which are not produced within, or under its institutional aegis. For some services there are no alternative productive processes, for many others substitutes exist. Visits to private physician offices and to outpatient clinics, diagnoses in independent laboratory facilities or in hospital laboratories, or even home care by private practitioners or by hospital staff in Progressive Patient Care programs are a few, but basic, examples of interdependence through substitutability in production. Interdependence with other elements of the medical care sector also arises through externalities in production, of which the principal example is the information generation and dissemination function of physician-hospital interaction, from medical training through attending privileges.

Interdependence with other production processes of personal care services and the degree of substitutability of these processes, varying with diagnostic categories, establish the production trade-offs between hospitals and all other technically feasible sources of services. For any given diagnostic category for which treatment substitutability is technically feasible, the interaction of five sets of complex factors determines which of the feasible modes of production will be chosen. The factors are: (1) the relative stocks of service capabilities and their relative prices, (2) the preference functions of potential patients, (3) the preference function of the medical decision maker, (4) the reward system facing the medical decision maker, and (5) the budget constraint faced by the patient. Postulating the medical decision maker's preference function to incorporate preferences over treatment options in a technical sense at any given level of the state of the arts, and assuming that the decision maker is the private physician, the choice between diagnosis in the office, on an ambulatory basis with the use of hospital facilities, or on an inpatient basis will result from the interaction of these five sets of factors and their realtive "weights."

Since our primary purpose is the analysis of hospital production processes, we shall not deal at length with patient and physician preference functions and their interactions. What we do wish to do, however, is to consider the hospital as a specialized yet integral component in the production of medical care services. The questions of hospital utilization, costs, efficiency, pricing, or functions cannot be meaningfully posed unless the hospital is seen as an important cog, but only a cog, in an interrelated system. As will be shown in the discussion of differential utilization and costs under varying institutional configurations, practice settings, and financial arrangements, demand for the services of hospitals, and their costs, are not independent of the above five factors.

It is important to realize, and to take into account explicitly, that the demand for and utilization of hospital services, for a given population and disease distribution, is not a single-valued function of medical knowledge, or of physician's preferences, or of the number of available beds. In many cases the chosen diagnostic or therapeutic process will be determined, to rephrase the formulation, by the availability of substitutes, their costs, and the nature of the rewards to both physician and patient.

To address the issues of hospital utilization, cost, efficiency, functions, and relationships to the other parts of the medical care system, it would be helpful to have an explicit model of the medical care sector.

To have an explicit model of the relevant sector means that we must be able to define the relevant sector boundaries in terms of the interdependence of decision-making units within the sector and their relationships to other sectors. It also means that we must be able to formulate precisely objective functions, production functions, resource and other relevant constraints, for each of the decision-making units. This necessitates specification of the expected shapes of the functions: the arguments and their relationships to each other must be made precise. Unless we are interested in purely heuristic or theoretical problems, the relevant variables and parameters of the model must be operationally specified: they must be empirically testable. And to be able to evaluate normatively the observed and now measured results, there must exist in explicit form a set of value judgments, a set of standards incorporating social, ethical, political, and economic values, by which the results can be said to be "good" or "bad." For while it is true that the proof of the pudding is in the eating, social policy results are often irreversible, hence it is advisable to make sure that none of the ingredients are toxic (170, p. 3).

The literature on hospitals yields no puddings; even ingredients are rare. And above all, there is no recipe. We cannot even be sure what the ingredients should be.

In her incisive look at the problems of public policy in the area of medical care, and of hospitals specifically, A.R. Somers (397) concludes that prior to any meaningful solutions the conceptual issues must be worked out and our understanding of the empirical phenomena improved. She lists ten areas which suffer from lack of conceptualization and valid empirical research. They are:

1. The definition of a hospital.
2. The definition of a hospital system.
3. Measures of hospital cost and productivity.

4. The relation of the hospital to other health services.
5. The accurate allocation of costs.
6. Comprehensive insurance coverage of ambulatory care.
7. Hospital-physician relationships.
8. Hospital labor relations and personnel policies.
9. Reimbursement.
10. Hospital liability.

"Clarification in *all* these areas is a prerequisite to any effective attack on the problem of hospital financing" (397, p. 353).

The Gorham Report, after a careful consideration of the problems of rising prices and costs, concludes that the major obstacle to analysis "is that there are no generally accepted measures of output, input, and productivity in the hospital sector" (271, p. 32).

We shall attempt to provide a framework for the analysis of the operations of short-term general (acute) hospitals and to review critically the burgeoning literature within this framework.

In chapter 1 we construct an analytic framework which stresses the multiplicity of demands facing the hospital as a diversified production unit at the heart of the medical care system. Unlike the analysis of other production units of the economy, we cannot posit the existence of a single objective in terms of profit maximization. Patients, physicians, administrators, researchers, teaching units, and the communities which support the hospitals financially may all envision separate and distinct goals to be attained by the hospital. In chapter 2, therefore, we consider *Hospital Objectives.* The analysis of production and efficiency requires that we have an operational definition of *outputs*, which we consider in chapter 3. Chapters 4 and 5 are devoted to the discussion of *productivity, costs,* and *efficiency*, with emphasis on the issues of economies of scale and efficiency. *Utilization* and *demand* can best be considered by keeping in mind that, unlike the demand for other commodities and most other services, the demands for medical care are often involuntary. The extent to which medical care is perceived as a "good" is debatable. That small portion of the services which is devoted to the prevention of illness or its early diagnosis is perhaps within the set of the usual economic "goods." But since our system is essentially oriented to crisis sickness care, the services may be seen not as "goods" but rather as necessary evils. Medical care, like television repairs and opening up the clogged drain, is not something people want because it is satisfying and enjoyable in itself. This is discussed in some detail in chapter 6. With increasing demands for hospital services and an increasingly larger share of the financial costs of operations being assumed by insurance carriers and public funds, the issues of *pricing* and *reimbursement* are central to the attempt to bring about efficient operations. Chapter 7 is devoted to these questions.

The urban government hospital system, the *municipals*, is characterized by all the problems associated with other types of short-term hospitals. But in addition to that, while they are encrusted with bureaucratic controls, subject to the whimsies of political organizations, generally considered a bottomless pit for public tax funds, they attempt to serve the medical care needs of the disadvantaged, the forgotten, the poor, the teeming urban masses of a suburban society. Chapter 8 is devoted to the special problems of municipal hospitals.

Our approach shall be to pose the issues in analytic terms. We shall posit the relevant questions to ask and we shall inquire what the existing literature has to contribute to their solutions.

We shall find that while no single book or article enables us to arrive at definitive answers, the literature as a whole permits us to phrase the proper questions.

Hospital Economics

1 The Framework of Analysis

> Man, in building theories, patches up his world image in order to integrate what he knows with what he needs, and he makes of it all (for he must live as he studies) a design for living.
>
> –E.H. Erikson, *Childhood and Society*, p. 414.

The Medical Care Decision Process

Consider that there exists some level of perceived need which eventuates in the potential patient's decision to seek care. Once that decision is made, contact with a primary provider is initiated. At this juncture the patient enters the formal medical care system, and the medical care process begins. We shall discuss this process in greater detail in chapter 6, so for now it is sufficient to consider that at the initial entry point there is some level of patient originated demand for services which is ipso facto met. An individual may translate his perceived need into effective demand simply by walking into an emergency room or an outpatient department. The patient presenting himself at the physician's office, the emergency room, or at the outpatient department will generate some minimal level of services by the receptionist, nurse, or diagnostician regardless of the outcome of the diagnostic process. The implied derived demands are for time intensive services at the least. If the symptomatology giving rise to the demand results in diagnostic services of whatever complexity, some production of outputs results. Minimally from the resource allocation perspective, but not so minimally from the psychological point of view, information is produced. At this stage of the process the initial medical decision is made.

It is the outcome of the initial medical decision process which determines the subsequent demands for services. A potential patient cannot have effective demands beyond the initial contact. He can only request, but not express an effective demand for, say, serum cholesterol tests or chest X-ray examinations. He cannot admit himself. The resource intensive services of the medical care sector are legally responsive only to demands translated by, legitimated by, or independently generated by the physician. Hence it is important to consider that while some minimal level of patient originated demands for services can be directly translated into effective demands, with its implied derived demands for medical care services, the overwhelming proportion of potential demands become effective demands, or utilization, if and only if legitimized by professional medical decision makers.

The initial medical decision may result in three outcomes: no diagnosis, diagnosis of a self-limiting condition, or a positive diagnosis of an acute or chronic condition. The first two outcomes (no diagnosis or self-limiting condition) either terminate the process of care if they satisfy patient expectations or trigger an iterative process if they do not. That is, if the potential patient for whatever reason does not agree with the diagnostic outcome, he may seek out a different primary contact and reenter the diagnostic process once again.

A probable positive diagnosis of a condition thought to be amenable to medical intervention initiates a stream of demands both for further diagnostic services and for therapeutic services. The nature of the outcome of this initial medical decision process is determined by five sets of factors: (1) the patient's medical condition, (2) the state of medical knowledge, (3) the patient's socioeconomic characteristics, (4) physician characteristics, and (5) alternative available supplies of medically appropriate services. Since it is these sets of variables that determine the demand for and utilization of hospital services, let us consider them in somewhat more detail by referring to their schematic representation in figure 1-1.

When the patient enters the medical decision process, presupposing his expectation that the system is capable of relieving his anxiety and of correcting his perceived imbalance (or dis-ease), his initial demand is for information.

We need not speculate here on the complex patient-physician interaction in terms of joint decision making, a subject inadequately studied and meriting much further research. It is useful to assume that the patient's entry into the system itself manifests his belief in the medical decision maker's ability to choose the medically appropriate course of action. The patient's belief is of a degree sufficient for him to delegate to the medical expert the function of choice making. This does not imply that congruence between medical expert and patient choices is totally maintained throughout the medical care process. Patient agreement and hence patient medical behavior may, and often does, diverge from the course of action chosen by the medical expert for economic, social, temperamental, cultural, or psychological reasons. Continued cigarette smoking and high fat and caloric intake are obvious examples. Nevertheless, it is the medical expert whose decision generates demands for medical services.

At any given time there exists a set of diagnostic and therapeutic processes, which are the equivalents of technical production functions, embodying the current state of knowledge.[a] The medical decision maker is the sole and unique participant in this process who has command of the state of knowledge. It is almost trivial but nevertheless fundamental to the understanding of the medical process to stress that it is the physician who alone can and must make the

[a]That there exists an optimal production function, that the medically "best" diagnostic and therapeutic processes are known, does not imply that they are universally known. The dissemination of knowledge in medicine is a not well-understood process.

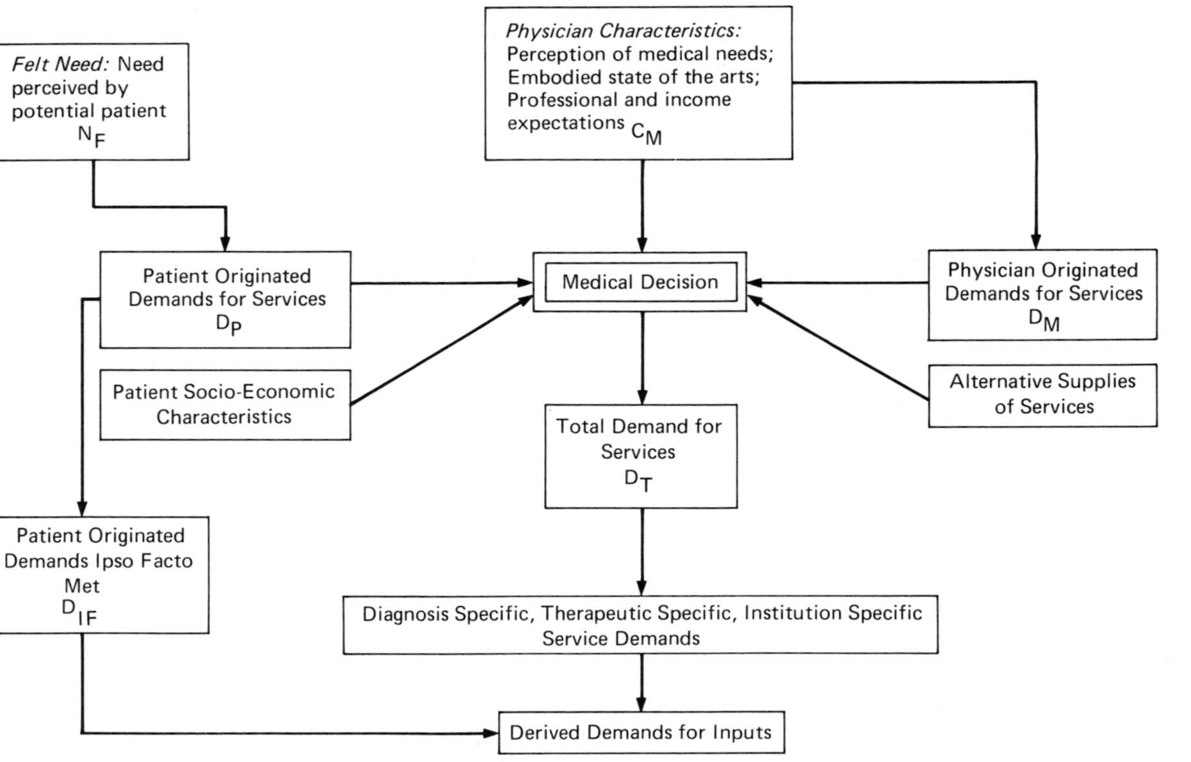

Figure 1–1. Five Sets of Factors Determining Initial Medical Decision Process.

choices which will result in the initiation of the flow of services.[b] His perception of medical needs, his ability to identify the services medically appropriate to those needs, and his knowledge of alternative courses of action constitute his basic contribution. Even disregarding for the moment the relevance of the decision maker's preference function, as opposed to his technical knowledge, it is important to stress that the choice of medically appropriate action is a probabilistic one.

The fairly recent development of increasingly powerful chemical, electronic, radiologic, and inferential diagnostic techniques facilitate accurate diagnoses. But even though the false negatives (no diagnosis when in fact a disease process is present) and false positives (diagnosis when in fact the identified disease process is not present) may be decreasing, in the case of many disease processes the diagnosis is still probabilistic. The therapeutic process is even more so. For while diagnosis is generally designed to attain disease detection, to identify the pathogen, therapy must be tailored to the pathogen embedded in the human host. Hence whether or not a given therapy is likely to be successful depends not only on the accuracy of the diagnosis, but on the individual patient's reaction to the prescribed regimen. His age, the simultaneous presence of other conditions, detected or undetected, his physical stamina, psychological state, social support, along with many other factors, influence both the choice of appropriate therapy as well as its efficacy. Therefore, the physician's ability to select the optimal therapy, even in the case of a clear and accurate diagnosis, is an important determinant of this dimension of the quality of care. Let us assume that in the idealized model of the technically perfect decision maker, the medically optimal choice is attainable with some high probability. This dimension of the decision outcome we call *patient focused*.

Were the physician's decision to result only in patient focused outcomes we might then assume, as we usually do in economic analyses, that the demand for services is exogeneously determined. That is, we could then assume that the physician performs for the patient the technologically constrained choice which the patient is unequipped to do. He could then be seen as decomposing into its elements the demand bundle presented by the patient, with the demand being independent of the objective function of the supplier. But the physician's decision results in outcomes other than those which are patient focused.

Assuming that the decision maker is not indifferent to the financial rewards, peer recognition, professional status rewards, community recognition, and so on, associated with alternative patient focused outcomes, it is reasonable to expect that his preferences in these respects, or his valuations of them, are relevant in

[b]We are using the term "physician" as a shorthand for medical decision maker. Other medical workers also perform the decision function if within a smaller choice set focused on a narrower range of issues. Further, the physician of course may and does delegate some decision functions, but at least in our society he retains the ultimate legal responsibility for the decisions and consequent actions.

understanding his medical decisions. Especially where alternative diagnostic and treatment processes are available and considered probabilistically medically appropriate, the chosen course of action is likely to be the one which the physician expects to maximize his preference function. It is at this point that the concept of *physician originated demand* becomes relevant. While we shall consider this point in greater detail within the institutional framework of the hospital, it is fundamental to the understanding of the total demand for medical services to point out that considerations other than purely patient focused medical ones play an important role in the formation of total effective demand for medical services.

The decision maker is likely to choose from among the available alternatives that course of action which he associates with the highest reward state to himself. Service demands may be originated by the physician for purposes of research, for teaching, for demonstrating high esoteric skill achievement, for status, and for increasing his income or decreasing his workload, or both simultaneously. None of these elements need be detrimental to patient focused medical outcomes. But they differ from them in that the desired results are expected to benefit primarily the decision maker. The shotgun approach to diagnostic laboratory procedures, admissions for treatment when ambulatory alternatives exist, complex surgical procedures of debatable therapeutic value (of which heart transplants are the example *reductio ad absurdum*) are some cases where patient welfare need not be the primary determinant.

The medical decision is subject to three types of constraints. In figure 1-1 we indicate two of these, the patient's socioeconomic characteristics and the availability of alternative supplies of services. Prior to discussing these factors, it must be considered that there exist a set of ethical, legal, and institutional factors which both help shape the physician's preferences and constrain his choice set. Legal prohibition of fee splitting, or the inability of one physician to charge another physician for referring patients, legal prohibition against the delegation of certain medical functions to persons who are not licensed to perform them are some examples of legal constraints. (We are not here concerned either with the rationale or economic irrationality of some of these prohibitions.) Many of the institutional constraints are presented in the context of quality control. Thus, required consultation prior to certain surgical operations, the medical record review prior to admission, and the clinico-pathologic conference, variously required in various institutions, while designed to increase or to maintain the medical quality of care, also serve as constraints on the medical decision. The practice setting, or institutional matrix of the physician, partly determined by his preferences, also, at the same time, acts to shape them. Even if we continue to assume that technical medical knowledge is uniformly distributed, both the perception of medical need and the relative weights of preferences on physician focused outcomes are likely to be influenced by the decision maker's professional and physical location. The physician in private fee-for-service solo practice with an established referral practice in a suburban setting is likely to make choices that will differ from those of an equally technically competent clinician on salary in a multi-specialty group practice. And their choices may both differ from the harried internist in the emergency room of a city hospital.

The patient's willingness and ability to pay himself or to have paid on his behalf by private or public insurance or other mechanisms is an important constraint on the medical decision. While this need not imply that this constraint is inflexible regardless of the patient's medical condition, where alternatives with different costs and prices exist, the financial considerations will be relevant. They will be relevant with respect to the intensity, complexity, and locus of services chosen.

The nature of insurance coverage, for example, is believed to have a significant effect on the choice of the locus of services. Health insurance which provides payment for diagnostic services performed on an inpatient basis, but not for the same services on an ambulatory basis, assuming that both alternatives are available, is likely to result in admission. A public program which provides payment for prenatal care in a physician's office, but not for the same care in a hospital outpatient department, is likely to influence both the scope and the place of service.[c]

In addition to the direct costs and prices, the patient's income security may also be relevant. One of the peculiarities associated with the consumption of certain medical care services such as inpatient care is that increased consumption of it, like that of leisure, not only reallocates the patient's income but, in the absence of income security such as sick pay, reduces it. Hence when alternative medical processes with different income losses (or opportunity income foregone) are present, they may well influence the outcome of the medical decision.

It need not be stressed that the patient's age, family status, education, and social status are variables relevant in the *physician's* choice of care pattern. We stress that they are relevant in the medical expert's decision since, as we shall see, in most of the economic analyses of demand for medical care they have been assumed to be relevant in patient generated demands. Should we, for example, find a higher rate of hospitalization for conditions manageable on an ambulatory basis for children in large families than for children in small families, or for children in lower income than in higher income families, the deductions that larger families have a higher demand for inpatient care, or that the demand for inpatient care is inversely correlated with family incomes are less plausible than the hypothesis that in the medical expert's opinion the appropriate care pattern is less likely to be followed in a household full of children with the

[c]Among the weird and wonderful provisos of Medicaid in Michigan is one which specifies that the payment for delivery will be made in lump sum form only and to private physicians only. Hence if a pregnant mother desires prenatal care, she must find a private physician who for the lump sum maternity payment also delivers prenatal care.

multiple demands on the parents than in one with fewer competing chores. Analogously for the lower income family. In either case, the observed demands for services are indeed related to socioeconomic patient characteristics, but not through the usually assumed differences in patient preferences. The implications of traditional demand analysis for expected utilization patterns will have to be modified under different pricing schemes faced by patients, as we shall see in chapter 6.

The remaining constraint on the medical decision is the availability of alternative supplies of services. The extent to which complex diagnostic facilities are available, as well as their costs to both the patient and the physician, is not independent of the extent of their use. The cost to the decision maker, of course, may be negative. It is not uncharitable to suggest that physicians who own diagnostic facilities are more likely to be extensive users of them. The various state laws prohibiting physician ownership of pharmacies and optometric dispensing facilities demonstrate the recognition of this interaction effect. The availability of hospital beds is not independent of the admission rate, as we shall see in chapter 6.

The availability of alternative supplies of services is determined not only by economic, institutional, and physical factors. One important aspect of availability is accessibility. As we shall discuss in chapter 8, racial, social, and psychological characteristics of both patients and physicians, as well as economic factors, help determine which among the physically available alternative supplies are in fact accessible, hence de facto available.

We have so far considered a general and aggregate model of the medical care decision process within which the medical decision maker plays the central role in determining the process and the implied demands for services. The total demand for services is generated both by patients and by medical providers. When the total demand set is disaggregated into its diagnostic, therapeutic, and locational components, it is clear that only that set of demands we have called *patient originated* directly result in derived demands for services without physician legitimization. Most specific diagnostic and therapeutic ambulatory services are physician originated. With the exception of perhaps cosmetic services, all inpatient services are physician originated. The demands for services and the corresponding derived demands for inputs are not therefore exogenously determined.

The central implication for the analysis of demands, prices, costs, and supplies is that rather than dealing with a recursive system in which the supply and demand equations may be independently estimated, we are faced with an interdependent system. Institutional arrangements, physician and patient preferences, the complexity of medical technology, and a multiplicity of substitutes with differential patient and provider rewards constitute a complex system of interactions which can best be thought of as a system of simultaneous equations.

We have so far stressed that the central decision-making role in the medical care system is that of the physician. He determines what services will be produced. Many diagnostic and therapeutic services can be and are simultaneously produced in private offices, independent laboratories, and the outpatient departments of hospitals. All inpatient care, by definition; many complex diagnostic procedures, those for example involving the use of radioactive isotopes; as well as many types of complex therapeutic processes requiring complex equipment, are generally produced in the hospital if on an outpatient basis. The source of the initial medical contact may be located in a private office, in a clinic, or in the emergency room of a hospital; further, many medical specialties, particularly those requiring highly developed medical technology embedded in equipment, are hospital based. What, then, is the hospital's role in this system?

The Hospital as the Fulcrum of Care

Considering the hospital as an organization of departments producing a flexible heterogeneous service mix, the interaction of factors in the medical care sector not only helps determine the rate of utilization of existing services, but, to some extent, the dimensions of the service mix itself. Thus can we understand the accelerated expansion of outpatient diagnostic and therapeutic services. In the other direction, the fairly recent development of home care by hospital personnel represents a shifting of some patient care functions from within to outside the hospital. The relationships are important, and our comprehension of the factors contributing to changes in treatment patterns is crucial to fruitful analysis. For not only is quality one of the dimensions of output, but since the hospital is the most resource-intensive of the alternative production facilities, it is also the most expensive. Hence differential utilization of alternative treatment processes is economically relevant.

The economic position of potential patients, that is, their budget constraints, as well as the relative prices of alternative services facing them, to a significant extent help to differentiate between private (non-profit, and proprietary) and public hospitals. While we shall define and analyze both private and public organizations later, now we wish to point out that as each member of the set of hospitals produces a heterogeneous service mix, the hospitals within the set are themselves heterogeneous. We shall not consider those that provide long-term care or which are specialized, that is, characterized by a narrow service mix, such as mental and tuberculosis hospitals. Within the non-federal acute hospital set, however, three distinct subsets are present: (1) the private hospital, (2) the public, or municipal, hospital, and (3) the affiliated teaching hospital, private or not. In reviewing the literature we shall discuss some of the differentials in terms of observed costs, and other variables. Here we consider that as the functions of hospitals in general overlap with those of other medical care providers, the functions of the three subsets of hospitals are also interdependent. Their interdependence is, in a considerable measure, attributable to the price differentials of their services and the differential budget constraints of potential patients. The well-established historical pattern has been the provision of services for paying patients in private hospitals, with some "charity" beds in the voluntaries, and public provision of services to the indigent in public institutions. Thus the demand for the public institution's services is extensively influenced by population patterns, income distribution, and alternative zero-price services. And to the extent that public programs have reduced or eliminated the price differentials facing potential patients in the private and public institutions, the specialized functional interdependence of the past has been transformed to result in the current period of chaos and questions. What is the role of the public hospital? And what should it be? To what degree are all hospitals public? What is, and should be the relationship between the hospital and the community?

Our focus is the role and operation of the urban public hospital. In terms of the demand for its services, and by implication, their nature, scope, and quality, it is an intimately related part of the hospital subsector and of the medical care sector in general. The analysis of its organizational, managerial, and sociological configuration might well proceed without considering its relationships to the other parts of the hospital subsector. For the purpose of *economic* analysis of its role, operation, and performance, the relevant sector is that composed of acute hospitals.

Since we are interested in the nature and impact of demand for its services on its performance and costs, we must also explore, however tentatively, the relation of the hospital sector to the rest of medical care. We have provided the economic rationale for it. From the content, or medical perspective, we add that the pattern of care for a given episode of illness may be comprised of three non-exclusive, iterable phases: ambulatory or office care, inpatient care, and post-discharge ambulatory care. Disease history and etiology, the state of the arts in diagnostic and treatment procedures, as well as the relative scarcities of diagnostic and therapeutic facilities on ambulatory and inpatient bases jointly determine feasible patterns of care. Variations in these factors, along with the uncertainty attached to medical outcomes, determine the repeatability of the inpatient phase for a given diagnosis. Some diagnoses generally do not require hospitalization (e.g., essential benign hypertension); others do (e.g., benign prostatic hypertrophy and malignant disease). For this reason, as well as to be able to identify the nature and appropriateness of services rendered patients, it would be desirable to have a model in terms of well-identified diagnostic categories.

Not in all episodes will all three phases be present. But with very few exceptions, at least two of the three will be. Observed differentials in hospital inpatient utilization in terms of admission rates and length of stay are tractable to analysis only within a framework that explicitly incorporates the economically relevant variables. In the analysis of hospital operations the existence of alternative diagnostic and therapeutic processes and facilities during the same or different phases of the episode of illness is economically relevant.

We consider the hospital to be an organization of a set of departments each producing a set of outputs, services. In analyzing the hospital as a producing unit we posit that it produces the following set of outputs:

1. Personal Medical Care—Patient Care
1.1 Ambulatory Care
1.2 Inpatient Care
    1.2.1 Direct Patient Care Services (i.e., nursing)
    1.2.2 Indirect Patient Care, Ancillary Services (i.e., pathology)
    1.2.3 Direct Patient Non-medical Services (i.e., "hotel" services)
    1.2.4 General Housekeeping and Maintenance Services
    1.2.5 Administrative Services
2. Community Medical Care—Ambulance Services, Social Work Services, Community Health Centers
3. Information Dissemination Services—Medical Staff Affiliation, Medical Seminars, Continuing Education
4. Teaching and Training Services—Intern and Residency Programs, Nursing School Programs, Medical Technician and Paramedical Training
5. Research in Medicine and Medical Technology

Were our focus the development of production functions for acute hospitals, each of the output categories would be further disaggregated and departmental outputs precisely specified, which we shall consider in chapters 4 and 5.

We shall hence refer to a hospital's "output mix" to differentiate it from what the literature calls the "service mix" or "service complexity," since that definition usually has relevance to our output category 1.2 (Inpatient Care) exclusively. We shall distinguish somewhat further output component 1.2.1, Direct Patient Care Services, along functional dimensions, namely, medical-surgical, obstetrical, and pediatric. Direct Patient Non-medical Service, category 1.2.3, will be further specified along accommodation dimensions: ward, semi-private, private.

Without considering for the moment by whom and by what procedures it is defined, we postulate that for each hospital there exists an Objective Function which it wishes to maximize, subject to a set of endogenous and exogenous constraints. What constitutes the argument of the objective function and which are the relevant constraints are the subject of much debate. Unlike the analysis of the individual profit-making firm, we can not assume an objective function expressed in terms of profit which the firm then attempts to maximize. Analogously to the analysis of individual consumption behavior, we assume that the hospital's objective function is complex. We assume that the objective function is expressed in terms of the quantity and quality of output mix, physical facilities, and prestige. The elements of the argument are assumed to have differential weights: the hospital may "prefer" higher quality to greater output quantity, or it may prefer increased physical facilities independently of its output mix implication to both.

Since we are not constrained by the mathematical complexities resulting from interdependence of elements within the objective function, and since it enables us to derive useful conclusions from the analysis, we assume that the quantity and quality of output mix and prestige are interdependent. This implies that the quantity and quality of the output mix incorporated in the objective function are partially determined by the weight given to "prestige," where that is defined as professional (medical) prestige, community approbation, and socio-ideological sanctions. "Institutional status" can be defined as its equivalent. We wish to consider explicitly, for example, that while inpatient care as a component of the product mix may enter independently into the objective function, ambulatory care, community medical care, and teaching and training services may enter, or if present be given perceptible weight only through their interdependence with the community approbation component of institutional status.

We shall not now consider in any detail how, through what procedures, and by whom the objective function is defined, partly because it is clear that here the distinction between private and public hospitals may be relevant. It might be suggested that the distinction between public and private may also be relevant in the definition of the content of the objective function. We are assuming that it is not. We shall show that an objective function of essentially the same content can be assumed for both private and public acute hospitals for two reasons. The tenor of socio-ideological sanctions and community approbation no longer distinguish significantly between private and public institutions. And second, two important elements in the definition of objectives, the physicians comprising the medical staff and the hospital administrator, have essentially identical preferences or values irrespective of their institutional setting. This raises the interesting sociological question of the extent to which professional and occupational status considerations outweigh organizational identification and in fact influence institutional goals. For economic analysis the relevant points are two: the impact of the physicians' preferences on the objective function of the hospital in terms of output mix, and the implied resource costs.

The hospital's objective function is maximized subject to a set of constraints. Some of the constraints relate to the quality of care, the manning and organization of certain medical departments, and other medical aspects for which minimum standards are established by the relevant bodies of accreditation. Since accreditation is a prerequisite for the maintenance of internship and residency programs, and is helpful in receiving certification for participation in public insurance programs such as Medicare and Medicaid, the criteria, while minimal, act as constraints on at least some aspects of hospital production.

Additional certification required for participation in the largest private insurance program, Blue Cross, as well as increasing facility regulation by public bodies, such as the regional planning agencies, impose additional constraints.

For simplicity and because it appears to permit useful analysis, we assume two financial constraints: maximum acceptable yearly operating deficit and a capital-budget constraint. That is, we assume that the objective function will be maximized subject to not exceeding some deficit perceived as acceptable (which constraint is therefore somewhat flexible) and an absolute limit on available funds for net investment. In the case of public hospitals, the acceptable yearly operating deficit may be defined two ways: the current value of expected possible supplemental appropriations, or, in "tight" organizations, zero.

The distinction between operating deficit and capital constraint, as we shall see, is required, since both private voluntary and public hospitals are subject to functional funding, the basic distinction being usually between operating and capital funds.

Since the hospital's objective function is assumed to be defined by some *n*-tuple of individuals with assumed different individual preferences over the elements of the objective function, the agreed upon operating objective function must be one which assures the hospital's internal viability. If the operating objective function does not satisfy the minimal preferences of one or more internal constituencies, either hospital operations will be altered or the objective function must be redefined. Should the cardiac surgeons, for example, have strong preferences for maintaining an open heart surgical team in conflict with the desires of the administrators and the board of governors, and should their preferences not be met, the surgeons may relocate and thereby severely limit the hospital's possible scope of services. Demands for private patient privileges by staff physicians, which may conflict with the wishes of the other constituencies, differing preferences of the administrator, of the staff physicians, and of the affiliated attending physicians over length of stay or the scale of operations of outpatient clinics, constitute examples of possible internal conflict.

It might be argued that the formulation of an objective function incorporating multiple non-harmonious individual preferences may be thought of as an example of "satisficing" (266a). Alternatively, it appears useful to consider that in addition to the constraints we have discussed above, the constraints established by realities external to the hospital, there are constraints which are internal to it. These internal or endogenous constraints are posed by the requirement that the objectives or preferences of all internal constituencies must be met at some minimum acceptable level. The possible configuration of the hospital's objective function, therefore, is constrained by elements internal to the hospital.

We have now posited that each hospital produces a multidimensional product mix, defined in terms of services, in such a way as to maximize its objective function subject to internal and external constraints. Note the implications: since economic efficiency, as opposed to technical or engineering efficiency, can only be defined in terms of some objective function, from the hospital's view that combination of inputs which permits maximization of its objective function, in terms of outputs and prestige, and only that combination, is efficient. Hence that pricing strategy which corresponds to the *hospital's* perception of an efficient output mix is the hospital's efficient pricing strategy.

Any congruence between the hospital's definition of efficiency and the economic concept of social efficiency results from the simultaneous presence of two conditions: (a) operation on an optimal production function, and (b) the marginal rates of substitution between the elements of the hospital's objective function are equal to, or are linear transformations of social marginal rates of substitution. The relative social valuation of outputs, in other words, must be the same as the relative valuations of output by the hospital. Since we assume prestige, or institutional status, and its interdependence with other maximands in the hospital's objective function, the implication is that *even if* the hospital were operating on an optimal production function, congruence between social economic efficiency and the hospital's perceived efficiency is, at best, accidental. We note that this deduction is independent of the absence of the classically required conditions for Pareto optimality (170). We shall show that the discussion of "Cadillac only" vs. "Volkswagon" medicine, "need vs. demand," quality competition and duplication of facilities, yield to the same analysis when viewed in terms of the divergence between the hospital's objective function and its definition of efficiency and that assumed by the individual analyst to represent the social definition.

In the absence of market signals of social valuation in a truly atomistic market of "buyers" and "sellers," in the absence of public definitions of social valuations in other than vague generalities, and in the absence of direct or indirect enforcement mechanisms of even such imprecise conceptions of social valuation, congruence between economic efficiency and hospital efficiency can only occur through a unique happenstance. Were social valuations precisely reflected in the prestige maximand of the hospital, that condition may result.

One implication of this analysis for the measurement and evaluation of efficiency in the hospital's production of services is now obvious: multiple criteria exist. A given hospital, or a set of hospitals, may be operating efficiently in the sense of maximizing their objective functions. The evaluation of their efficiency in economic terms, independent of the hospital's objective functions, requires the assumption that some social welfare function, or set of relative social values over hospital services, exist. Economic analysis can assist the hospital in attaining higher levels of maximization through the use of more economically efficient processes. But higher levels of efficiency in terms of the hospital's objective function may yet result in lowering efficiency in terms of social values. Those seventy-two hospitals in the State of New York which had cobalt bombs in 1965 may each have maximized their individual objective functions. They may even have done that in a technically efficient way. But since no more than fifty cobalt bombs would have been required to meet the medically determined needs of a population seven million larger than that of the entire state, while a municipal hospital was closed for lack of funds and others were accommodating inpatients in corridors, it is not very likely that resources were efficiently allocated (66, n. 36, p. 199).

Attempting to maximize the objective function subject to the assumed constraints with existing production facilities, the hospital will produce a set of outputs, which we have defined as a service mix. We shall not here consider further or alternative definitions of output. It is clear, as we shall show, that different conceptual formulations are not only feasible, but required for different analytic purposes and necessitated by varying models of the production and consumption of health care. Output definitions in terms of process, intermediate products (or value added), final consumption and investment goods, or "product characteristic" are all tenable if within the given theoretical framework that definition is logical. In a construct which considers "medical care" to be that set of services and commodities which result in improved health levels (the end-result approach), however defined, and which views the physician as the central decision maker, or the essential "entrepreneur" who in producing medical care chooses from the set of available alternative resources in the production of medical care, the hospital's outputs are logically intermediate goods, measurable by whatever dimension the *physician* considers to be their relevant characteristics. That is, for a given diagnostic category, if the physician in this formulation considers the essential output of the hospital in "producing care" to be simply bed rest and close observation, "patient days" is an appropriate dimension of intermediate *output* to measure. If, however, all professionally provided medical care is seen as a set of inputs into a healing process with the patient as the producer of "health," and if one of the dimensions of the healing process is time, the "patient day" is an *input*. Patient days, admissions, and discharges are the generally used definitions of hospital output which we view as vague proxies for a multidimensionally variable mix of services.

Depending on the accepted definition of the output mix, we have to identify the relevant production function or functions, which specify, for desired levels of outputs however defined, the optimal feasible combinations of inputs required. Given input proportions and input prices we can then calculate the cost of producing observed levels of output as well as estimate changes in cost components resulting from changes in the levels of output and the scale of operations. That is, for a specified output mix we can calculate the costs of production with existing input capacities, their prices, and the technologically determined input combination alternatives, and estimate cost changes resulting from changes in each. We should be able to identify both the short-run and long-run cost structures of different levels and rates of production.

The model of the medical care decision process presented in the first section of this chapter identifies the physician's central role in generating demand. In the specific case of demand for hospital services, we posit that the total "demand for hospital services" is the sum of four distinct yet interrelated demand sets.

Consider first that the demand can represent demand for services for the treatment of conditions varying in severity along a continuum from elective to emergent. We may argue conservatively that both the income and price elasticities of patient originated demands decrease rapidly with increasing case severity, attaining zero in cases of emergency. It is less theoretically polished but more realistic to suggest that in the presence of some rather significant subset of medical situations the economic choice algorithm is irrelevant.

Given the variation in case severity, which may be differentially evaluated by the patient and the physician, the bulk of the demand for services are physician originated. Hence the four components of demand for the services of the hospital: (a) patient originated elective, (b) patient originated emergent, (c) physician originated elective, and (d) physician originated emergent.

The analytic framework for considering relationships between demand, utilization, and "need" as defined by potential patients, direct medical care providers, and funding bodies, and their impacts on the level of operations, output mix, and costs of hospitals, as well as the feasibility of alternative pricing systems, requires this elaboration of demand formation. We consider the differential four-demand construct, since we hypothesize that for the analysis of efficient output levels, efficiency-pricing, output mix complexity, and the relationships between hospital outputs and those of the rest of the medical care sector, the "demand for hospital services," or as it is usually considered, utilization, is too broad, too heterogeneous an aggregate, composed of segments expressed by both potential patients and physicians and varying in elasticity. Of course one might argue that transportation is transportation, and for some analytic purposes it is. But for others the distinction between bus and private automobile transportation, between private automobiles and bicycles, or between Cadillacs and Jeeps is significantly relevant and must be explicitly expressed. The importance of the physician's decision, of the role of condition severity, and of differences in observed utilization rates of hospital services make our distinctions of demand by source of origination and underlying condition severity both relevant and significant.

Additional complexities in demand analysis stem from the central role of the physician. The hospital's objective function, externally generated demand for its services, demands internally generated for patient care services as well as for research and teaching activities, relative demands for non-hospital based patient care services, and the definition of the medically relevant production function to produce the output mix implied by this set of demands all are interrelated. They all have at least one element in common: the central decision-making role of the physician.

Implications for Analysis

In the rest of this book we consider in some detail aspects of this complex system and the physician's central role in it. The complexities of interdependence between, for example, supplies and demands is brought about by a variety of factors, among which the assumed behavioral relations are of primary significance. The behavioral relations are assumed in this form because we expect that they reflect, to a degree necessary for our analytic purposes, the conceptually observable behavioral relationships as they exist within the institutional network we wish to examine. This suggests that the observed interactions are not solely the results of technological interdepence, but are principally influenced by institutional arrangements: the social, economic, political, ideological, and legal factors that shape the nature of the medical care system, in addition to its technology, give rise to the interdependencies. Viewed in this light, it might be said that experimentation with institutional arrangements different from the usual solo fee-for-practice medicine, such as prepaid, comprehensive group practice, is an attempt to eliminate some of the interdependencies we posit, as well as their economic costs. For example, the attempt in such a setting to limit or neutralize physician focused outcomes by removing monetary rewards from the provision of specific services, or the choice of certain types of patterns of care, can be seen as an attempt to reduce physician originated demand to that set solely determined by patient focused considerations. A clear example of this is the attempt to limit hospital admissions to cases where the patient's medical condition clearly requires it, that is, when ambulatory substitutes do not exist, whether or not the admission would serve the physician's non-medical preferences by reducing his workload, increasing his income, or both. The establishment of formal hierarchical decision patterns, channeling potential patients through decision points determined by medical workers of increasing specialization from paramedical assistants to, say, urologists is an attempt, among other things, to reduce the high level of physician generated demands associated with specialists. In fact the gamut of proposals for the establishment of Health Maintenance Organizations, prospective budgeting for hospitals, the establishment of patient panels for hospitals, as well as for the various degrees of rationalization, planning, and public control embedded in various national health insurance schemes may be seen as attempts, however tentative, so to restructure the institutional arrangements in the medical care system as to increase those interdependencies which are likely to lead to the provision of better care for more people and to reduce or eliminate those interdependencies which lead to inappropriate utilization, low quality, and high costs.

Summary

To recapitulate, we have established an analytic framework for the purpose of examining the operations and problems of acute hospitals. In our framework the model of the medical care decision process pinpoints the central demand determining role of the physician. The hospital is viewed as a central part in an interrelated medical care system. While substitutes for some of its products exist, it is the sole supplier of a large set of services to the entire population and the sole source of care for significantly large population subsets. In this regard, we shall show that to the extent the problems of urban public hospitals constitute a special set, those problems arise not only from the forces acting on the medical care system alone, but also from that aggregation of conditions which have led to the urban crisis.

Postulating an objective function in terms of output mix, output quality, and prestige, we assume that the hospital will attempt to maximize that function subject to endogenous and exogenous constraints. Responding to internally and externally generated demands, the hospital will produce an output mix with its existing production processes at relative prices it assumes will yield optimal results in terms of its own objective. We have discussed some analytically interesting deductions. We have abstracted from some problems by drastic, but useful postulates.

Our framework will enable us critically to review the selected literature and to interrelate its disparate parts. For if the hospital sector is heterogeneous and atomistic, the literature is an accurate reflection of it.

2 Hospital Objectives

What is a hospital and what are its objectives? After considering various definitions, we shall conclude that it is a complex organization attempting to maximize its objective function. Unlike the case of most other economic production units, the firms, its objective function can not be defined simply in terms of profit maximization. Hence we proceed to attempt to identify how its objective function is formulated and the terms in which it may be expressed.

We shall find that while there is less than a general agreement among the analysts on what it is that the hospitals seek to maximize, there begins to appear something like a consensus that the physician's decision-making role in the medical care process and the hospital's constituencies' desire for prestige are the important if not unique determinants of its objective functions.

The relation of the hospital's objectives to those of its communities raises additional questions, all of which are less than clearly understood.

The Hospital as a Complex Economic Organization

The literature does not present a unified definition of the organizational unit of analysis. It has been defined simply as a "producing unit" (133, p. 7), as "a place for more or less total care where various technical or other highly complicated interactions or procedures may occur" (96, p. 77), as the socially provided workshop of the physician, either "free" (374, p. 112) or merely "private" (401, p. 51), or one which the physician uses to maximize his own income (325, 438). Alternatively, it has been viewed as a "secondary office" for the private physician (153, p. 49); "the central core of medical intelligence and activity" (378, p. 10); a "communications network" (445); more drastically, in terms of current functions, as simply the emergency room: "the emergency room *is* the hospital" (326, p. 326); or the "family M.D." (56). A.R. Somers suggested that a multidimensional definition is required in terms of "minimum services and facilities, organization of the governing board and medical staff, provision for quality and utilization review, and determination of service area" (397, p. 353), in addition to other aspects such as ownership. This multiplicity of contradictory definitions stems, to a significant extent, from the diversity of analytic foci.

Which of the definitions is appropriate depends both on the kinds of questions to be asked and the framework within which they are posed. For the purposes of cost analysis it is meaningful to define the hospital as a "producing unit." A study of changes in inpatient and ambulatory utilization rates in an urban hospital may require definition in terms of interdependence with the rest of the medical care system, as a fulcrum of activities. The economic analysis of the efficiency of hospital operations placing central emphasis on the physician's role may consider the hospital as a "workshop." A sociological perspective, or an analytic framework that focuses on the relationships between internal interaction and organizational behavior, may well view the hospital as a "social system" (433; 16, p. 81-2). Definitional difficulties arise either when the definition is inappropriate for the purpose at hand, or when the process of definition itself substitutes for analysis.

The generalized definition of the hospital as a complex organization attempting to maximize its objective function through the production of a multidimensional output mix subject to internal and external constraints and demands, permits analysis to concentrate on its economically relevant individual components.

Objectives of the Hospital

That the hospital's objectives are complex and multiple in nature was early recognized by Codman (82), and elaborated and extended by MacEachern (262). They both posited a fourfold definition of functions in terms of (a) care of the sick and injured, (b) medical education and the maintenance of medical standards in the community, (c) prevention of disease and the promotion of health, and (d) the advancement of medical research. Writing as a physician well before the development of the concepts of externality and interdependence, Codman placed heavy emphasis on what he called the "important by-products" (82, p. 494). The "product" of a hospital, in terms of the number of patients treated, cannot be meaningfully discussed in the absence of criteria for evaluating the results of treatment, hence, he suggested that the quality of care, in terms of end-results, is an important aspect of both hospital production and of objectives directly. But since, in his argument, the quality of treatment is a function of medical knowledge, which in turn is determined by the level of medical education in the hospital, where medical education includes the continuing interaction between the hospital and the private practitioners in the community, the quality of care is seen to possess the by-product of community impact. Certain of community impact as one of the major objectives, he posits two alternative means to achieve it: having one or more hospitals in each community with salaried, full-time staffs to "set an example for the practitioners to follow," or to encourage hospital-oriented practice via an expansion of attending privileges (82, p. 494).

The definition of objectives is rather generalized and, along with Sloan's similar discussion some forty years later (392), is somewhat vague about what it is that is being discussed. That is, it is not clear whether the functions, or objectives, defined are those that *exist*, or those that *should exist*. In fact, Codman, MacEachern, and Sloan, each concerned with similar problems at different levels of analysis and at different historical points, are representative of the rather superficial, somewhat propagandistic, and logically opaque discussion, often confusing that which the hospital does with what, in accordance with some undefined and unarticulated set of values, it should do. While the hospital's "obligations to the entire community" are often stressed, the obligations are not precisely specified, not their means of attainment delineated. Codman may be the exception who recognized that since both incentives and legally imposed duties are absent, the specification of objectives or functions at this level could more appropriately be termed a discussion of ethical systems, of values.

There are two fundamentally different possible approaches to attempting to derive objective functions for hospitals. One is to assume that, analogously to other economic productive units, the hospital's objective function can be expressed in one or another variant form of the profit maximization hypothesis. The variants of the profit maximization hypothesis have taken many forms from "utility maximization" to "cash flow maximization" (100, p. 31). Perhaps the most prolific and imaginative student in this area, Karen Davis, has advanced, in a number of interesting and speculative papers, a plethora of variants of the profit maximization hypothesis. She finds some empirical evidence to validate the cash-flow maximization, utility maximization, and the net revenue maximization hypotheses (100, p. 30; 101, p. 3; 98). The studies, however, assume that the outputs of the for-profit and not-for-profit hospitals are the same, while even the data presented in the studies demonstrate the tenuous nature of this assumption. For the year 1969, for example, while 71 percent of the not-for-profit hospitals had blood banks, only 47 percent of the for-profit hospitals did so. The ratios for the presence of pathology laboratories are the same, indicating not only a significant difference in the scope of services and hence the composition of the patient day, but in the quality of care as well. The attempt to demonstrate that the price-average cost is a function of demand and supply factors, which would lend credence to some form of the profit maximization hypothesis, has to be accepted with the degree of skepticism engendered by R^2's in the range between 0.12 and 0.45 in regressions, where the values of the dependent variable are not presented (101). That the profit maximization hypothesis is not easily validated should not be surprising, since questions about its tenability even in the manufacturing sector have been frequently raised.

A fundamentally different approach is to assume that the objective functions in the not-for-profit sector are generally different, expressed in reward terms other than profit, and then to identify these terms.

The economists' attempt to define operational objective functions in this context exhibits some limited advances toward clarity. Long and P. Feldstein

(257, p. 119) would not go as far as Kaitz (204, p. 2), who considers the hospital to be an "anomaly from an economic and managerial point of view. . . . somewhere between the price-oriented private sector and the tax-oriented public sector." They agree, however, that the objective of profit maximization is inappropriate and would substitute for it the somewhat less specific notion that "hospitals seek to optimize some complex, differing, and for most institutions, ill-defined goal subject to certain financial constraints," which is not further elaborated. Neither this formulation, nor P. Feldstein's earlier one that hospitals "wish to maximize social welfare subject to the restriction of recovering their total cost of operation" (139, p. 66), is operational or theoretically convenient, since neither permits the analysis of observed hospital behavior in terms of unambiguous, stated, objectives.

The attempt to derive analytically useful definitions of the objective function has proceeded in terms of the quantity and quality of output. At its simplest level the hospital's objective function is assumed to contain a single maximand, the number of patients treated during some time period (216, p. 121). But even here it is not quite clear whether it is simply the number of patients that is to be maximized or the average daily census, or to what extent both measures are proxies for gross revenue. The confusion is represented in one of the frequently recurring expressions in the professional hospital literature, "a filled bed is a billed bed."

Assuming, however, that the number of patients treated is the maximand, it is sometimes realized that this does not obviate the need for some weighting mechanism. It has been suggested that the apparent objective is "to maximize the weighted number of patients treated (per period of time), the 'weights' being the professional prestige of the doctors attending them" (339, p. 480). While the precise meaning of this formulation is not clear, it appears to imply that one of the maximands is professional prestige itself, as reflected through the "prestige" of the attending physicians. If it can be further assumed that the professional "prestige" of the individual physician, or, in particular, that aspect of "prestige" which appears to be desirable enough to be used as a weighting scheme by the hospital, is partially or fully determined by his education, certification, professional position, attending privileges, and practice history, then it can be inferred that, at the least, "prestige" and the expected quality of care are not independent. Somewhat more positively, it can be argued that the "professional prestige of the doctors attending" is an indirect indicator of the expected quality of care to be provided by them.

This formulation of the objective function is insightful since it appears to hint at the recognition of the physicians' central role in its specification. A related if somewhat different hypothesis in terms of "conspicuous production" promises to be even more fruitful, even though the empirical evidence amassed for its validation is less than convincing. Lee, in an elegant and imaginative paper, suggests that the hospital production process and the ruling objective functions can best be understood in terms analogous to the Veblenian concept of conspicuous consumption (236). Each hospital considers itself to be a member of some group of hospitals which it considers to be its peers in terms of the scope of services, prestige, reputation, and excellence. To maintain membership, it must engage in the production of services in scope and quality dimension equivalent to or similar to those produced by its peers and must do so in a manner that makes it known. Hence it will tend to attempt to maximize its "conspicuous production." It would be both fascinating and useful to employ this hypothesis in the investigation of the dissemination of knowledge and the so-called duplication of little used but prestigious facilities. It might also be useful to consider this hypothesis in the debate about the role of quality in the objective function.

Quality as such has been explicitly incorporated by Long (256). He advances the interesting argument that while the level of quality at any given time acts as a constraint, increases in quality above the observed level enter the objective function. The implication is that the marginal rate of substitution between observed quality and quantity of output is zero, but some substitutability between increases in quality and increases in output quantity exists. The analysis, however, is inhibited by no specification of "quality." Rice, in an otherwise rather inadequate attempt to substantiate the quantity maximization hypothesis, advanced the useful distinction between amenities and medically required treatments (346). Arguing that some trade-off between quality and quantity of output may exist, Rice argues that the quantity maximization hypothesis refers exclusively to the medically required outputs and not to amenities, whose production is subject to profit maximization. The implication appears to be that the quantity-quality trade-off is relevant to medically required outputs only, while the production of amenities does not directly enter the objective function in any of its dimensions.

Newhouse (304, Appendix 3-1) develops a tentative, yet so far most explicit, model of the hospital as a non-profit organization trying to maximize an objective function, whose arguments are both quality and quantity, subject to a budget constraint specifying the maximum acceptable deficit. Quality is denoted by an unspecified "vector of characteristics" and quantity by simple unweighted patient-days. Assuming the existence of several quality vectors at any given time, each with its specific cost analogue, he posits that "the hospital decision-maker chooses that quality vector which maximizes quantity . . . at a given price" (304, p. 47). This assumes that while more than one quality vector may have the same cost analogue, the decision maker restricts himself to that set which maximizes quantity for the given cost level. In other words, while a number of quality standards may have identical cost coefficients, there will exist one, and only one, among the set for which the quantity of output will be at the maximum, and that is the one chosen. This has two important implications: (a) with each quality vector there is associated a given level of cost, and (b) any increase in quantity, with constant quality, and *vice versa*, is attainable only at a higher cost.

Since for each quality vector there is a corresponding, precisely specified cost analogue, Newhouse can then proceed, in his analysis, to measure quality by observed cost, for given levels of the quantity of output. Quite distinct from the economic arguments about the proper measures of quality and of changes in quality, this assumes a monotonic relationship between quality and cost and disregards the difficulties involved in what has been referred to as "over-utilization." That is, if medical criteria for diagnostic and therapeutic processes can be established, as they have been (see 116; 119; 146; 322; 369; 372), observed variation in quality can be expected around those criteria in both directions. In the absence of such criteria it is not known whether observed higher levels of "quality," as indicated by more intensive use of laboratory procedures and reflected in higher costs, which in Newhouse's formulation would denote an increase in "quality," correspond in fact to increases in the quality of care or to medically unjustified over use of convenient, income-generating services. That, however, is not the end of the difficulties, for Newhouse then proceeds to assume that the demand schedule facing the hospital is not only significantly downward sloping, but that increases in the quality of services provided will shift it outward. The assumption appears to be that an increase in the quality of the hospital's output will increase the demand for that hospital's output. Without further justification, the assumption appears to be rather extreme, but nonetheless it enables Newhouse to deduce formally that which others have averred: that hospitals wish to maximize their long-term growth, they wish to "prosper and expand" (340, p. 58).

Newhouse shows that, given his assumptions, the hospital's production possibility contour, in terms of quantity and quality of output, can be determined and that in combination with the increases in demand resulting from increases in the quality of output, a production point will be chosen at which no further trade-offs between quantity and quality will yield increased revenues. On the assumption that higher revenue-yielding production sets can be achieved either through internally generated funds or through deficits, the direct implication is that production will take place at the least cost point: for any given quantity-quality mix, that production process which generates the highest net revenues is desirable. This attempt at pseudo-profit-maximization is implicit in the assumption that the hospital's production possibility locus can be shifted to higher and higher revenue producing planes. The "profits" earned, therefore, can be used to shift out further the quantity-quality transformation curve. Since the "profits" earned are inclusive of deficits, up to some constrained amount, this also implies that in organizations where deficits can be covered there will be a positive incentive to generate them.

Newhouse concludes from his analysis that a number of conditions prevent the achievement of optimality,[a] chief among them an insufficient variation in available quality levels. While quality variation is observable, the overall levels of quality are too high, and at any rate higher than they would be if hospitals were profit maximizers. He argues that "from a normative standpoint one would desire that the hospital produce all qualities (all products) which were profitable when price equalled marginal cost, just as a profit maximizing firm would" (304, Appendix 3-1, p. 53). He is probably correct, and fortunately so. We refer the reader to chapters 6 and 8 for a discussion of quality, and its variation.

In addition to this assumed prejudice against quality differentiation, the entry of third-party reimbursement permits the hospital decision maker to shift the quality-quantity production contour to the point where no additional changes would yield the decision maker any increases in satisfaction. That is, Newhouse assumes that the decision maker's objective function is locally satiable: his objective function can be satiated by producing a quantity-quality mix, at the cost of increased insurance premiums, but at no cost to himself, above which he is indifferent to any increases in quantity or quality.

So far his analysis is very similar to that of the non-profit firm by Baumol and Bowen (41) who, however, do not assume local satiation and hence are forced to conclude that ". . . the objectives of the typical non-profit organization are by their very nature designed to keep it constantly on the brink of financial catastrophe, for to such a group the quality of services which it provides becomes an end in itself. . . . These goals constitute bottomless receptacles into which limitless funds can be poured" (41, p. 497). There are other, more fundamental differences between Newhouse on the one hand and Baumol and Bowen on the other. Newhouse does not discuss the nagging question of externalities, and, as we have seen above, evaluates observed and expected behavior in terms of Pareto Optimal conditions. It is precisely the absence of such conditions (e.g., lack of consumer information, non-optimality of income distribution, interdependence between internally and externally generated demands) which prompt Baumol and Bowen to argue that:

> . . . Nonprofit organizations as a group share at least two characteristics: (1) they earn no pecuniary return on invested capital and (2) they claim to fulfill some social purpose. . . . Any group which sought to fill no social purpose and earned no financial return would presumably disappear from the landscape (41, p. 497).

[a]His definition of social optimality is ". . . the outcome observed in a market dominated by knowledgeable consumers which functioned so as to satisfy their tastes (assuming the income distribution is optimal)." Appendix 3-1, p. 58, n. 1. This criterion is of somewhat questionable applicability in a sector where none of the conditions are met. Hence the evaluation of observed outcomes in terms of such a criterion is debatable. It reminds one, in fact, of Margolis' well-known dictum a propos another economist that "his approach is natural to economists—a perfectly competitive utopia which fails and therefore necessitates the sinful tampering by government." It gets to be rather difficult to observe outcomes in perfect markets dominated by knowledgeable consumers anywhere, particularly in the service industries, and nowhere more than in the medical care system.

The implication is not that the "claimed" social purposes are fulfilled, but rather that both the "social purposes" and the "claim" to attain them are considered legitimate, or at least legitimate enough to facilitate the survival of the claiming organization.

It has been argued that the profit motive in the hospital sector would be the answer to their problems. The non-profit hospitals are now only so in name and take their "profits" in terms of "prettier secretaries, thicker carpets, less intense efforts to oversee routine activities, and, most notoriously, the duplication of expensive equipment such as heart-lung machines in order to enhance the prestige of their institutions and themselves. Planning is not the way to cope with this problem, competition is" (32, p. 127). The profit-making hospital would invest in equipment "only if the demand for its services were large enough to make it pay off." If such a purchase did not pay off, that would mean that the "need" is simply too low for it.

Discussion of the hospital's objective function, as by Newhouse, is useful only for the limited purpose of evaluating hospital performance in terms of its own desiderata. Neither its objective function nor its performance can be evaluated in the absence of some social welfare function, or, at least, some clearly stated social goals. Since profit-making (proprietary) hospitals do exist, accounting for 6 percent of the beds in all non-federal acute hospitals in 1968 (189, 1969, p. 475), it would appear that both the social purpose non-profit hospitals' claim to fulfill and their claim to attempt to fulfill them are legitimated by some social values not attained or not attainable through the market sector.

The fundamental limitation of attempts to evaluate objectives and behavior in the absence of clearly stated explicit social values is illuminated by the Piel Report. The argument is clearly and forcefully made that the definition of objectives for municipal hospitals in terms of the quality of care and the efficiency of its provision is partial at best, since it excludes a most important component from the standpoint of community needs: "what is not provided because needs are unmet and unrecognized" (326, p. 337). The question is not which concept of social values is tenable, acceptable, or desirable. It is rather the assumed values not made explicit, as in Newhouse, that the level of medical need for personal care reflected in individually expressed demand is the level to be satisfied, masquerading as economic efficiency criteria. This necessarily flows from an inadequate understanding of the medical care system in which the consumer is seen as the basic decision maker originating demands and choosing between alternatives. Hence no attention is paid to the central role of physician, as if the patient could simply admit himself or as if he progressed through the usually assumed economic choice paradigm when faced with the prospect of lung cancer. And even if he did so, it assumes that he should. This might be called the Frostian social welfare function, since, according to Robert Frost "The most inalienable right of man is to go to Hell in his own way."

This assumption, and its implicit logical consequences, is not the only source of analytic difficulty. The notion of a single "hospital decision maker" is an additional one.

Beginning at least with Codman (82, p. 495), the complexity of decision making in the hospital has been recognized, if not incorporated into the analysis. Penchansky and Rosenthal, in an elegant paper, suggested a basic dichotomy (325). They suggest that the hospital provides the capital inputs into the production of treatments in which the attending physician performs an important role. The capital thus provided is social capital, in the sense of social funding, which increases the private productivity of the physician. The productivity of such social capital, however, is not reflected in capital earnings, but is rather captured by the physician. The physician, if he is an income maximizer, has every incentive to increase social investment in facilities which increase his private (personal) productivity and therefore his income. The objectives of the hospital, therefore, are strongly influenced by the private preferences of physicians. Stevens, along somewhat similar lines, has argued that "the view of the physician as an independent professional operator who uses hospital facilities is central to the conceptualization of hospital management structure" (407, p. 12).

Both the Penchansky-Rosenthal and Stevens formulations can be subsumed under our proposition that the majority of demands for hospital service are physician originated. Whether to maximize their incomes by the use of social capital or to shape the hospital to their private professional needs, the physicians as central decision makers in the process of care will attempt to shape the hospital's objective function to their purposes. Even Newhouse's criticism, inappropriate though it is, fits within the rubric. For if physicians and other internal constituencies define objective functions so as to maximize their own private rewards, these rewards may be in terms of esoteric equipment, recondite skills, and conspicuous procedures, which may, in some technical definitions of it, result in high quality medicine, if not in high quality of medical care.

Not only the special interests of the physician have been recognized, but also the possible conflicts among different sets of decision makers resulting from the division of authority, both legal and professional in nature, over medical and non-strictly medical functions (304). This is assumed to lead to lack of clear definition of objectives in even relatively narrow terms.

It has also been suggested that for purposes of management and goal definition the hospital is best viewed as being presided over by a triumvirate: the board of directors or trustees, the staff and attending physicians, and the administrator (219, chapter 9). Stevens has maintained that each of the "different components of the management structure may entertain different and sometimes not compatible objectives" (407, p. 8). This he considers to obviate the possibility of deducing behavioral hypotheses from motivational postulates, as, for example, the postulate of profit maximization facilities. Why this is so, or should be, is not clear. It may well be that the objective function, as we posited it, is complex and interdependent. That, however, does not logically preclude either the inference of objectives from observed performance or the attempt to establish the objective function directly. Stevens, however, does not undertake that attempt and falls back on the earlier formulation of the central role of the private practitioners, who, in their assumed attempt at income maximization, "want the use of these facilities as a necessary adjunct to their own business operations" (407, p. 19).

If the literature on the objectives of hospitals agrees on a central point, it is that the objectives are vague, ill-defined, contradictory, and sometimes non-existent (326, p. 531; 401, pp. 214-15).

There is some support that both quantity, in terms of services provided, and quality enter explicitly into the hospital's set of goals. There is no clear statement, and little or no attempt at either precise definition or analysis of the relevant dimensions either of quantity or of quality. No distinction appears, in that part of the literature dealing with the hospital's goals, between inpatient and ambulatory care. Nor is there a discussion of how these two basic types of aggregate output mixes interact with each other in the treatment process and with alternative sources in the relevant community, or market.

At least some of the literature tends to support the hypothesis that the objective function incorporates, however imprecisely, the element we have called institutional status: this is reflected in the concern with the attending physicians' prestige, with that undefined vector of quality characteristics, and with "conspicuous production."

There is at least some consideration of the relevant constraints, which tend to be taken as either the maximum acceptable deficit (Newhouse) or left undefined (Stevens, p. 7, n. 5). To the extent that a separate capital constraint is considered, it is assumed that "the independent hospital behaves as though capital had a zero price and invests funds regardless of the rate of return to the community" (256, p. 213), a rather good restatement of the "bottomless pit" hypothesis of Baumol and Bowen.

While there is scant agreement on what hospitals attempt to maximize, on what they should attempt to maximize, and how both relate to social goals, there begins to appear some consensus among the analysts that the profit maximization hypothesis is not appropriate. The imaginative if tentative attempts to hypothesize objective functions in terms of conspicuous consumption, quantity-quality trade-offs, physician prestige, and physician income maximization all tend to suggest that the postulate of physician generated demand is worthy of research.

The analyses of hospital objective functions that appear to be promising consider the hospital to be a part of the medical care system. There is not a sufficiently accurate understanding of the nature of the relationships between the hospital and the other segments of the system and there has been little conceptual and less empirical work in this area. Analyses of physician decision making as it helps determine hospital utilization on both outpatient and inpatient bases is required if we are to have the ability to predict with some degree of accuracy expected utilization rates.

The relationship of the objectives of the hospital's *internal* constituencies to its potential patients, or *external* constituencies, is not merely an additional conceptual conundrum, but a politically live and socially explosive question. Increasing demands for "community control," increasing objections by both patient groups and by some physicians to considering patients as "teaching materials," increasing demands to involve the acute hospital in the preventive and maintenance aspects of medical care, and the rising chorus of demands for public accountability imply that the analysts of hospital operations should address seriously the question of how hospital objectives are established, by whom, and for what purposes. For it is only in terms of those objectives that we can analyze the efficiency of their operations and the appropriateness of their outputs.

In the next chapter we consider the difficult question of how the hospital's outputs can and should be defined and measured.

3 The Hospital's Outputs

The hospital, a complex organization at the fulcrum of the medical care process, is the major institutional producer of medical care services. Our objective is to analyze how well hospitals attain their objectives and the social objectives of maintaining or attaining satisfactory health levels. Health, needless to say, is not produced in hospitals; illness remission is. To address the questions of how efficiently, with what costs, with which configuration of resources this process of illness remission is brought about, we must be able to identify what specific outputs are produced. Many if not most hospital cost studies have floundered on the appropriate definition of those outputs whose costs are to be measured.

In this chapter we address the issues of output definition useful for the analysis of costs and production. It is the complexity of the medical process and the multiplicity of its services in the absence of a common denominator that make output identification difficult. Several recent approaches in terms of case mix specification, diagnostic categories, and a medical value index, have the promise of providing the output identification required to focus on the economic issues of production and efficiency.

Approaches to the Definition of Relevant Outputs

In economic theory final output is that which yields satisfaction to the consumer. The role of the consumer in converting products and services purchased in the market into levels of satisfaction is not considered. It is assumed that his preferences are expressed directly over the commodities and services per se. Preferences, in other words, are directly for goods. This implies that "if a man becomes a more efficient consumer and requires a smaller quantity of a given good to achieve the same level of satisfaction as before, that either cannot or should not be measured" (225, p. 85). More lately, it has been argued that commodities and services are basically bundles of characteristics and it is the consumer who transforms the sets of characteristics from possibly different commodities, into satisfaction yielding activities (229). Therefore, the argument proceeds, output should be defined not necessarily in terms of its physical dimensions, but rather in terms of those "characteristics that the buyer is really seeking" and that thereby "we will catch the output-increasing effects of quality change and the better will be our measures of output" (225, pp. 90-91).

For medical care, and hospital production specifically, it can be argued that the consumer receives satisfaction from expected improvements of his health.[a] In this formulation, the consumer does not purchase, say, two office visits, five days of hospital care, three X-rays, and sixteen tablets of antibiotics, but rather the expectation that his level of health will be improved. Disregarding "painful" aspects of the treatment process, the consumer might well be indifferent to the specific combination of the various medical units of service, or to any of its components.

The output of the medical care sector, therefore, is best reflected by the satisfactions consumers derive from improved states of health. The argument, advanced by Fuchs in several places (see e.g., 157; 160; 161), that health levels are determined by a variety of factors, environmental, economic, demographic, and cultural, in addition to medical care, is from this point of view irrelevant. That health levels are not uniquely determined by medical care services does not negate the proposition that preferences are formulated in terms of health levels, and not in terms of specific services or commodities. (For an attempt to develop an integrated model of the determinants of health levels, see 25.)

Such satisfactions are not directly measurable. In markets where optimality conditions exist to a sufficient degree, it can be assumed that relative preferences, as reflected in marginal rates of substitution, correspond to observed relative prices. Without an explicit and direct measure of consumer satisfactions, therefore, prices can be used to indicate relative preferences. This may not be the case in the medical care sector. As Cohen has said: "Certainly in the non-competitive, non-profit, consumer ignorance filled, insurance influenced world of the demand for hospital services the values of services are not proportional to their prices or to their average cost" (86, p. 4). If prices of individual output components are not the appropriate measures of their values to the consumer, the validity of the definition of output in terms of its physical dimensions is also in doubt. Kravis has recognized this explicitly by saying that "as soon as we begin to ask significant questions–as we have been doing in the medical care area–we are forced to get closer to welfare oriented measures of output. . ." (225, p. 92).

While no specific measures of this nature have been developed, or even attempted, the groping towards output definition in terms of episodes of illness, health levels, and end results are moves in that direction.

In the literature of medical care, and of hospitals in particular, the definition of output is not only unclear, diverse, conflicting, tautological and ephemeral, but, according to Fuchs, "there is as yet no agreement as to what, in

[a]The definition of "health" is complex. For the present purpose, it is used to mean the highest attainable level of functional ability, given the state of the medical arts. For a detailed discussion, see chapter 6.

principle, should be measured . . ." (159, p. 126).[b] Mann and Yett maintain that the "basic conceptual issue is the specification of the time dimensionality of output. Is it a stock or is it a flow?" (265, p. 196). The definitional problem is complicated by the diversity of patient originated and physician originated demands facing the hospital, as well as by the multiplicity of functions performed within the hospital.

Viewing the hospital as an organization of departments producing a multiplicity of services, some of which are direct medical patient care, some ancillary services, and some hotel type services, the fundamental conceptual question is not one of time dimensionality nor of "what should be measured." The basic issue is the purpose for which the measure of output is required. If hospitals, as has been suggested, attempt to maximize their objectives defined in terms of the number of patient days per year, then for the purpose of evaluating how well they succeed the appropriate definition of output is in patient days. If physicians are seen as coordinators of medical services, medical entrepreneurs, the hospital's products are intermediate outputs to be defined in terms of those characteristics which the physician considers as his relevant inputs. This may be patient days, or the number of laboratory and other ancillary services, or nursing care. If the purpose of the analysis is the determination of the social efficiency of medical resource allocation, the relevant outputs are those that contribute to increases in health levels, or more specifically, the end results of treatment processes for defined diagnostic categories. It is the lack of conceptual clarity, the absence of modeling, the confusion of patient and physician roles, which has permitted the development of multiple and inconsistent definitions of output and as a corollary, the imprecise and sometimes tautological measurement of costs. (For an incisive review of the difficulties of defining output and for some suggestions for improvement, see Somers and Somers [3], as well as Lave [233].)

The literature presents six basic approaches to the definition of hospital output:

1. Patient days, weighted or unweighted
2. Hospital services
3. Episode of illness
4. End-results and health levels

[b]Fuchs argues further that "conventional measures of medical care output such as physician-visit, or a hospital day, are patently unacceptable to economists because they come close to measuring input instead of output" (159, p. 126). His incisive and stimulating discussion of the theoretical issues does not inhibit him from presenting in the same article empirical analysis in which total national expenditures in current dollars are used as a measure of output, and the deflated dollar figures as measures of "real output" (159, p. 117).

5. Intermediate inputs
6. Composites of one or more of the above

We shall discuss these in turn.

Output as the Patient Day

The number of patient days, or sometimes, the number of discharges, are generally used as surrogates for output (350, p. 213). The distinction between adult and pediatric, and within adult, between medical-surgical and obstetrical, is often not made, although sometimes it is suggested that patient days ought to be classified in terms of the "intensity of treatment" (176). The difficulty of using patient days or discharges, alternatively or simultaneously, is pointed out in a U.S. Army study which found that, at least in military hospitals in the United States, the labor input associated with admission and discharge is "equal to approximately ten times the manpower value of one day of inpatient care" (1, p. 47).

The difficulties in measuring output as patient day stem from several factors, all related to the fact that the "patient day" is a gross aggregate.

It can be shown that associated with each inpatient stay there are three distinct types of services: admission-specific, stay-specific, and diagnosis-specific. *Admission-specific* services, such as chest X-ray examinations and blood tests, are independent of the diagnosis on admission or discharge or of the length of stay. *Stay-specific* services, such as routine nursing care and hotel type services are determined by the length of stay, again largely independently of the nature of illness. *Diagnosis-specific* services, such as laboratory, inhalation therapy, physical therapy, surgical operations, vital functions monitoring, radiation, and other specialized services are determined neither by the act of admission nor by the length of stay but by the suspected or defined diagnosis, modified by case severity.

Stay-specific services, nursing and hotel type, may be quite adequately captured by unweighted patient days. Admission-specific services, however, will not be accurately reflected unless patient turnover is explicitly considered. And to the extent that the ancillary, specialized, service intensity of care exhibits a degree of heterogeneity among and within diagnostic categories, ten days of patient care delivered in the same hospital during the same time interval to two different patients, one with cerebral hemorrhage and the other with a broken leg, will correspond to different sets of services, with different capital and labor intensities.

One possible approach to capture the heterogeneity of the patient day is to adjust for case mix variation. The case mix, in terms of diagnostic categories, is an attempt to capture what we have called diagnosis-specific and case severity-specific services variations. The classification is generally some revised, aggregated, version of the internationally used disease classification taxonomy, known as the International Classification of Diseases Adapted for Use in the U.S., or ICDA. The ICDA classification of diseases, based on topographic and etiological considerations, is designed for biomedical research purposes. As such, "Diseases are accepted as entities . . . when an identifiable set of causes, and an understandable chain of pathogenic mechanisms can be invoked to explain a collection of signs, symptoms, and laboratory measurements of individuals" (422, p. 42). Use of the ICDA categories to construct case mix measures to capture service variation in the patient day assumes that to each of the diagnostic categories there corresponds some specified set of medical services. For purposes of economic analysis of production and costs, the ideal classification of patients would entail the construction of "isoresource" categories. That is, the patient load should be disaggregated into subgroups within which all patients receive the same amounts of the same services, thus representing equal derived demands for hospital resources. It has been suggested by Lave and Lave that a reasonably close proxy of isoresource classification may be attained by using "broad ICDA groupings" (231, p. 18).

In an independent and almost simultaneous effort Dowling followed a similar procedure. In the context of a linear programing approach to hospital production analysis, he constructed a matrix of 55 ICDA diagnostic categories by fourteen medical service departments to estimate the flow of specific services to specified diagnoses. He found the input coefficients to be reasonably accurate and fixed, implying that the diagnostic groupings were such that within each "patients . . . [are] homogeneous with regard to their use of medical services. . ." (120, p. 110). In this promising approach to disaggregating patient day, M. Feldstein has developed a similar but broader measure (133, chapter 2, esp. pp. 24-25). Since his objective is to measure interhospital cost differentials, his problem is to develop a measure of output of the highest attainable degree of homogeneity. He defines output both in terms of patient days and in terms of patients treated, controlling alternatively, for case mix, facility and service complexity, and the actual numbers of special services performed. In each case the assumption necessary to attain homogeneity of output is that the services actually delivered to patients are very much the same, if not identical, once case mix, or service complexity, are controlled for. Most specifically in the third case, where the actual numbers of services delivered are controlled for, but in the other two as well, the implicit assumption must be made that the same set of services delivered to different individual patients result in the same "output." To the extent that considerations of quality, patient demographic characteristics, and patient satisfactions are left out of account, Feldstein's measure of output is more properly a measure of intermediate inputs. Further, since neither the number of patients nor the number of patient days appears to be corrected for discharge status, that is, one cannot distinguish between discharges to other hospitals, to nursing homes, to the home well and alive, or to the morgue, it must be assumed that discharge status is homogeneous among hospitals. Outpatient care is explicitly excluded from the definition of output.

P. Feldstein developed perhaps one of the first weighted patient day measures (139). He attempts to measure "adult patient days of service per month." Recognizing the difficulties arising from differential case severity as well as from diagnostic versus therapeutic admissions, for which he cannot correct, he tries to relate departmental costs to patient days. Even though the attempt is less than successful, this is an explicit recognition of the implied relationships between patient days and departmental activity.

While recognizing all of the difficulties in using patient days, Lave and Lave (234) attempt to avoid them by assuming that in its relevant dimensions the output mix of a given hospital is constant over a relatively short period of time. They then proceed to estimate costs in terms of patient days. In their interhospital comparative cost analysis the vector characterizing hospital-specific product mix is not used, thereby ignoring the problem.

Stevens (407) not only uses patient days, but confuses output with capacity. He maintains that he uses "direct measures of output (capacity) in terms of beds and patients days. . ." (407, p. 2). Let output per period of time be Q_t and capacity, the level of output at the minimum point of the short-run average cost curve, Q_t^*. Alternatively, capacity may be defined as that level of output which the decision maker considers to be the desired level of maximum output per time period. In either case, only if $Q_t = Q_t^*$ is it meaningful to use "output" and "capacity" interchangeably. In other words, if, and only if, the level of observed output corresponds to that level produced at the minimum of the short-run average cost is output the equivalent of capacity. If the average cost curve is L-shaped, or a very shallow U, output and capacity may overlap for wide variations in output. Additionally, the concept that patient days are the appropriate measure of output is not much less precise than the notion that "beds" are the appropriate measure of capacity. They are both gross measures and inconclusive.

> . . . Danger and inconclusiveness have hardly been avoided by measuring prices and output in terms of units such as a "physician's visit" or a "hospital day"; it is no more justifiable in principle to take these radically changing services as units of output than it would be to take, for example, an "aluminum sheet" as the unit, regardless of changes in its quality and size (225, p. 91).

Output as Services

In an attempt to recognize the service-mix variation by diagnosis (133, chapter 2), by length of stay (195), and by type of hospital (84; 85; 86; 368; 46; 47) output has been defined either as the sum of weighted services or as patient days, weighted by service intensity.

Cohen defines output as the sum of weighted services, where

W_i = weight of *i*th service

Q_i^k = quantity of *i*th service in the *k*th hospital

S^k = service output of the *k*th hospital.

Output is then defined to be $S^k = W_i Q_i^k$ (84; 85; 86). The Q_i are defined as weighted operations (1/3 minor plus major), deliveries, EKGs, blood transfusions, outpatient visits, diagnostic X-rays, adult and pediatric days, etc. Cohen considers these services to comprise the set of intermediate outputs over which the hospital decision makers have some choice (86). The service outputs are directly measured in physical units. The attempt to incorporate quality differentials, consistent with his delineation of output, is ingenious, but somewhat troublesome. He assumes that there is a strong positive correlation between the quality of care delivered to the patient and the degree of accreditation and affiliation of a hospital, and further, that the quality differential can be represented by an arbitrary factor assigned to the sum of weighted services, output. That is, he assumes that the average output unit of the affiliated hospital is either 10, 20, or 30 percent "more care," depending on the degree of affiliation, than that of the non-affiliated hospital (86, p. 13).

The basic difficulty with the definition of output as the sum of weighted services is the appropriate weighting factor. Cohen weighs each specified service unit, Q_i^k, "by its estimated average cost," on the argument that while from the standpoint of demand analysis weighting by costs is not particularly relevant, "in the revenue constrained world of the supply of these services, relative average cost will be an important determinant . . . of which services to offer and how much of each" (86, p. 3). This of course assumes that the attending or staff physician will prescribe treatment patterns on the basis of their relative costs, which is an interesting hypothesis, still to be tested. The basic question is the purpose for which this definition of output is appropriate. Cohen uses it to measure the interhospital cost differentials of service bundles. For that purpose his innovative and valiant effort is negated on two grounds: statistically one would expect a high degree of autocorrelation between output weighted by cost and cost itself. Logically, he is testing a tautology. Contrary to his statement, therefore, that his $R^2 = .992$ between "adjusted output" and average cost is surprising, anything much less than that would be amazing (84). Nevertheless, he does attempt to develop a more inclusive and a more meaningful definition of output, including outpatient visits.

The attempt to develop an output measure in terms of weighted services by Saathoff and Kurz is somewhat similar (368). They define output in terms of adult, pediatric, and newborn patient days, outpatient services, and four other basic services. In this inventive method the weights are based on "logical time and cost." Thus, adult, pediatric, and newborn days are taken as a standard; surgical and obstetrical days are assigned a weight of 0.2. There is little discussion of the origin of the weights, and they recognize its arbitrary nature.

A somewhat similar procedure is recommended by the American Hospital Association (8). With the objective of developing statistical and accounting data for management purposes, they recommend that the output of each department within the hospital be defined in terms of those services which the given department renders to the other departments. The concept of intermediate inputs is implicit. The unit of service by which departmental output is to be measured varies with the department, from the number of meals and pounds of laundry for the dietary and laundry departments, to the number of weighted operations, or time used for the operating room. Since the objective is to develop measures that accurately reflect the volume of services produced by each department, the approach does not explicitly consider a weighting scheme. However, since for the medical departments the units of suggested service is either in terms of the numbers of operations, treatments, or procedures, or the time dimension of service, an implicit weighting mechanism is present.

Kovner has developed a detailed weighting scheme for specific services comprising ambulatory care. Each of the well-defined process steps, such as history taking, prior evaluation of records, etc., is identified with a high degree of specificity and assigned a relative weight. The weights themselves are multidimensional, based on the professional qualifications of the individual performing the service, the health status of the patient (case severity), and the estimated difficulty of the diagnostic or treatment procedure. Based on an investigation of the medical content of outpatient visits to Southern California Permante Medical Group facilities by members, Kovner develops marginal weights for each of a large number of narrowly specified procedures (223). The observed procedures so weighted are aggregated into an index, which he calls the "Identifiable Medical Procedure."

This is a bold and conceptually appealing attempt at specification leading to better, and quantifiable, measures of medical services output, which, theoretically, should be applicable to inpatient care as well. The multidimensionality of the index, and its independence of diagnosis specificity, would make tractable some of the major problems, such as the presence of multiple diagnoses per admission.

In his study of interhospital cost differentials Berry is concerned with a measure of output that avoids the difficulties stemming from product heterogeneity and quality variation (46:47). He is, therefore, not concerned with the development of a comprehensive concept of output, but rather a more narrow one. On the crucial assumption that hospitals with identical facility-service mixes produce patient days homogeneous in service intensity, he groups hospitals into sets of identical service-facility capabilities. For each such set of hospitals with identical service and facility capacities, he then defines output to be patient days. He indicates his awareness that the existence of identical facilities does not indicate the extent to which those facilities are utilized nor the relative interhospital differentials in service intensity, and that therefore the jump from facility homogeneity to product-mix homogeneity is a rather brave one (46, p. 135). His basic assumption, that hospitals with identical facility-service mixes produce patient days homogeneous in service intensity, or identical case mixes, is directly tested in the so-far most extensive study of the relation of case mix to hospital characteristics.

In the literature it is generally agreed that variations in case mix indicate the lack of homogeneity of output across hospitals. The most frequent method used to correct for product heterogeneity is to group hospitals by facility/service complexity, most often measured as the number of services and facilities the hospital has. Other characteristics, such as whether it is a teaching unit or not, and location, are also thought to bear on its case mix.

Lave and Lave analyzed 249,696 patient records generated by the Hospital Utilization Project from sixty-five hospitals for the second half of 1968, as well as time series data from nineteen other hospitals for six preceding semiannual periods. The forty-eight most commonly occurring medical diagnoses and the thirty-six most common surgical procedures, thirty of the latter weighted by the Blue Shield Relative Value Scale, are investigated. Lave and Lave found that while a relatively "small subset of diagnoses and of surgical procedures . . . account for a large proportion of all cases in the sixty-five hospitals studied" (231, p. 37), not only is there a large amount of variation in case mix among hospitals, but *less than half* of such variation is "explained" by the traditionally used institutional characteristics. Their analysis lends considerable support to some of the commonly used assumptions about the relationship of surgical complexity to hospital characteristics. They show that "health centers" (in this case the teaching hospitals of the University of Pittsburgh Medical School) not only have more surgical cases than other hospitals, but perform significantly more complex procedures and significantly fewer simple procedures than the average hospital, while at the same time the proportion of their medical case mix accounted for by relatively common diagnoses is very much lower than that of average hospitals (231, table 11, pp. 30-31). The precise evaluation of these results is made somewhat difficult by the absence of partial coefficients.

The coefficient of the most commonly employed variable, number of services, attains significance in only one of the six sets of equations presented: where the dependent variable is the average surgical complexity index. That is, neither the proportion of common diagnoses, the proportion of surgery, or of simple and complex surgery, appears to be related to the number of facilities in the hospital.

Lave and Lave's results indicate strongly that the number of services and facilities, as well as other characteristics such as "advanced teaching," can not be meaningfully employed as proxies for case mix. Cost analyses of so-called "homogeneous" groupings by such characteristics, therefore, implicitly rely on an output measure which varies across the hospitals. Further, while a number of students have recognized that quality is an important dimension of output and that the quality of services rendered (both in terms of technical quality and medical appropriateness) is therefore a relevant output dimension, no attempts have been made to capture the quality dimension explicitly. One of the results of not explicitly including quality in the analysis of productivity over time is to bias the results. Lamson has shown that the exclusion of the quality vector from output definition introduces "a large downward bias to the resulting output time series," yielding, therefore, a low estimate of productivity (228, p. 302).

Approaches to the definition of output in terms of service units aim either at inclusivity (definition of output as the sum of services) or exclusivity (output as a homogeneous patient day). No agreement on the proper weighting scheme for the services included has emerged, and with the possible exception of Kovner's work, none is in sight.

Output as Treatment of an Episode of Illness

So far but two attempts to define output in terms of the episode of illness treated have seen print. Scitovsky in her path-breaking, if unfollowed, study is concerned with the measurement of the cost of treatment for specific illnesses over time and not with the definition of output (377). She considers five illnesses, acute appendicitis, maternity care, otitis media in children, fracture of the forearm in children, and carcinoma of the breast, and studies their cost of treatment over a fourteen year period. Implicit in the work, however, is a definition of output in terms of treatment process for well-defined diagnostic categories. She explicitly recognizes that while quality is not controlled for, nor identified, to the extent that changes in quality have taken place over time and are reflected in the treatment processes studied, they are included in her measure (377, p. 1194).

Since the episode, in this definition, is inclusive of all relevant phases, ambulatory, inpatient, and post-discharge, the hospital's output would comprise a set of specific intermediate inputs into the treatment process. While from some points of view this may not be acceptable, from the standpoint of the efficiency of resource allocation and economic welfare it is both relevant and stimulating. It also accords well with the proposition that consumer preferences are expressed in terms of expected results, and not in units of individual medical care services.

Ro and Auster, in an effort to develop an efficient pricing scheme for hospitals, consider a similar definition of output in explicit terms. They define the hospital's output to be the "number and categories of episodes of illness given adequate treatment" (351, p. 178). The terminology is somewhat less than precise, for from their discussion it is clear that what they have in mind is the inpatient phase of the complete episode. While the concept is intriguing, it is not developed. "Adequate" and "successful" are used interchangeably (351, pp. 178, 184), but both terms are left undefined. Quality differentials are not taken into account, nor can they be assumed to be incorporated in "adequate," since length of stay is also not considered. Perhaps both considerations are obviated by their remark that the approach "would require narrow diagnoses, fairly standardized treatment, and a clear differentiability of costs where two illnesses coexisted: the degree of homogeneity of illness is an important consideration" (p. 184).

Output in Terms of End Results or Health Levels

If indeed the ultimate objective of the medical care system is improvement in health levels, that is what output measures ought to be concerned with. It is well known that health, no matter how defined, is not and cannot be produced by the medical care sector alone. A sickness-oriented system such as ours produces not health, but disease remission. To the extent that disease remission (and prevention) contribute to increased health levels, the output of the system, and hence of the hospital, is its contribution to the successful termination of illness episodes.[c] This is recognized by several students, but there is disagreement on whether or not such measures of output are feasible.

Granting that current definitions of output in terms of patient days, weighted services, etc., do not reflect the effect of hospital production, Somers and Somers argue that "it seems virtually impossible at the present time, to find any index of health, either for the individual or the community, that can be specifically attributed to hospital services" (401, p. 230). May, on the other hand, suggests that while for a variety of purposes other definitions of output may suffice, "for the purposes of the development of public policy with respect to the entire health services system, the appropriate definition of 'output' may very well involve health levels, morbidity and mortality rates, or some other as yet undeveloped measure of health and welfare" (268, p. 58).

Sanazaro and Williamson suggest the development of hospital specific end-result measures in terms of altered status, symptoms, and functions (369). Chiang and others developed rather precise indexes of health status, but none so far can be directly related to the effects of hospital services (77; 184; 185).

Perhaps the most sophisticated and promising approach is the one by Fanshel and Bush in which both state of health and illness severity are decomposed into a continuum of function/dysfunction and the transitional probability of moving

[c]For a stimulating theoretical discussion of this issue, see 314. A contrary view, that in terms of "health production" the contribution of the system is zero, see 408.

into a different state along the continuum within a specified time period. It is noteworthy that this index, the Health Status Index (HSI), is based on societal judgments of appropriate and desirable functional states for individuals (129). (For further discussion of health indices, see 167; 239.)

The paucity of work on end-result measures of hospital production in terms of improved health status is the result of a variety of factors. Failure of imagination is only one. Perhaps equally important is the dominant notion, appropriate for a smoothly operating market system, that relative prices do accurately reflect relative individual satisfactions and the private and social valuations coincide. In the absence of significant externalities, with an acceptable degree of price-competitive market behavior, and an income distribution if not optimal at least tenable, the consumer is taken to be sovereign. He expresses his relative valuations in the competitive market place, and the market place responds. It is therefore neither analytically required nor ideologically permissible to develop direct measures of either consumer satisfaction or of market performance in terms of end results. If consumer preferences are taken to be sovereign, and if those preferences can be efficiently translated into effective demand, no need for direct measures of performance exists. Medical care services, in this view, are no different from other services and commodities. If some problems do exist, they are attributable not to the fact that somehow the demand for radiation treatment for cancer may be intrinsically different from the demand for color television sets, but rather to the fact that physicians behave "as if the provision and sale of health services were somehow different from the provision and sale of other things consumers want" (32, p. 127).

Consumer ignorance, the absence of price competition and of free entry into the market, atomization of the producing sector without any invisible hand to coordinate it, differential accessibility by income, color, and location to a set of services proclaimed to be "rights" would suggest that market criteria are deficient. If public policy is to be concerned with the efficient allocation of medical care resources, some measures of results in terms of health levels and consumer satisfaction are required.

Output as an Intermediate Input

As suggested in the discussion of the objective function, whether the hospital's production is seen as resulting in final or intermediate products is determined by the analytic framework at hand. If we consider that the final product of the medical care process is the provision of the highest attainable level of health, given the state of the arts, it is clear that the output of the hospital is more precisely an intermediate input into this process. Hospital production, in this nexus, is but one of the stages of production, and its contribution can properly be called "value added."

Considering the physician to be performing the coordinating function in the process of diagnosis and treatment, May has suggested that the hospital's output "is in effect, sold to the physician who uses it as a raw material in the production of his services to the patient" (268, p. 58). Though this formulation is somewhat tenuous, at least legally, it does focus on the intermediate nature of hospital production.

It might be argued that the question of whether the outputs should be considered final or intermediate is scholastic at best. When the cost of outputs is considered, below, it does raise the issue, for example, of the proper consideration of length of stay. Disaggregating output into its direct patient care medical and hotel components, the question of whether stay-specific hotel type services are in fact final outputs or intermediate inputs used in the process of care, largely determines whether an additional day of stay is a contribution to output, or a more extensive use of inputs. The analysis of interhospital or interregional differences in length of stay for the same or similar diagnoses, depending on how stay-specific hotel type services are defined, can conclude that a longer length of stay corresponds to the production of larger output or, conversely, to an inefficient production of the same output with more resources. As will be seen in the discussion of cost analysis, this question is both difficult and important for the definition of the efficiency of hospital production.

Output as Composite Units

Ingbar and Taylor, in a complex statistical study of hospital costs in Massachusetts, used a veritable smorgasbord of output definitions ranging from patient days to laboratory activities, X-ray activities, maternity activities, medical education, and ambulatory care. All definitions were deflated by "available bed days" and measured by surrogate variables estimated by factor analysis. This approach does not by itself guarantee conceptual advances, since the principle for accepting the most relevant definition of output is the degree of its correlation with observed average costs per patient day (195).

A somewhat similar composite is developed by Ro (349), who uses the number of days hospitalized, the weighted sum of services delivered, and the amount of the patient's bill as his measure of output. The basic distinction is that this composite is patient oriented: directly and indirectly Ro attempts to measure as output that which is delivered to the patient. Output is conceptualized as that set of services which the patient "consumes" (p. 297). Aside from the rather questionable value of his statistical analysis,[d] and his idiosyncratic assumptions such as that the existence of outpatient clinics in a hospital

---

[d]Ro fits least squares single regressions to data on 9,000 patients in 22 hospitals in the Pittsburgh area for the year 1963. While most of the signs of the coefficients appear to be what one would expect theoretically, in no case does he attain an r^2 greater than 0.23.

indicates that staff and attending physicians "adhere to the concept of integrated care" (p. 300), his attempt at an integrated definition is stimulating. Certain difficulties remain, however, such as the necessary assumptions that for each diagnosis there is one prescribed set of treatment procedures, and that each treatment process is composed of a uniquely defined set of services.

The attempt to construct accurate cost studies by the U.S. Army has resulted in the development of the concept of output as the "Composite Work Unit" (1). The patient day is taken to represent the standard, or "normal" day of care, with a weight of 1, and other aspects of care are rated on a scale of 1 through 10. Thus both the event of admission and that of birth is assigned a weight of 10. Since the newborn is apparently not counted in Army hospitals as a patient, this may be more reasonable than appears on the surface. Outpatient visits are explicitly considered, and assigned a weight of 0.3 (1, p. 47). This attempt at a better measure of output is less than successful, since the patient day is taken to represent a homogeneous output mix in terms of service intensity.

Conclusions on Output

The discussion of the representative literature on the concept of output warrants a number of conclusions. Perhaps the primary one is that there appears to be no agreement, either on a conceptual or merely definitional level, among those who have most intensively studied the economics of hospitals on what the appropriate measure of output is, or should be. The analyses are not only fragmented, partial, inconclusive, and often theoretically empty, but there is little evidence of recognition in the body of the analyses of the multidimensionalities discussed in the preambles.

There is little or no discussion, for example, of one of the basic dimensions of output: quality. M. Feldstein, in his otherwise incisive study, argues that "Measuring the quality of medical care remains an unsolved problem. If useful quality indices are ever developed, a new dimension could be added to the assessment of hospital costs" (133, p. 25). He then proceeds to assume away quality differentials. Ro considers quality relevant, but then equates the quality dimension of output with the existing "scope of services" (350, p. 210). Cohen, on the other hand, takes not the scope of services, but the degree of hospital affiliation as his "measure" of quality (86, p. 13). For hospitals with the same service-facility mix, Berry assumes that higher costs indicate higher quality (46, p. 127). The role of quality will not be discussed at this point, but the indicated approaches to it in the literature are symptomatic of the general confusion.

The view of the hospital as a complex organization producing a variety of services, as we have suggested in chapter 1, is not generally recognized in the empirical studies. The focus of the analyses is on the production of inpatient care. Hence the service flows are those directed at inpatients. The simultaneous production of ambulatory care, the rendering of services to emergency room and clinic patients by the same departments which produce an overlapping set of services for inpatients, means that there are competing demands for their outputs from within the hospital. The laboratories, radiation departments, as well as many of the medical departments, such as internal medicine, obstetrics, pediatrics, and ophthalmology, provide both inpatient and ambulatory services. Hence, however one wishes to or can technically define their outputs, the exclusion of outpatient services means that they are only partially identified. Additional complexity is engendered by the recognition that patient directed services do not exhaust the complete output set. Research and teaching activities absorb a significant proportion of staff time in many hospitals. Informal educational activities provided to community physicians, other community services such as ambulance, social services, and outreach, vary from hospital to hospital. But in an increasing number of them they also constitute outputs. Of all these activities unrecognized in the attempts at output definition the provision of ambulatory care, as we shall demonstrate in chapter 8, is by far the most important in terms of resources used and services provided.

It is useful to consider the various hospital outputs as they are related to the major productive units in the hospitals. We have suggested that the outputs are multidimensional, comprising direct and indirect patient care, research, training, and training associated outputs, as well as community-oriented outputs. If we consider the service departments in which the services are produced, it is apparent that the direct and indirect medical service departments originate service flows into the two patient focused operations. As we show in figure 3-1, inpatient services interact with ambulatory services in at least two ways. First, given existing service capabilities, there exist some trade-offs between inpatient and outpatient services. This is not generally considered in the literature's analysis of outputs, or of costs. Yet it appears obvious that to the extent the inpatient and ambulatory functions generate derived demands for the same service departments, their mutual existence ought to be expiicitly recognized. Further, the hotel type services (food, laundry, janitorial), while flowing exclusively, or almost so, to the inpatient functions, also represent resource demands which compete with the resource requirements of the medical service departments. The appropriate view of the hospital is one which recognizes the multiplicity of its products, whether defined in terms of services, patients treated, end results, or health levels contributions. This formulation also reinforces the suggestions, in chapters 1 and 2, that the objectives the community hospital attempts to maximize are at best complex and subject to conflicting internal and external objectives and preferences. The discussion of outputs should recognize, and empirical research should explicitly incorporate, the multiplicity of patient and non-patient focused outputs and their competing demands for the use of hospital resources.

It seems reasonable to conclude from this examination of the status of output

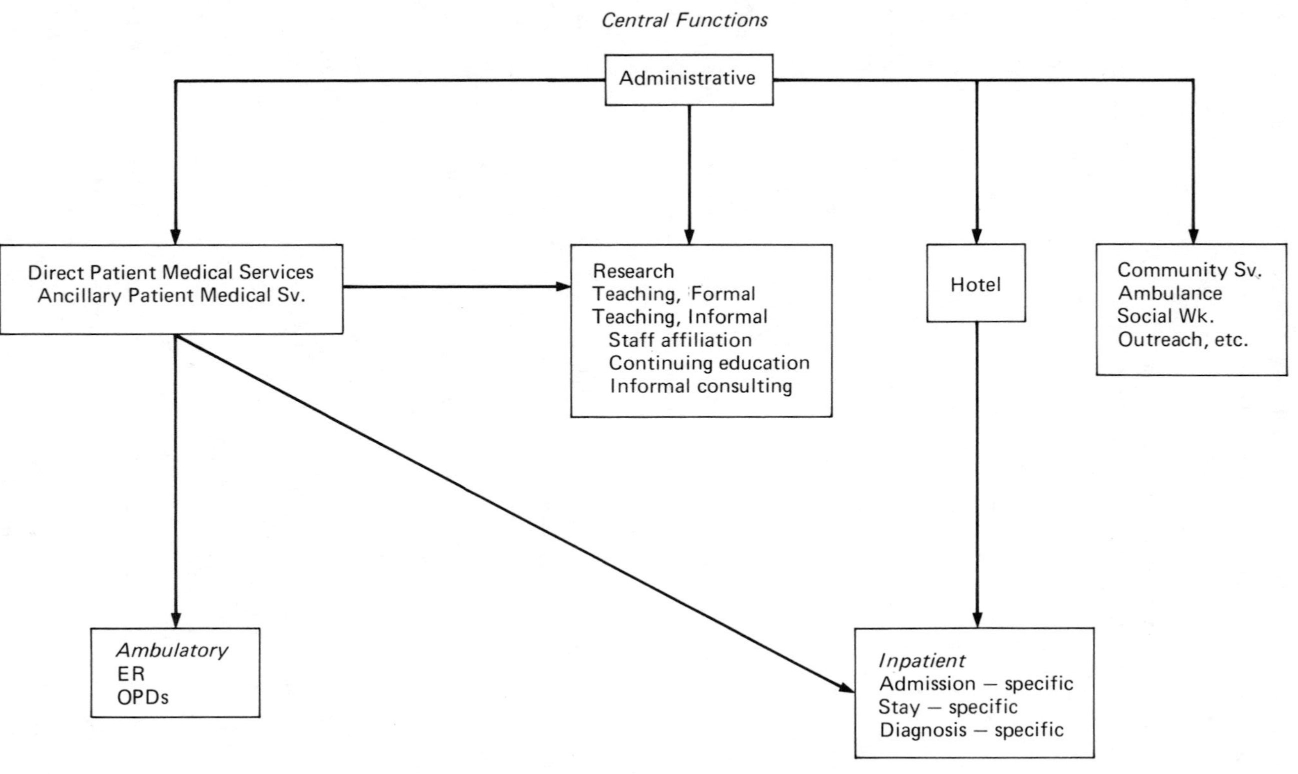

Figure 3-1. Hospital Outputs.

analysis that, while fragmentary and partial, promising approaches have recently appeared. The detailed case mix studies, the attempts at diagnosis-specific service identification, and Kovner's construction of the Identifiable Medical Procedure index represent not only significant analytic advances, but potentially provide better bases for what we wish to do: to analyze the productivity, costs, and efficiency of hospitals.

4 Productivity and Efficiency

> A majority of social scientists agree, "in effect, that all value judgments but one are outside the business of the social scientist: the one exceptional value judgment is the so-called 'pig principle', that more is better, so an economist's concern is with efficiency."
>
> —Sidney S. Alexander

Assessment of the efficiency of the hospital sector would be facilitated by an understanding of the technological and economic processes of production within the individual institutions. Productivity and efficiency can best be analyzed in terms of the technical and economic production relationships, summarized in the production function.

In this chapter we first explain and discuss the nature of the production function, distinguishing between technological and economic concepts of efficiency. We then consider the part of the literature which has attempted empirical identification of production functions in hospitals. Productivity and efficiency are concepts that may be differently applied to various aggregates of production units. After discussing the general issues of productivity and efficiency, we turn to the analysis of the productivity of inputs, stressing the importance of labor input productivity.

The empirical studies in the field demonstrate the difficulties in identifying the various factors to which productivity and efficiency differentials may be attributed. Since one of the major reasons for the relative absence of fruitful empirical studies is the apparent lack of appropriate analytic models, we next consider the theoretical bases applicable. In this section we show that the distinctions between economic and technical efficiency can be analytically made and empirically applied. But considerations of productivity and efficiency in the individual institution are not the whole issue. We also have an interest in assessing the efficiency of the hospital sector, emphasizing the factors that may lead to the generally assumed state of inefficiency. This is the subject of the last section.

We shall find in this chapter that while the empirical work is not yet complete, in the sense that we do not yet have adequately accurate representations of the production relationships, the recent application of linear programing techniques appear to yield promising results. We shall further find that the state of conceptualization is now probably sufficiently ready to permit the initiation of analytically meaningful empirical work. The discussion of the state of efficiency and of the factors relevant to its consideration for the system as a whole are less well developed, partly because there is scant agreement on what "efficiency" ought to mean, and for whom.

The Production Function and Efficiency

The production function specifies the physical relationship between outputs produced and the inputs employed in their production. It is an expression between quantities of outputs and quantities of inputs. It may be given by a single point, a single continuous or discontinuous function, or by a system of equations. In general, we deal with a simple, continuously differentiable function in two or three inputs and one or two outputs.

In its simplest form, assuming only one output, and only two inputs, x_1 and x_2, used in its production, the production function is symbolically expressed by

$$q = f_1 (x_1, x_2).$$

Here q denotes the rate of output and x_1, x_2 the rates of inputs per unit time, with both the output and the inputs expressed in physical units. In general, four basic assumptions are made about the production function: (1) The first assumption is that for any combination of the inputs, x_1, x_2, there is one, and only one, output level: that it is a single-valued function. (2) The second general assumption states that the production function is a smooth and continuously variable function. That is, it is assumed that from any initial input levels, it is possible to vary at least some of the inputs, singly or in combination, by very small amounts, and that the resultant change in output will also be gradual and continuous. The economic significance of this assumption is its specification of the possibility of input substitution: the inputs can be substituted for each other gradually and smoothly. (3) The third assumption states that depending on the time frame of analysis, at least some of the input factors may be invariant, or fixed, and then relates to the nature of the continuous variation in output resulting from the variation of the inputs that are not fixed, the variable inputs. This is the source of the "law" of diminishing returns, more properly termed the "hypothesis" of variable proportions. (4) The fourth assumption is usually stated in implicit form only, namely that the single value q associated with any input combination values, x_1, x_2 is the *maximum* technically feasible value. In explicit form this states that the production function is not only the technical relationship between the outputs produced and the inputs used in their production, but the *best* technical relationship. It is assumed, in other words, that the production function reflects not only the technologically *possible* input combinations, but the *best* of the possible technological combinations. In this sense the production function is assumed to presuppose the attainment of technical efficiency and to incorporate it. It is generally this assumption which then leads to the statement commonly found in any economic text that the production function is an "engineering datum," that it is a "technical, not an economic problem," or "a datum of analysis."

It is more realistic and analytically useful to make an additional assumption: (5) At any given time there exists a set of possible production functions with differing degrees of technical efficiency, that is, for any given level of the output q, there exist a multiple of input combinations, embodying different levels of technical knowledge. This recognizes that "technology" in any time period encompasses a variety of technically feasible production processes. A production unit, which is the subject of analysis, may not be employing the technically most efficient production function for a variety of reasons.

To begin with, the production function available to the producing unit, in our case the hospital, is constrained in the short run by the resources of the hospital. The technical relationships between input combinations and output levels represented by the production function are those between *specific* inputs and specific outputs. At any given time the hospital may not have available to it the inputs *specified* in the technically best production function. When the literature, and especially the criticisms of the operations of urban hospitals, attributes "inefficient" hospital operations to antiquated buildings and facilities, to the inadequacy of current equipment, and the lack of medically useful equipment, the meaning for the purposes of production analysis is that the inputs required for the attainment of technically efficient production are not present.

The best an existing producing unit can do, given some fixed inputs, is to use the technically best production relation, given its inputs. At this level, the identification of the best attainable technical production relationships (always keeping in mind the constraints established by the existing fixed inputs) is an engineering function. That is to say, if we are concerned not with *planning* a production unit but with the *operation* of an existing one, the problem of achieving a technically best combination of inputs, given that some of the inputs are fixed and in place, is one for engineers.

This problem in hospitals is complicated when the outputs are defined in outcome terms. To suggest that there may exist different input and technical production configurations to produce clearly developed X-rays is to pose a relatively simple engineering problem. But if we consider that the product is a successfully treated episode of illness, the outcome is always probabilistic and hence the objective is to find that technically feasible input configuration which maximizes the probability of a successful outcome. This implies that while the assumption of "homogeneous" or "invariant" or "fungible" outputs associated with different production functions may conveniently be made and then quickly forgotten in the analysis of some product outputs, all of whose dimensions can be specified, considerations of the effect of different technical combinations of inputs on the differential probabilities of successful medical outcomes must always be kept in mind. But even if we assume away the difficult issues imposed by the world of uncertainty in which hospitals operate, there are additional reasons why the technically best input combinations may not be present.

The combinations in which inputs can be used, that is to say, the substitutability among inputs, is constrained not only by technical factors but by institutional, professional, and social factors as well. Particularly in hospitals, where the largest component of input costs is labor costs, the non-technical constraints on the use of labor inputs which limit the attainable technological combinations of them must be recognized.

If the "output" is the treatment of a patient with the diagnosis of recent myocardial infarction, the "inputs" of physicians, nurses, nurses' aids, dietary and laundry facilities, chest X-ray, blood chemistry, E.K.G., possibly monitoring, inhalation therapy, and "days in bed" are all used. Clearly the services of nurses and nurses' aids are to a significant extent technically substitutable for each other: the R.N. can make the bed herself, or himself. The services of physicians are also technically substitutable for those of nurses to a significant extent: they too can make the beds, administer pharmaceuticals, take the temperature. And to some, but more limited, extent, the services of nurses are technically substitutable for those of physicians: they can both take the pulse rate, administer I.V., run the E.K.G. But nurses' aids, and most nurses, cannot read and interpret the E.K.G. or the chest X-ray. Further, at least during the diagnostic process, some services are substitutable for others, but not all are substitutes for each other. If the exact quantities of each of the inputs required to produce a "successful" treatment were known, a rough production function would result. If the substitutabilities among the various inputs were also known we would have a very acceptable production function. However, the extent to which the various labor inputs of different professional standing, technical training, and organizational status are substitutable for each other is determined by a complex set of role definitions which severely limit the technically feasible range of substitutions.

This issue in production and productivity may be seen from two perspectives. In one, we can posit that there are institutional, professional, and social constraints which establish the boundaries within which the technologically best combination of inputs, or production function, can be attained and that the objective is to identify and then to implement that production function. In the other view, the objective is to identify the best technical production function without considering non-technological constraints on the use of labor (and other) inputs and then to attempt to change the existing institutional and professional constraints which prevent its operationalization. While both of these perspectives are somewhat simplistic, they partly account for the very different evaluations of productivity in hospitals one finds in the literature.

A third reason for the absence of the technically best production function is that technological information is not free. At this point we are skirting an additional major concept, that which distinguishes between *technical* and *economic* efficiency.

If at any given time and for a given range of outputs there exists a multiplicity of input combinations, there exists one, and only one, input combination such that for the range of outputs the inputs are minimized: the technically efficient production function. Each input has a price and relative input prices vary. Therefore, given the degree of technical substitutability between inputs as reflected in the production function, and their relative prices, at any given time and for any given range of outputs there exists a set of input combinations which are least costly: the economically efficient production function. This may also be called the least cost combination of inputs, or factors.

Gold is a better conductor of electricity than copper, and copper better than aluminum. The *technically efficient* way to transport electricity overland would be attained with the use of high tension wires made of gold. They tend to be made of copper, and lately of aluminum. When inputs have prices, and alternative technically substitutable inputs have different relative prices, the *economically efficient* production process is that which, for a given value of output, minimizes the cost of inputs used to produce that output. The logical corollary of this states that the economically efficient process is that which, for a given cost of inputs, maximizes the value of output: "the biggest bang for a buck." That is to say, the technically best combination of inputs may not be the economically best combination. We shall come back to this distinction later. For now, consider that if technical information is not costless, the identification of the technically best production function itself becomes an economic question. It is traditional to consider this question as a subset of the larger questions revolving around the identification of the economically best production function. Consider that information is not free and that, therefore, the identification and implementation of the economically best (the least cost) production function involves technical information costs. We must then compare the present discounted value of the cost *saving* attainable from introducing the economically efficient production function and the information cost incurred in its identification and implementation. To be able to make the calculation, both the information costs and the expected cost saving resulting from the efficient production function must be known. But the *expected* cost saving will partially depend on expected production levels and on the time horizon, or the length of time during which the production function is to be used. Both of these variables can be known only probabilistically, where the probabilities are determined not only by changes in all those variables that influence utilization rates, but also by the rate of change in the applicable technology. Assuming, however, that acceptable information on all these variables is obtainable, the economically rational decision would be to incur information costs in an amount up to and including the present discounted value of expected cost savings.

We may summarize our discussion so far by stating that at any given time there exists a set of technologically feasible input configurations, of varying technical efficiency, for the production of some well-defined outputs. Of this set, we are interested in that particular feasible one which for a given desired level of our well-defined outputs minimizes the input costs: the least cost production function. We have stressed the necessity of defining "technological" feasibility broadly to include social, professional, and institutional factors.

The two basic approaches to the identification of the production function in the economic literature have been *statistical* and *engineering*. In the statistical approach we attempt to identify the production function indirectly by studying an appropriate sample of costs and outputs from which a cost function is estimated. Given the successful identification of the cost function, we can then derive from it the underlying production function. In the engineering approach the focus is on the detailed description of the production relationships in physical terms. The emphasis is on the use of engineering data to develop a technical production function directly, from which, given input prices, resource constraints, and desired outputs, we estimate the implied cost functions.

Production functions may be studied at differing levels of aggregation. The production function of a single department may be identified. This has been the approach of administration-oriented systems analysts using the analytic and research techniques of operations research. The production function for a single hospital may be identified and, further, the production function for aggregates of hospitals may be studied. "A production function for acute hospitals can be a useful tool for studying several practical problems: economies of scale, optimum input proportions, and the measurement of productive efficiency" (133, p. 90).

While much operations research work has been done on individual hospital departments, or even on smaller units, in terms of identifying nurse staffing patterns, radiology department scheduling, and related aspects of hospital operations, they have not considered the hospital as an organization of interdependent producing units and hence their results are of questionable value even for the limited purposes for which they were designed. There have been few attempts to study production functions in the hospital as a whole. We next consider two such attempts.

Estimated Hospital Production Functions

The major attempt to estimate production functions for hospitals was undertaken by M. Feldstein. Defining the hospital's output to be the sum of weighted case categories, with relative average costs as weights, he experiments with various configurations of three basic aggregate production functions (Cobb-Douglas, and C.E.S. and the Leontieff). The basic difference among the three functional forms relates to their different assumptions about the elasticity of input substitution, assumed to be fixed for each input in the Leontieff, to sum to one in the Cobb-Douglas, and to be parametric in the C.E.S. After various forms of input specification, and the use of different estimating techniques appear to yield few satisfactory results, this effort is abandoned in favor of a more generalized model (133, p. 120).

The "more general model of production relations" is a recursive system of five equations in beds (B), medical staff (M), drugs and dressings (D), nursing (N), and housekeeping (H) as inputs. Of the five inputs only *B* and *M* are exogenously determined, or constrained, beds by existing physical facilities and medical staff by the staffing rules applicable in the British National Health Services (from where the data originate) and the existing supply conditions. Drugs and dressings inputs are determined by the two constrained inputs *B* and *M*, while the levels of the other two factors are not considered to influence output levels, but are to be determined by the intensity of hospital operations itself, the level of output. Thus of the five inputs, output is determined by only three, *B, M,* and *D*, while the other two *N* and *H* are output determined. While beds are measured in physical units, all other inputs are measured in money terms as expenditures. Output, as in the other models, is measured in terms of weighted case categories. Hence both the measures of inputs and of outputs are highly aggregative.

In the five equations model then, output is seen as determined by the three inputs of beds, medical staff, and drugs and dressings, of which only *B* and *M* are fixed. The results show slightly decreasing returns with increasing output scale. Output, however, could be increased by a reshuffling of inputs, with less nursing and housekeeping activities and increases in the medical staff (133, p. 123). Whether the tentative nature of the analysis justifies the policy conclusion that "A general expansion of the medical staff and a reallocation in favor of larger hospitals seems warranted" is debatable (133, p. 123).

The conclusion is also baffling in view of the fact that, given the nature of the model, the inputs to be minimized (nursing and housekeeping) are endogenously determined: their levels are a function of the size of hospital output. That they are endogenously determined implies that there exists some technical relationship between their use and some dimension of output, whether captured in the definition used or not. Hence a reduction in the output-determined inputs implies a change in some dimension of output. If that dimension is considered relevant, what the model predicts is that for some other input combination more of a *different* output could be produced. Only if the output dimension changed is considered undesirable or irrelevant is Feldstein's conclusion valid. Hence the meaning of his statement that "the possibility of increasing hospital output by decreasing the amenity standard becomes clear" (133, p. 123) implies that he considers "amenity standards" to be an irrelevant dimension of output. In that case his conclusion is valid. However, since his definition of output excludes any consideration of other quite relevant dimensions of output, such as the quality of care and discharge status, it is also obvious that output measured in patient days, weighted or not, could be substantially increased by stacking patients in wards, two to a bed.

What would be desirable is a less aggregative production function, a production function of treatment. This would entail the specification of medical and hotel type services by diagnostic category for a successful termination of the inpatient phase of an illness episode. In its absence one can only speculate on the substitutability of such aggregates as "beds" and "medical staff": more complex cases may require higher numbers of time-intensive procedures, such as complex blood chemistry or BMR surveillance, and fewer medical-staff intensive inputs, resulting in longer stays and lower medical staff inputs. Other types of case complexity may require the opposite combination. Feldstein's analysis, therefore, is an interesting and careful exercise in econometrics, with some misspecification of output, but its operational fruitfulness as he cautions, is yet to be demonstrated.[a]

An attempt to identify a much more disaggregated production function of the medical services in the hospital has been undertaken by Dowling (120). Considering the hospital to be a multiproduct firm composed of a series of departments, analogously to the model we propose in chapter 1, the focus of the study is narrowed to the production of medical services for inpatient care. Output is measured by patient case load decomposed into fifty-five diagnostic categories, each equally weighted on the assumption that the hospital's objective is to maximize its total patient care. The inputs are specified in engineering terms and measured in the appropriate physical units as services flowing to patients in the different diagnostic categories. The model is a linear programing one in which it is assumed that the input coefficients by diagnostic categories are fixed. That is to say, the basic assumption, whose applicability is later tested, is that to each diagnostic category there corresponds a well-defined and invariant medical service mix in terms of nursing days, specified operations, prescriptions, laboratory tests, etc. The next step is to specify the functional relationships between the service producing departments and the patients by diagnostic categories to which the services are rendered, the hospital's technology matrix.

The technology matrix is initially specified by fourteen medical service departments and fifty-five diagnostic categories and the input-output coefficients are estimated by regression techniques.[b] The absence of available data for

[a]This reminds one of the aptness of Leontieff's dictum: ". . . in all too many instances sophisticated statistical analysis is performed on a set of data whose exact meaning and validity are unknown to the author or rather so well known to him that at the very end he warns the reader not to take the material conclusions of the entire 'exercise' seriously" (238, p. 3).

[b]The initial fourteen services specified are: nursing and intensive care unit, measured in patient days, blood units, ECG examinations, IPPB treatments, laboratory tests performed, intravenous fluids administered, prescriptions, X-rays, deliveries, and oxygen, anesthesia, operating room and recovery room services measured in hours (120, p. 154).

two departments (p. 178) limited the analysis to twelve types of services. Tests for the linearity of the coefficients revealed that in the case of three additional departments (inhalation therapy, ECG, and IPPB) the input coefficients did not meet the linearity assumptions, leaving the model with eight specified inputs.

In a linear programing approach, the problem is to estimate the input coefficients, specify the outputs, and, given the constraints on resources (input capacities), estimate the optimum feasible outputs in terms of the number of patients in the specified diagnostic categories that can be treated. That is, both the optimum volume and diagnostic mix are estimated as well as the trade-offs among the various diagnostic categories that can be accommodated.

Using an argument similar to Feldstein's (133, pp. 120-24), Dowling assumes that the so-called minor departments do not have rigid capacity limits and hence they do not act as constraints on output. He considers that of the eight departments for whose outputs the coefficients can be accurately estimated and accepted to be linear, only five enter the production process. Output, in diagnosis specific patient days, is therefore seen to be a linear function of five departmental service inputs: nursing days, laboratory, radiology, delivery rooms, and operating rooms (120, pp. 177-83). The capacities of the departments producing these services are estimated by considering both physical and institutional constraints, such as "normal" weekly periods during which operations are carried out. After trying various specifications of the linear programing model, Dowling concludes that the study hospital "operated at from 78.5 to 85.1 percent of optimum efficiency" (p. 228), that is, that it could have treated significantly more patients without exceeding its capacity.

Perhaps the most interesting finding of this study is that specification four of the model, which considers institutionally (or what Dowling calls "experienced") constrained capacities and where the minimum permissible solution values for outputs are constrained to the actual number of patients by diagnostic category treated during the study year (p. 206, ff.), the major binding constraint is the number of operating room hours (p. 211). That is to say, while in actual terms the hospital produced some 15 percent below its feasible optimum output, *had* it been on its production possibility surface, the constraint with the highest shadow price would have been operating room hours: for each unit increase in operating room hours 0.76 more patients in the surgical categories could have been treated. In general the findings on the other constraints (pediatric, medical-surgical, psychiatric, obstetric, and newborn patient days), while more disaggregated and hence more specific, are in accord with Feldstein's finding that the constraints are imposed by beds and staffing, while laboratory tests, drugs, X-rays and other ancillary services are nonbinding.

Dowling's formulation is both ingenious and potentially fruitful in demonstrating the approach to a detailed specification of the production processes within the hospital. But, as he recognizes, a number of problems remain. One major problem, to those who are interested in the quality dimension of medical care, is that that dimension is not captured. In further attempts with the linear programing approach, quality should be incorporated into the output. Further, there are some serious difficulties with the assumption that in the hospital's objective function all treatments to patients, regardless of their diagnostic class, are weighted equally. This is recognized by Dowling and discussed at length by Feldstein, who demonstrates that the use of different weighting schemes (equal weights, by duration or by average cost of stay) yield very different results in terms of what the binding constraints are (133, p. 180).[c]

While an understanding of production functions would be useful in the analysis of hospital costs, appropriateness of input proportions, economies of scale, and the resource costs of alternative kinds of outputs, we have seen that in the economic literature on hospitals there have been few attempts to identify directly and to analyze the properties of the hospital's production function. Nonetheless, there has been much discussion of both productivity and efficiency as well as of the role of input productivities. Next we turn to the discussion of the issues of productivity and efficiency.

Productivity and Efficiency

Recalling our discussion of the production function, factor *productivity* may be relatively simply defined: in any process using one or more inputs and yielding one or more outputs, that increase in net positive output(s) attributable to a unit increase in one input, holding all other inputs at a constant level, is the (marginal) productivity of the input increased. We say "net positive" since one or more of the outputs may be "negative," undesirable. An increase in smoke, sewage, etc., should be counted with negative weights, or be counted as inputs. The average amount of output(s) attributable to the average amount of each input is that input's average productivity: that is, the total amount of output(s) attributable to the total amount of a given input, divided by the total amount of that input used. When many outputs are produced and many inputs utilized, precise empirical productivity estimation may be difficult, made more so by the existence of joint products, externalities in production, joint inputs, indivisibilities, etc. In theory, however, the productivities of the individual factors of production are knowable. But to know them the production function must be specified. It is the production function that relates to each quantity of output, per unit of time, the quantities of required inputs, their proportions, and their substitutabilities, or elasticities of substitution.

Many of the difficulties in analyzing productivity, or even identifying it, arise from the lack of conceptual agreement on the appropriate definition of outputs and inputs. It is not clear, for example, whether physician productivity should be conceptualized in terms of "output per physician hour" or "physician

---

[c]An interesting linear programing approach is also outlined in Ref. 33.

output per year."[d] If the physician's output is considered to be patient visits, then it seems clear that we would wish to maximize patient visits per hour (which would correspond to increasing the physician's productivity per hour) and the number of physician hours per year (which would correspond to increasing his or her production). Should his output be conceptualized as an input into the healing process and as *the* constraining resource, then presumably we would wish to maximize physician output by substituting other resources for it to the extent feasible. In the latter case we would wish to maximize his productivity in terms of his contributions to the medical treatment process and the relevant time dimension would be the assumed number of hours per year physicians are willing to work. In the absence of a production function clearly defined in inputs and outputs, discussion of productivity is difficult.

The discussion of the production function also pointed out that at any given time a set of production functions is likely to exist. The *technically efficient* production function is required: the minimum set of inputs required to produce a successful treatment. Then a given treatment process could be assessed in terms of its *technical efficiency*: is it using the technically efficient set of inputs?

Neither inputs or outputs, whether priced or not, are free. Inputs have explicit, and sometimes indirect, costs attached to them. Any output resulting from their use, therefore, whether that output carries a price or not, has a cost. Its resource cost is the cost of inputs used. Its opportunity cost is the value of other output(s) that could have been produced (with the same inputs) instead. The value of the output may be greater or less than the sum of the costs of input factors used to produce it. In a reasonably well-operating market system the problem of calculation is simply solved: if what people are willing to pay for the output(s) is greater than the cost of inputs used to produce it, that difference, net revenue, returns, or profits—we are not now concerned with what it is called or who gets it—is an indication of the amount by which the value of output(s) exceeds the value of inputs.

When an efficiently operating market system does not obtain to generate the signals by which to assess the economic efficiency of operations, alternative systems are required to valuate the outputs.

In the absence of a system to valuate the outputs, economic efficiency and efficient pricing strategies are not only indeterminate; they are indefinable. And any system which specifies a set of relative values for the outputs, and who is to get them, will have implicit in it both the economically efficient methods of production and pricing.

If the relative values of the presence of open-heart surgery facilities and of well-baby clinics are those established by the cardiologists in a hospital, the presence of unused heart surgery facilities and masses of unexamined poor babies are consistent with the concept of economic efficiency. Private pediatricians in the community may well view this as efficient as well.

[d]I am thankful to Uwe Reinhardt for the suggestion of this example.

As we have pointed out before, not only the presence of an objective function which valuates outputs is required, but the knowledge of *whose* objective function counts. If we assume that the objective functions of the private pediatricians in the community count, in the previous example—and assuming, perhaps, a not overly untenable set of values—the presence neither of well-baby nor of open-heart surgery facilities may be economically efficient; an enlarged pediatric ward might. To push this example one step further, should the preferences or objective functions of indigent families with small children count, the existence of the well-baby clinic might well reflect the efficient allocation of resources; not only what is produced, but also who gets it counts.

Overall economic efficiency is attained when resources cannot be reallocated in such a way that the changes in the resulting output levels yield an increase in the satisfactions of those whose preferences are to count: efficiency in production and in distribution obtains.[e]

Our review so far has shown that neither private nor social preference functions, or objective functions, have been acceptably specified, or even defined, in terms of what hospitals do or ought to produce. We have also shown that there is no general agreement on how to count, or measure, that which is being produced. Even disregarding the absence in the literature of the discussion of ambulatory services, indirect costs, and opportunity costs, we shall also show that there is no agreement on how to specify the costs of that which is now defined as the relevant output set, or the conditions under which the costs are incurred. Neither cost nor production functions have been acceptably specified: those that are specific are clearly unacceptable and those that are at least theoretically plausible are much to vague. It is in view of this that the discussion of the extant concepts of hospital productivity and efficiency must proceed.

One of the first results of this lack of clarity is that while "efficiency" is a beautiful thing, beauty is in the eyes of the beholders, each of whom view it through a prism—but not all prisms are the same.

The Gorham Report concludes:

At present, hospitals have inadequate incentive to be efficient. They are not under strong pressure from patients, because a substantial part of the patients' bills are paid by third parties. Third parties have usually reimbursed hospitals for cost incurred without pressing for greater efficiency. Hospital administrators often lack the training required for effective management. The medical staff of the hospital often presses the hospital administrator and Board of Trustees for acquisition of the latest medical equipment without regard to the cost implications involved. Trustees are often subject to pressures imposed on them by the

[e]For a full discussion see Graff (170), and Baumol (38). For discussions of the efficient allocation problem in the absence of accurate prices or where social and private valuations diverge, see Ciriacy-Wanthrup, (79); Freeman (151), Hirshleifer (188); McKean (293); and Williamson (434).

community and medical staff. Even where the incentive does exist, initiation is often beyond the resources of an individual institution (271, pp. 7-9).

Or consider the following extensive quotation from the Gardner Report:

Imagine that a visitor from Mars, intelligent but unfamiliar with such earthly problems as illness, happened into one of our hospitals and engaged the administrator in conversation.

"What is the purpose of this fine institution?" asked the visitor. The administrator explained that persons disabled by illness or injury come here for the most searching, skilled examinations and judgments to determine precisely what is wrong and apply measures, often requiring great delicacy and wisdom, to combat the disability.

"Ah, and as the man in charge here, do you make all the judgments and order these procedures yourself?" the Martian inquired.

"By no means," replied the administrator. "That is the function of persons called physicians, who qualify for these tasks by long periods of intensive training and observation."

"The physician, then, must make many decisions that determine how your resources are used and what work your people do," the visitor observed. The administrator acknowledged that this was an understatement, if anything, since the physician also decided which patients to admit, and when to dismiss them.

"And where do these important persons stand in your organization?" asked the Martian.

"Actually, they stand outside the organization," the administrator explained. "They are engaged and paid by our customers, as you might say, and they must observe certain organizational rules, but the fact is that the institution itself, by tradition, must not interfere or seek to influence their decisions."

"But you must be joking!" the visitor exclaimed. "As anyone can plainly see, such an arrangement would be impossible to manage."

The administrator acknowledged that it wasn't easy, and the visitor was heard to say to himself as he departed, "Impossible—or very, very expensive!" (378, p. 20)

One of the most highly regarded experts in the field, D.W. Anderson, has a different view:

. . . I certainly subscribe to the belief that the health services system can benefit from the strengthening of the managerial corps and managerial concepts. Tremendous resources are at stake that require the attention of a managerial elite. It is my observation, however, that the emerging managerial elite and the elite of the recent past do not understand the applicability to a health service system of the managerial techniques and concepts characteristic of modern industry. I refer here to the administration of professionals, patients, and a social system, and not to the cut and dried bookkeeping and hotel aspects of the system. The latter can certainly benefit by tidy administration with respect to billing, food service, management of non-professional personnel and so on. I would hope, however, that we are moving in the direction of management concepts that are peculiar to the health services system and that are more analogous to concepts familiar to universities and research organizations than to industry. Sophisticated managerial theory reflects a growing realization that there is a range of managerial styles related to types of enterprise. This is relatively new to the health field. Hence, I tend to fear the premature and naive application of managerial concepts appropriate in industry to health services (16, pp. 81-82).

Considering the approaches of some of the economists, perhaps Anderson is justified in his fear of "the premature and naive application of managerial concepts appropriate in industry to health services."

The goal of maximum efficiency is dual in nature: to maximize the occupancy rate while minimizing the risk of being unable to meet the demand for beds. The optimum combination is a criterion of efficiency and, as such, it minimizes unit cost. In terms of business management, this is essentially an inventory control problem—a balancing of the inventory carrying charges against the cost of being unable to meet orders. (Ro, 350, pp. 190-91)

The primary inputs required to produce an output of treated patients are space, equipment, personnel, and materials (*sick patients* and hospital supplies). The first two of these inputs are already located at the site of production (hospital) while the latter two must be transported to the hospital. (Schneider, 370, p. 155, emphasis added)

The cost that it is worthwhile to incur to prolong life is a partial function of prior investment in the formation of human capital. *Other things being equal*, since society loses more from the extinction of more highly valued lives, it would pay it to devote more resources to the preservation of those lives than to less highly valued lives . . . Mankind is a durable good subject to physical depreciation the rate of which can be kept in check by maintenance and repair expenditures. *On economic grounds, approximately the same rules that govern when to maintain and when to scrap machine capital and that determine the optimal rate of maintenance expenditures for machine capital also apply to human capital.* (Rottenberg, 362, p. 111, emphasis added)[f]

Aside from the fact that it is usually assumed that people have preferences and that machines do not, there is, of course, some conflict between viewing

[f]In terms of the social efficiency of research, it may be worthwhile to note that the "research" which considered sick patients as material inputs was funded by the National Institutes of Health, while Rottenberg's opus was supported by the Social Science Research Council.

potential patients as hunks of embodied human capital on the one hand, and, on the other, as "material" inputs along with hospital supplies. The concept of efficiency as the "maximum occupancy rate" avoids this problem, but not by much. For, again of course, to attain efficiency we must minimize inputs, hence a hospital 100 percent occupied with healthy people would minimize the "material" "sick patient" input.

It may be suggested that these examples are somewhat extreme, unrepresentative. In terms of their ethical assumptions, that is correct. But they represent well that "premature and naive application of managerial concepts" that Anderson warns against. They also represent quite well the analytic chaos which fills the theoretic vacuum.

With few exceptions, there is general agreement that "efficiency," no matter how defined or undefined, is either partially or completely absent. The presumptive causal factors are many, as the Gorham Report and Gardner Reports indicate. The lack of a profit motive and of monetary incentives are usually cited as major reasons.

Our just preceding discussion indicated that efficiency is a relationship in outputs and inputs: for economists, technical productivity and economic productivity are its two intertwined elements. A complex of other factors, such as organizational, managerial, motivational, are all related to each other–and to efficiency. Economists tend to subsume such factors under the rubric of "entrepreneurial factors." It is the entrepreneur who, with technical assistance from engineers and managers, combines resources in the most efficient manner he is capable of, and reaps the private benefits in terms of profit.

The discussion of efficiency to follow will adhere to the inherent logic of the theory of production, which we presented in a most adumbrated form. We shall consider input factors, factor combinations, productivities, and then, efficiency.

Factors of Production and Productivity

> Alice had been looking over his shoulder with some curiosity. "What a funny watch!" she remarked. "It tells the day of month, and doesn't tell what O'clock it is." "Why should it?" muttered the Hatter. "Does *your* watch tell you what year it is?"
>
> –Lewis Carroll, *Alice in Wonderland*

The largest single cost component in hospital is labor costs.[g] It is generally assumed that the single most important source of hospital inefficiency is to be found in the simultaneous productivity lag and wage increases of labor (e.g.,

[g]For the most comprehensive summary of previous manpower studies see Appendix VI, "Major Studies of Manpower Requirements for Health Services, 1930-65," p. 265, Vol. II, Ref. 340. For the most comprehensive critical review of research and literature in the area see Butter (68).

397, p. 358). These are attributed to a variety of factors: "archaic licensing regulations and professional mores, . . . unassimilated revolution in hospital labor relations, . . . lack of flexibility in labor use, . . . increased unionization . . . " (397, p. 358). There is little or no discussion of labor-input output relations in a technical sense: no attempt to isolate even an impressionistic production function. That this would be feasible has been demonstrated in studies of "optimal" care and their labor requirements by skill level. The "Yale Studies" are an outstanding example of this (128, 372, 373).

The demonstration of labor productivity lag has proceeded in vaguely specified output and input units. Klarman (217, p. 110) and M. Feldstein (133), among others, cite the now classic study by Lytton (260) as evidence of productivity lag. "That hospitals lag in productivity gains is supported by one of the few studies of productivity (defined as output per unit of labor input) that compares trends in hospitals and in other service fields . . . This explanation has serious implications" (Klarman, 217, p. 110). Lytton considered "labor productivity" in federal agencies. Among others, the hospital system of the Veterans Administration is considered. Output is defined as unweighted *patient days* and the labor component of input as *personnel.* What Lytton then shows is that patient days per personnel has not increased over time. This result is well known. However, this is not even an approximation to a measure of either productivity or of productivity change over time since: (a) the output is defined in terms of a complex and unspecified aggregate; (b) any change in any of the undefined output dimensions, such as length of stay, quality, case complexity, patient demographic characteristics, disease distribution over an extended period, will change "output" but will not be reflected in the "measure"; (c) the composition of "personnel" is not known, and it also may have changed; and (d) service intensity and complexity is not specified, and we know that that has changed. Lytton's study merely says that "patient day" per "personnel" has not changed. To consider this as a measure of labor productivity is absurd: with 100 percent increases in patient turnover and in case fatalities and no increase in personnel, "patient days per personnel" can be shown to have increased 100 percent.

Fuchs estimates that labor productivity has increased somewhat over time, but by less than in the rest of the economy. For the period 1929-1965, his measure of "output" is deflated national total dollar expenditures. Labor input is again personnel, now appearing as "per man" (159, p. 117). The increase in "real output per man" is shown to be 0.9 percent per year. The same criticisms apply, but in somewhat stronger terms. Changes in the patterns and outcomes of hospital care between 1929 and 1965 make shambles of his measures of "real output" and "input."[h]

"All forms of covariance regressions analyzed show that the labor productivity measure is consistently the most important factor explaining cost differences" (sic) (Ro, 402, p. 255). What this means, and how it differs from Lytton,

[h]For a discussion of such changes, see Ref. 9 and 402.

is hard to tell, since "the labor productivity measure used in this study is simply the reverse of the staffing ratio–employees per bed . . . " (p. 256). It may well be that this "measure [is] often used by hospital administrators as a quality index" (402, 256), but since it measures the labor intensity of beds, and not of care, it may be negatively related to the quality of care. The nursing-home "industry" is an example of this. The number of beds per employee, Ro's measure of "labor productivity" which "explains" cost differences, is highest in long-term psychiatric institutions, which are not that much different from jails–except that the inmates serve indeterminate terms. Whatever factors or tendencies it measures, labor productivity is not one of them.

However labor productivity is defined, the argument is often advanced that decreasing hours and increasing wages imply higher costs (397; 219; 217; 340, esp. pp. 255-56). In several places Klarman has suggested that decreases in hours worked necessarily lead to decreases in productivity (219; 217). While this is certainly a truism as long as productivity is measured in "personnel per patient day," it is contrary to general U.S. national trends in manufacturing, where labor productivity has been more accurately measured. Denison, in fact, has shown that decreases in the work week have been associated with increases in labor productivity (108).

Not technical productivity lags, but rapidly increasing wages are held to blame by others. Since no measures of physical productivity exist, the argument is that "efficiency" must have decreased as a result of wage increases in excess of that in the rest of the economy. The comparisons are at times fallacious, as when hospital wage changes are compared with those of "full time employees for all industries" (340, Vol. II, p. 255).[i]

The theory proffered to explain higher than average wage increases in hospitals may be called "the closing of the gap" theory. The basic argument is that wage rates and working conditions in hospitals have been traditionally lower than those in industry in general. Unionization, and presumably greater horizontal labor mobility, have resulted in the gradual elimination of the hospital-industry differentials. Since hospitals had to "catch up," so to speak, increases in wages paid by hospitals had necessarily to rise faster than some national average. The "gap" has not been closed yet: there was still, in 1963, a "depressed state of hospital wages" (165, p. 293). This "depressed state" has been attributed to the "eleemosynary nature" of hospitals (337, p. 127). For this argument to hold it must be assumed either (a) that horizontal labor mobility exists but that employees are themselves at least partly motivated by "eleemosynary" tend-

[i]The usually careful Gorham Report makes the same error (271, pp. 28-31). If comparative studies are to have significance, comparable industries must be compared. The "rest of the economy" includes all technologically advanced capital-intensive industries. A possibly meaningful bases for comparison with the medical care sector, or with hospitals, would be legal services, or education. But no reliable measures for those sectors exist either, and probably for the same reasons.

encies—they could have moved, within skill categories, to higher paying jobs out of the hospitals, but preferred not to, or (b) that little horizontal mobility obtains in that segment of the market from which hospitals draw their labor force. It may also be that, at least in the recent past, both mobility and organization were absent in that pool of black and Spanish-speaking workers from which urban hospitals tend to recruit an overwhelming proportion of their low- and semi-skilled employees.

The precise identification of both the physical productivity of labor and of wage changes is indeed important. It is implicit in the statement that capital productivity is equally important. To the extent that the hospital sector uses resources in common with the other sectors of the economy, or to the extent that the opportunity costs of personnel in hospitals are wages and earnings in other sectors, if the other sectors demonstrate a secular increase in productivity, while the hospital sector can be said to have stable or lagging productivity, it is clear that general labor cost increases equivalent to the labor productivity of the growing productivity sectors will be easily absorbed in those sectors, without necessitating price increases, while they will impose cost increases in the lagging or stable productivity sector proportional to the share of labor in total costs. That is, growing productivity will be reflected in increasing wages in general, but if hospital productivity increases are small or non-existing, increased wages will result in increased costs. When the total operating cost is some 60 percent labor cost, this is no small problem.[j]

As suggested in our analytic discussion in the first section of this chapter, one of the many obstacles in the way of "efficient" specialization of functions and changes in labor inputs of various skills in hospitals is the strong status hierarchy. The constraints on labor substitutability imposed by status, institutional, and professional considerations may not be unique to the hospital sector, but they are probably the strongest here. Professional role definitions are not only well known but an important part of the training process as well as of the organizational rationale of medical care institutions.[k] Wessen, for example, has identified no less than twenty-three occupational status groups, ranging from the "janitor" at the bottom to the "visiting staff physician" at the top (433, p. 450). Since specific tasks are associated with given occupational categories, and since each of the occupational categories occupies a distinct rung on the hierarchical ladder, the reallocation of tasks is inhibited. Additionally, in the other sectors of the economy individuals occupying positions requiring low educational and/or skill levels may rise to higher levels through on-the-job-training, within certain limits of course. This job-related vertical labor mobility is encouraged and supported by both institutional ethos and consensus ideology, not to mention

[j]For an extended discussion of this issue, see Baumol and Bowen (41, pp. 499-501), and Baumol (39).

[k]But see Ref. 366 for a discussion of some possible changes.

Horatio Alger.[l] In the professions in general, and in hospitals in particular, such vertical mobility is neither encouraged nor legally permitted. No L.P.N. can become an R.N. without additional formal training and no O.R. nurse, no matter how proficient or experienced, may perform surgery without both formal training and legal sanction in the form of licensure.[m]

If the literature on labor productivity in the hospital is poor, that on the other factors of production is almost nonexistent. Some discussion of the sources of capital funds is present (for example, 286; 258; 389). It is informative in terms of the sources of funds, but generally purely descriptive. It is usually assumed that "the hospital will use whatever capital is available . . . " (256, p. 13).

Three interesting lagged-investment models of hospital capital investment have been developed by M. Feldstein, Ginzberg, and Kelman (135; 166; and 205). Both Feldstein and Ginzberg view the demand for capital as a function of the difference between the hospital's desired number of beds and its actual number. Kelman, on the other hand, considers external demand determinants, such as socioeconomic factors, and the availability of substitutes in terms of extended care facility beds as the principal independent variables influencing the level of the hospital sector's demand for capital.

Muller and Worthington, in an interesting longitudinal study, consider investment behavior. They conclude that "68 percent of the variance in annual real investment is explained by three factors: yearly changes in an output index, yearly changes in the ratio of semi-private days to admissions, and an allowance for a distributed lag in carrying out desired investment projects" (285, p. 3). Since "output" is defined to be admissions plus X-rays, laboratories, audit operations, all per admission, what they really measure is investment related to all inputs. One would expect, therefore, a better fit than what they find (p. 18). This is indicated by their finding a better fit when output is defined simply as admissions. While informative, the paper tells us little about capital productivity, which is not within the authors' purview, but which for purposes of investment analysis is quite relevant.[n]

Some aspects of capital financing will be discussed below, under reimbursement schemes.

In view of the fact that the production functions, either in physical or financial terms, have not been identified, it is interesting that some discussions have proceeded on the assumption of fixed input proportions. That is, it is

[l]He, of course, while rising rapidly and high, did so by a combination of luck and gumption. It's hard to train-on-the-job to rescue rich old men, or their pretty daughters. But mythology and its interpretation are reflections of ethos.

[m]For a good general discussion of manpower-organizational issues see Darley and Somers (56). See, in general, Apple (19).

[n]See Ref. 166 and 205 for other studies of hospital investment behavior as well as for references.

assumed that the proportions of labor and non-labor inputs are invariant with respect to hospital size or to treatment. An experienced hospital administrator has suggested that "increased efficiencies can be achieved primarily by improved utilization of a person's time through better scheduling of activities" (199, p. 62). Examples of making a "person's time" more productive include the introduction of scheduling of physician bedside visits and reducing the travel time of physicians resulting from the multiple staff appointments or admitting privileges. It is suggested that the physician should concentrate all his patients in one hospital (p. 64). This assumes that the crucial factor is the physician input, which may be the case. However, since physician services are separately billed for and not generally considered *hospital* costs, this appears to be an argument for the hospital as the doctor's "workshop."

Capital-labor substitution is not only considered not possible, but technological change is seen to be labor-intensive.[o] Since hospitals are labor-intensive and new technology demands more capital which is also labor-deepening, no prospects are seen for increases in productivity (217, pp. 237-39, and references cited). That is, a high proportion of inputs used are labor inputs. The introduction of additional capital not only does not replace labor, it requires proportionately more of it. The "more labor" may mean more bodies at the same skill level, or more frequently, more bodies embodying more knowledge.[p] As the director of a famous New York City hospital has said: "Unfortunately, however, most of the complex new diagnostic and treatment devices require more and better-trained technicians than the old diagnostic and treatment methods did" (405, p. 220). There is scant agreement on whether this is reflected in the cost data of diagnostic and therapeutic services. Klarman argues that the highest increases have been observed in the costs of laboratories, radiology, and operating rooms (219, p. 464; 217; p. 247). Cohen, on the other hand, maintains that at least for the period 1962-65 (and also in New York City), "the average costs of all services *but* laboratory examinations and blood transfusions increased" (86, pp. 13-14, emphasis added). He finds that, on the contrary, the highest percentage increases took place in "routine adult and pediatric days and emergency room treatment." (Ibid.) Alternatively, and not on the contrary, it may well be that there is no disagreement: "adult and pediatric patient days and emergency room treatment" are highly service-intensive. Thus if Klarman is correct and Cohen's specification of output a bit vague, it may well be that the costs of "adult and pediatric days and emergency room treatment" have experienced the highest cost increases *because* the costs of the ancillary services have increased at the fastest rate. A well-known economist once said that if the facts don't fit the theory, the facts are wrong. Of course, if there is no theory, any fact will fit. Even the fact that sick patients are "material inputs."

The discussion of the empirical analyses of factor productivity has demon-

[o]For some considerations of possible substitutions, see Refs. 105, 106.

[p]For a detailed discussion and an example, see Ref. 221.

strated that while there is a general presupposition that the source of the perceived lagging productivity is to be found in the hospital's inability to substitute capital for labor, productivity studies have not so far demonstrated this. It may well be that we are faced here with an example par excellence of Baumol's dual labor productivity theorem. Since labor cannot be displaced by capital in the medical treatment process, and since the introduction of new processes are even more labor using than the ones they displace, the productivity of labor in hospitals necessarily lags behind those sectors where it can be replaced by other inputs. Whether this is so or not is still to be answered by empirical research which employs identified production functions in terms of outputs defined in all their relevant dimensions, including quality. Further, one should make a distinction between historical experience on the one hand and what may be technically attainable were the binding institutional and professional constraints to be relaxed.

The empirical literature represents essentially ad hoc approaches and anecdotal reports. For a theoretical and analytically powerful discussion of productivity and productivity change in hospitals we turn to Professor M. Feldstein once again.

The Theoretical Analysis of Productivity and Productivity Change

If it is true that any group of three economists will have at least four contradictory theories, it is also true that any four medical economists are likely to have none. Professor Feldstein's attempt at theorizing must be viewed in that context. For while his conceptual framework(s) are not immediately obvious, and though he is by no means second, he tries harder.

As discussed above, M. Feldstein defines output as the weighted number of cases where the weights are the relative average costs of case types (133, p. 31). The theoretical argument supporting this procedure is important: his indexes of "costliness" and "productivity" depend on it.

The argument is that relative average costs can be considered proxies for social marginal rates of substitution between cases treated. While this is a very elegant argument indeed, it is tenable only if we postulate that relative *average costs* are linear (or at least monotonic) transforms of relative *marginal* social *values.* It must be assumed, that is, that the relative observed costs of treatment accurately reflect relative social valuations of those treatments: if the cost of a cerebro-vascular episode in an 85-year-old man is three times as great as the cost of an episode of acute appendicitis in a 15-year-old boy, the social values implied state that the first treatment is "worth" three times as much as the latter. This implies "society" would be willing to exchange three acute appendicitis treatments in 15-year-olds for one cerebro-vascular episode treatment in 85-year-olds. The relative social values determine the trade-offs. This is the precise meaning of taking relative average costs as representations of marginal social rates of substitution.

"Marginal social values of the individual cases" are identified as the relevant weights (133, p. 29). "The relative values to society of the different cases produced at hospital *i* may be measured approximately by the relative marginal costs of those cases elsewhere in the hospital system" (p. 30). "Unfortunately we do not have information about the relative marginal costs of different case types. We must go one step further and replace relative marginal costs with relative average costs . . . This cannot be justified by arguing that equilibrium conditions assure that relative average costs are the same as relative social values. Rather we assert as a plausible and useful assumption that society might value the cases of different types produced in a particular hospital in proportion to the average costs of producing those cases elsewhere in the hospital system" (p. 31).

A propos this procedure, it may be appropriate to call on Leontief once again:

Uncritical enthusiasm for mathematical formulation tends often to conceal the ephemeral substantive content of the argument behind the formidable front of algebraic signs . . . By the time it comes to interpretation of the substantive *conclusions*, the assumptions on which the model has been based are easily forgotten. But it is precisely the empirical validity of these *assumptions* on which the usefulness of the entire exercise depends (238, pp. 1-2).

The "validity" of an assumption is not testable. Since this is properly in the area of welfare economics, a quotation from Graff may be appropriate:

It is in practice, if not in principle, exceedingly difficult to test a welfare proposition. . . . The consequence is that, whereas the normal way of testing a theory in positive economics is to test its conclusions, the normal way of testing a welfare proposition is to test its assumptions. . . . In positive economics we can often simplify our assumptions as cavalierly as we please, being confident in the knowledge that their appropriateness will be tested when we come to apply the conclusions inherent in them to our observations of the world about us. In welfare economics we can entertain no such confidence. The result is that our assumptions must be scrutinized with care and thoroughness. Each must stand on its own feet. We cannot afford to simply much. Nor can we blindly hope that two erroneous assumptions will somehow "cancel out" and produce an acceptable conclusion—whereas in positive economics this procedure is as common as it is essential. There the proof of the pudding is indeed in the eating. The welfare cake, on the other hand, is so hard to taste that we must sample its ingredients before baking (170, pp. 2-3).

In whatever form the assumption is made, relative average costs must somehow be taken to represent relative marginal social valuations if Feldstein's analysis is to hold. Otherwise his index of "costliness," C_i^*, cannot be constructed (133, pp. 31-33). Costliness is defined to be the ratio of costs observed in hospital *i* (any given hospital) to the national average cost for the same set of outputs, the same cases. In a most elegant formulation, Feldstein then shows costliness to be a function of the relative efficiency with which factors of production are used (P_i^* or "productivity") and the appropriateness of input, or factor, proportions (I_i^*). We will not discuss the derivations in detail here. They are correct logical deductions from the assumptions of a social welfare function, and the relationship between relative social marginal rates of substitution and observed average costs. Given the assumption, the rest follows, in a beautiful way.

It is important to keep in mind that the concept of relative costliness of producing a given set of outputs in a given hospital is determined by the degree to which that hospital's production processes diverge from the observed national average efficiency. Efficiency, the resultant of factor productivity and factor proportions, or alternatively, input levels and input combinations, is the precise analogue of our previously posited distinction between observed and efficient production functions. It is a useful analytic tool.[q]

The distinction between costliness and productivity focuses attention on the multitude of factors that may result in inefficiency. But note, as we have stressed all along, "efficiency" is defined in terms of some objective function, in this case an assumed welfare function. It bears repeating that while we may entertain some doubts about how that welfare function is postulated to be revealed, without *some* set of assumed, postulated, hypothesized, or observed objective function the concept of "efficiency" is the smile on the face of the Cheshire cat.

Feldstein applies his construct and finds that about a third of the hospitals, sixty-six, have estimated costs by case type which differ from the estimated average costs by more than 10 percent (133, p. 43). Further, he finds that productivity is better correlated with costliness than with input efficiency: the relation between productivity and input efficiency is "quite weak" ($r = 0.048$) (p. 48). Variations in costliness are attributable to variations in productivity (P_i^*) (133, p. 48). Since input efficiency, or appropriateness of input proportions (I_i^*) measures to what extent the "right set" of inputs are purchased, and productivity (P_i^*), the extent to which the purchased inputs, "right or wrong," once purchased, are efficiently used, the two need not coincide.

Consider the argument in terms of Professor Feldstein's Diagram 2.1 (133, p. 32), reproduced here, in modified form, as figure 4-1. There are two inputs, X_1 and X_2, employed in the production of some output Q, both measured as flows

[q]It must also be kept in mind that some of the other assumptions required, such as that all hospitals face the same input prices, may be appropriate for Feldstein's data, the N.H.S., but not for the U.S. Recall also that capital costs, costs of ambulatory services, and all quality dimensions of output are also assumed away.

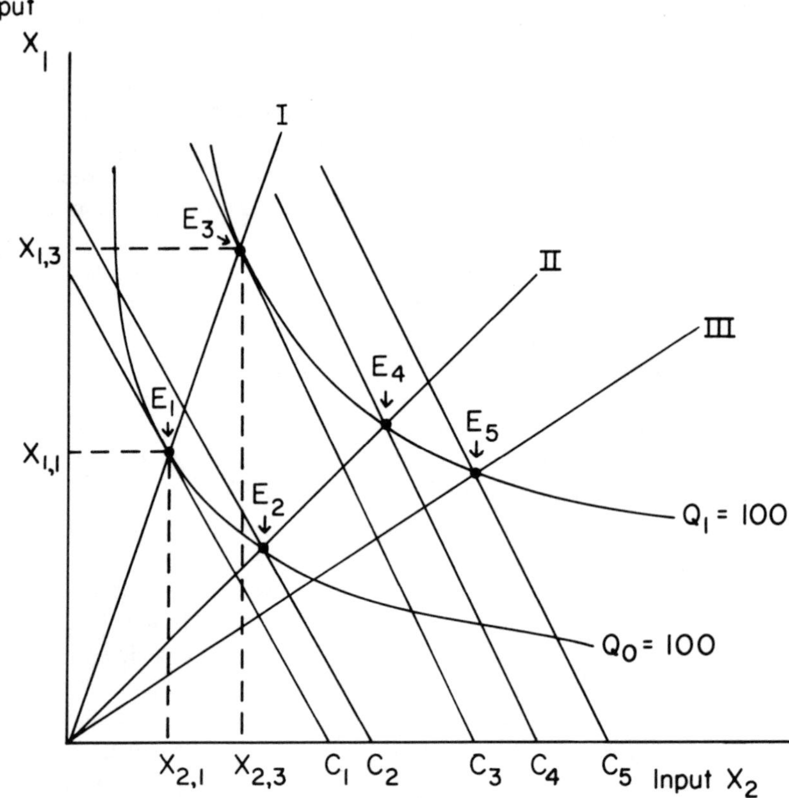

Figure 4–1. Costliness, Appropriateness, and Efficiency.

per unit of time. Both of the isoquants, Q_0 and Q_1, represent the same output rate, say Q = 100. Each of the isoquants represents the technically possible input combinations to produce the specified level of Q. If each isoquant is considered to represent a slice of the production function, it is immediately obvious that the production functions they represent are not equally technically efficient since Q_1, for all possible input combinations, requires more of each of the two inputs to produce the same rate of output than Q_0. If for purposes of the ease of diagrammatic representation we assume constant returns to scale, we can denote three possible input combinations by the production rays labeled I, II, and III, and assume that "a proportional increase in the distance from the origin along a ray corresponds to an equiproportional increase in the hospital's output" (p. 33). Given the input prices for X_1 and X_2, the total costs of each of the (considered) input combinations to produce Q = 100 are represented by the isocost lines C_1 through C_5.

Now we can consider four possibilities: (A) a hospital may be operating on a technically inefficient production function and employ an economically inefficient input combination (E_4 and E_5); (B) a hospital may be operating on a technically inefficient production function but employ the economically efficient input combination (E_3); (C) a hospital may be operating on a technically efficient production function but employ the economically inefficient input combination (E_2); and (D) a hospital may operate on the efficient production function employing the efficient combination of inputs, it is then efficient both technically and economically and is using the least-cost combination of inputs (E_1).

Let us first suppose that we observe two hospitals, one operating at point E_2 and one at point E_5. Both are producing the same output, Q = 100, at very different costs. The difference in total costs, or "costliness" (C) of the hospital operating at point E_5 can be expressed as C_5/C_2. With the construct in figure 4-1, we can now ask to what the observed cost differential may be attributed. It is clear that the hospital at E_5 is using a technically inefficient production function, and that the one at point E_2 a technically efficient one. If the hospital with the technically inefficient production function were using an economically more efficient input combination, such as that corresponding to E_4, it would be using a more "appropriate" input combination and could thus reduce its costs to C_4. This observed cost differential, therefore, can be attributed to the inappropriateness of the hospital's input proportions, denoted *I*, which is equal to C_4/C_5. Using the same input combination on the technically efficient production function would get the hospital to E_2. The cost differential between C_4 and C_2, therefore, is attributable to its lower technical productivity, denoted by P = C_4/C_2. Costliness, in this analysis, is the resultant of two factors: the technically inefficient production function and the economically inappropriate, or inefficient, input proportions employed.[r] The hospital at point E_5 corresponds to our case (A) and that at point E_2 to our case (C). While case (C) or point E_2 is less "costly" than case (A) or point E_5, neither is least costly, given its technical opportunities.

If the hospital with the technically efficient production function were to employ the most economically appropriate input combination (Case D), it would operate at point E_1, with the least total cost of C_1. If the hospital with the technically inefficient production function were to employ the most economically appropriate input combination, given its (technically) inefficient production function, it would be at point E_3, with its attainable least total cost of C_3. Consider three examples.

1. An 800 bed acute hospital may be performing laboratory tests manually. If autoanalyzers exist, the hospital can be said to be on the "wrong" production

[r]Feldstein then shows that $C = P \cdot 1/I$ (133, p. 32). Only trigonometry is required for this derivation.

function. If the laboratory technicians and existing equipment are used in the "best" possible way, to produce the most that they can be expected to produce during a given time period, factor productivity may be at the highest. The hospital would be at point E_3. (Case B)

2. An equivalent 800 bed acute hospital is performing laboratory tests on an autoanalyzer. The hospital can be said to be on the "right" production function, using the efficient production function. If the technician feeds in the wrong samples, or the generating plant runs the voltage up to 300, or the results are misread, or the technician responsible for the analyzer goes home at five in the afternoon, and noon on Sundays, input productivity may be low. The purchased factors are not most productively used. The hospital would be at point E_2. (Case C)
3. The equivalent acute hospital uses the technically efficient production function and employs the economically appropriate input combinations. There are no inefficiencies and it operates at point E_1, for the least total cost of C_1. (Case D)

The objective of efficiency is to get the "right" production function used with the most economically "appropriate" or productive input combination. Why may this not occur?

Consider first that information is costless. If technical information is free, why would any hospital opt to produce on the inefficient production function, Q_1? For four possible reasons: (1) the hospital is ignorant of the existence of Q_0, it simply does not have the free technological information; (2) it has an objective function which is resource intensive, i.e., it prefers to employ more resources for purposes of "conspicuous production"; (3) the specified production functions disregard the institutional and professional constraints and hence it may be that Q_0 is not attainable to the hospital; and (4) inputs are incompletely specified since the hospital at E_3 using $X_{1,3}$ and $X_{2,3}$, could proceed to E_1, using only $X_{1,1}$ and $X_{2,1}$, less of each output, if that option were known to it cost free. Hence it is possible that at least one of the inputs represented as variable is fixed or that there is some other input(s) not considered.

What if information is not free? If what we have defined in the discussion of production functions as information costs do exist, then this is an invalid comparison of production functions. If in fact both of the inputs are variable as here assumed, the move to the efficient point (E_1) would be justified if the present discounted value of the cost differential between the two positions (C_3-C_1) for the expected length of future operations is more than, or at best equal to, the information cost required to move to E_1. Some or all of these factors may in fact be present in actual hospital operations.

This somewhat lengthy discussion of the analytics reflects a belief that the construct is indeed useful in helping to think about the complex nature of productive efficiency in hospitals. Though the analytics are stimulating and are likely to lead to much further research, the empirical findings attached to it are less convincing.

Feldstein finds the weakness, or one could say non-existence, of the relation between productivity and input efficiency surprising. In an ad hoc argument he maintains that it is attributable to the duality of decisions: the "inherited pattern of past allocation" and administrative decisions determine which inputs will be purchased. "The productivity with which resources are used is more likely to be determined by medical and nursing staff . . . " (p. 48). The duality is appealing and buttresses the arguments we previously advanced about possible conflicts in objectives on the parts of the individual members of the triumvirate. But nonetheless, the conclusion is not quite acceptable, for the opposite one is just as logical: the administrator may be more interested in how productively resources are used and the medical staff in what complex, even if unneeded, facilities are built.

In general, the results and the conclusions must be accepted with reservations. Given limitations in data availability and validity, the fact that some of the independent variables used to estimate the measures of costliness, efficiency, and productivity are themselves the dependent variables in other estimating equations, that many of the coefficients in the costliness regression appear not to be significant (e.g., for gynecology the coefficient is −10.79, its standard error is 21.47 [p. 40]) would indicate the presence of multiple and indeterminable biases. Therefore, while in principle "Costliness, productivity, and input efficiency are . . . indices of hospital performance in the selection and use of resources" (p. 50), one should be rather careful to "proffer" them (the word omitted in the above quotation) as guides to action. This welfare cake may not go down too well.

The question of technological change has been touched upon briefly, and implicitly, in the previous discussion of the labor implications of more intensive capital use. We touch upon it again, both because it is an important subject and also to provide another example of "the premature and naive application of managerial concepts appropriate in industry to health services."

The disaggregation of innovation into *process innovation* and *product innovation* is well accepted. The first refers to a change in the production process itself, the attainment of a more efficient production function. By the second is meant the production of a "better" product.

In another place, M. Feldstein has made the distinction between process innovation which alters the treatment process but leaves "the effectiveness of treatment unchanged while reducing cost" (134, p. 144), and product innovation which alters, improves, the effectiveness of the treatment.

In the absence of empirical evidence, the proposition is advanced that process innovation is more likely to occur where there has been no product innovation: where treatment effectiveness is constant, the treatment process itself is likely to be made less input-intensive, less costly. This extension to the medical process of an accepted if troublesome theorem from the analysis of industrial production is dubious at best.[s] If we agree, as we must, with Feldstein's own emphasis on the ubiquity of uncertainty in this field, then it follows that the "effectiveness of treatment" is itself probabilistic.

In a surgical case we may define the "product" as a corrected case with no infection or other iatrogenic complications. For example, in communicating hydrocephalus in children, the product may be defined as the correction of hydrocephalus by the implantation of a valve-regulated venous shunt (258; 312). The "success" of a treatment, in terms of the probability of the patient surviving the operation for, say, five years, is a complex joint probability in part of (a) the introduction of infection during surgery; (b) the correct and precise location of the occlusion causing the symptomatology; (c) the introduction of infection during the diagnostic and post-operative management phases; (d) the probability of correct valve function; and (e) the detection of occlusion at either end of the shunt prior to cerebral damage.

A recent innovation in diagnostic and post-operative management is the location of the occlusion and monitoring of the distribution of cerebro-spinal fluid by a process which obviates ventricullography. The new process eliminates the need for a tap and the disturbance of intracranial pressure, thereby significantly reducing both the probability of introducing infection and the probability of intracranial pressure disequilibrium, both during the diagnostic and post-operative phases. It is clear, therefore, that the probability of observing a successful treatment is increased (5; 126; 249; 253). Only by defining the "product" as "successful treatment" *without* an attached probability can innovation be termed "process innovation." The length and frequency of hospitalization for post-operative management are reduced, and hence costs are also reduced. But since, as we have seen, the new process also reduces a number of risks, it simultaneously increases the likelihood of a successful treatment. Therefore, it can be properly termed "product innovation."

In medical procedures this is by no means unique. Quite the contrary. Changes in treatment and diagnostic procedures are generally introduced not for their resource-saving effects, but for their patient-saving effects. They are introduced because they are expected to yield an increase in the probability of obtaining successful treatment.

Certain changes in institutional arrangements, or innovations such as a shorter stay with more extensive home care, may properly be analyzed in terms of process innovation as opposed to product innovation. In general, however, it is at best a dubious and often invalid distinction which would misconceive the innovating process, and in addition, bias downward measured productivity change. In terms of our discussion of productivity, not only the inputs must be

[s]Troublesome, because in all complex production processes it is rather difficult to change the process of production in any significant way without ipso facto changing some dimension of the product.

completely specified but the outputs as well. And in all their relevant dimensions. The assumption of homogeneous outputs is only justified if the quality dimension, of which the probability of a successful outcome is perhaps the fundamental one, is controlled for. Unfortunately, no such studies exist.

We have seen in this section that the hospital's productivity may be usefully analyzed in terms of the production functions and the appropriateness of input proportions. Inefficiencies in the hospital may be attributable in this analysis to the absence of a technically efficient production, to the use of economically inappropriate input combinations, or to both. In the next section we consider the broader questions of efficiency as they are related to the incentives operating on hospitals and to their objective functions.

Efficiency

> The age of chivalry is gone; that of sophisters, economists, and calculators has succeeded.
>
> –Edmund Burke

> The first lesson in economics is: Things are often not what they seem.
>
> –Paul A. Samuelson

The theory of consumer choice has been called the irrational pursuit of unreachable rationality. The literature on efficiency might be termed the inefficient search for undefined efficiency. We have seen some definitions of "efficiency" as it is used in the literature in the section "Productivity and Efficiency" above. Approaches to "efficient pricing" and "efficient resource allocation," crippled as well they may be by the absence of any precise knowledge of what is being produced with what, will be discussed in chapter 7, in the contexts of pricing and of reimbursement.

The rest of the literature on efficiency offers conflicting views. Efficiency as "maximum occupancy rate" (350, p. 190) is clearly unacceptable on any ground. Fitzpatrick, Riedel, and Payne distinguish between "effectiveness" and "efficiency." Effectiveness is defined in terms of the hospital's ability to deliver the complete service spectrum: ". . . the most effective hospital can take care of any patient, with any diagnosis, requiring any service" (146, p. 499). Efficiency has something to do with costs: "If the effective hospital is also efficient, it will render its services at the lowest possible cost." (Ibid.) "Effectiveness" as it is defined implies that a hospital system does not exist, that each unit is not only separate but autonomous and unsubstitutable; that there is no, and no possible, coordination, and that there are no economies of scale. This is recognized by Skinner (391, p. 848). Without further specification, little can be made of this distinction, for such "effectiveness" implies that the sixty bed county hospital, regardless of its location, ought to be equipped with a linear accelerator. In terms of our early discussion of the objective function, the statement, however, is interestingly revealing. The search for this kind of effectiveness leads to and accepts one of the favorite "causes" of the critics of inefficiency: duplication of facilities.

That "duplication" exists is not debatable (see, e.g., 66). By duplication is usually meant the simultaneous existence of facilities in excess of demand for the actual use of their services. The outstanding example is that of heart surgery: "Of 327 hospitals equipped for open-heart surgery, 41 percent performed fewer than 10 such operations per year and an additional 37 percent performed between 10 and 49 per year" (2, Vol. II, p. 55). This means that 77 percent of all hospitals with facilities to perform open-heart surgery performed less than one operation per week. By 1969, 16,000 open-heart surgeries were performed and the number of hospitals which performed less than one per week rose to 86 percent. Only in 14 percent of the hospitals reporting the performance of open-heart surgery was the operation performed at least once a week on average (330). For closed-heart surgery, of 777 hospitals equipped to perform it in a recent year, in 30 percent, or 256 hospitals, not a single one such operation was done. Of those that performed at least one during the year, 87 percent did less than one per week (2, Vol. II, p. 55). The suggestion is made that between 200 and 250 hospitals so equipped would be sufficient for the country as a whole. The suggestion is strengthened by the expressed relation between frequency of use and technical competence, or the quality of care: "Hospitals in which cardiac surgery is done once every two weeks or once a month cannot hope to maintain the competence and experience of a well-trained team" (2, p. 56).

Note that we defined duplication as "facilities in excess of demand for the actual use of their services." It could be argued that the existence of facilities even if not used is efficient (a) from the hospital's perspective and (b) from the community's standpoint.

If, as it has been suggested, the objective function which the individual hospital's decision makers attempt to maximize does include some element such as professional or "institutional prestige," from that point of view "duplicative facilities," if they yield such prestige, are not inefficient. If price competition is frowned upon and the "blue ribbons" are awarded for "image" or "prestige" (91, pp. 60-61; and 236), "duplicative facilities" may be used as bait to attract the desirable specialists in the community to a particular hospital. If, in addition, the staff and visiting physicians insist on "effectiveness" as shown by the presence of a complete service-facility mix, other decision makers may have no choice. In either case the presence of "duplication" from the standpoint of the individual hospital may not be inefficient, given the system. And if the presence of the facility increases the probability of receiving a federal research grant, the hospital may view it as very efficient.

If such facilities are the sine qua non for attracting and maintaining in the community a specialist or specialists whose services would otherwise be unavailable, it is not obvious that such duplication is inefficient. If indeed the only way a community can have available to it the services of cardiologist(s) is to have heart surgery facilities, even if not used, then such facilities are to be viewed as the "price" (or more properly "reservation price") that must be paid. The toy department on the first floor of the department store which attracts the customers may well be a "loss leader," but inefficient it is not.

If a teaching program is considered desirable by the hospital as well as by the community for its external benefits in terms of intern and resident provided patient-services and quality effects, and if cardiac surgery facilitates affiliation, it may not be viewed as inefficient by the community. Should the community's social system discourage extended family separation, it may place a high value on facilities which maintain the patient within the community, even if that facility is seldom used.

This is not to argue that duplication is not, or may not be, an indication of serious misallocation of resources. It is to argue that in an imperfect system, the correction of any given imperfection may lead to worse, rather than to better results.[t] "Tinkering" or "incrementalism" in a disorganized system, where many if not most of the conditions for the attainment of economic efficiency are absent, is a feasible approach only if all of the direct as well as indirect effects of such piecemeal interference are predictable.

The complexity and imperfection of the system reduce the likelihood that the effects are in fact predictable. The reasoning does not imply that therefore no attempt at the correction of imperfections is feasible. What it does imply is that to attain efficient allocation and distribution, large scale, system-wide rationalization may be required. The reasoning also points out the necessity of having some dominant objective function in whose terms the "efficiency" or "inefficiency" can be assessed. The implied argument in the "duplication" discussion is twofold: (a) the hospital's objective function is not to be considered dominant—from the "social" point of view duplication is a waste of resources; (b) the hospital's objective function is dominant, but the hospitals go about maximizing their objectives in an inefficient way—less than some minimum use of facilities leads to "improper" use. In either case, so the argument goes, the "excess" facilities are a waste: in the first case the solution is complete elimination, in the second, interhospital coordination.

From the overall point of view, the entire discussion of "location," "planning," "regionalization," "comprehensive regional planning," and the development of hospital councils can be viewed as various attempts to attain a "better" distribution of resources socially, demographically, and areally. The resources to be efficiently allocated, however, are usually viewed in terms of hospital resources per se; technical, social, medical, and economic interactions between

[t]For the classic statement and analytic proof of this theorem, see Lipsey and Lancaster, (251).

hospital facilities, on the one hand, and alternative sources of care, on the other, are either not recognized at all or are assumed away. The significant exception is the literature on prepaid groups, some of which will be discussed in the context of demand and utilization in chapter 6.

P. Feldstein distinguishes between "effectiveness" and "efficiency," defining the first as the minimization of the "cost of an illness episode," and the second as minimization of the "cost of hospital care for given levels of care" (137, p. 17). This differentiation is not only valid but useful: when viewed as a separate entity without interconnections with the rest of the medical care sector, the achievement of hospital "efficiency" may still result in the socially inefficient use of resources. In this definition social efficiency is termed "effectiveness": resources are most effectively used when the "cost of an illness episode" is minimized. This is explicitly recognized by Auster and Ro, who state that: "Ultimately, the only way to produce the fullest efficiency of treatment involving various types of care facilities is to offer consumers total care through the integration of all phases of health care, including outpatient and out-of-hospital care" (351, p. 186).

That this is recognized by the Health Insurance Association of America as well is implicit in the recommendations of its Committee on Medical Care Economics, that more emphasis in coverage be placed on ambulatory, home, and preventive care, as well as on the performance of certain services on an ambulatory basis which are now provided on an inpatient basis (183). It is clearly recognized that a shift from inpatient to other forms of care would reduce the most resource-intensive, and hence costly, component during an episode of illness. Their recommendations for operations to be maintained on a seven day basis, as well as the sharing of certain equipment and functions (such as purchasing), imply a realization of the desirability of a greater degree of coordination and planning for the more efficient use of resources.

That excessive concern with efficiency in an area where precise knowledge does not obtain in terms of outputs may lead to undesirable changes in some dimension of those outputs is well put by Somers and Somers:

> . . . If such pressures result in relaxed standards of admissions, or influence the length of stay or the use of diagnostic and related procedures, the result would be higher total cost to the community and the individual patient, even though the cost to the hospital per patient day would be lower (3, p. 13).

The "areawide" planners and "rationalizers" consider inefficiency to be endemic to the *system of hospitals.* The analysts of costs locate inefficiency within the *individual hospital* unit itself, attributing it to two fundamental causes: the non-profit nature of the institution and hence the absence of financial incentive, and decision-making managerial inefficiency resulting from fragmentation of authority as well as from inappropriate reward systems. To anyone acquainted with some of the problems of central planning, particularly the role of incentives in meeting planned production quotas, the arguments seem both familiar and not very sophisticated.[u]

A respected expert in the field concludes that "because blue ribbons are not awarded to the most efficient hospitals, the hospital is tempted to seek prestige rather than economy.... The search is often for the best image rather than for efficiency" (Brown, 91, pp. 60-61). This is most generally attributed to the fact that hospitals are "not for profit."[v]

> The prevalence of nonprofit enterprises implies that incentives for efficiency are absent (Berry, 46, p. 125).

> Attempts at reform have been seriously handicapped by the hospitals' eleemosynary tradition and financial structure (Somers and Somers, 401, p. 98).

> It is . . . an industry in which support by taxation or private philanthropy diminishes financial pressures and in which public opinion opposes profit (Weisbrod, 431, p. 18).

The "inefficient" are further protected from "competition" by barriers to entry *because* they are non-profit (304, Appendix 3), or because of financial barriers (431). The stress on quality also inhibits competition, it is argued (304, Appendix 3, and see references). Less stress on quality would bring about "efficiency" and "more care," hence "Let's Make Volkswagen Medicine Compulsory" (see 157 p. 110). Similar to the "bottomless receptacle" argument is the idea that financial incentives will not bring about efficiency: ". . . Monetary rewards, in the form of any excess of income over costs, will find their way into additional investment in facilities or higher salaries, thus raising costs for the next go-around, unless controlled by external regulation" (Somers and Somers, 401, p. 193).

Alternatively, and/or additionally, it has been suggested that organizational factors are at the bottom of "inefficiency." (Note that in none of these arguments is "efficiency" meaningfully, or at all, defined.) This is at times located in the divided authority system:

> For example, nurses are the hospital's employees and, therefore, accountable to the administrator. But they are responsible to the doctor for the individual

[u]It is interesting, and perhaps indicative of the monastic nature of the discussion of planning, incentives, and prices that no advantage has been taken of the extensive literature on precisely these points by economists concerned with these issues in their non-medical care applications. As an example, see the analysis of prices and incentives by the Polish economists Wakar and Zielinski (424), and by Montias (279 and 280). For a comprehensive discussion of these as well as other planning questions, and for references, see Montias (279).

[v]For a view that attributes most if not all of the difficulties in the hospital system to a lack of informed price competition, see Ref. 32.

patient—meaning many doctors at once—in their medical duties (Somers and Somers, 401, p. 52).

The supply response of the hospital sector is predicated not upon some not-for-profit motive of the hospital as an enterprise *per se*, but rather upon the for-profit motives of the individual practitioners who want the use of these facilities as a necessary adjunct to their own business operations (Stevens, 407, p. 19).

On this last point the previous discussion of the objective function is relevant.[w]

Some acute analysts suggest that the source of the "efficiency difficulties" are not to be found in individual management or management structure. They recognize the logical difficulties of assuming that the *content* and *nature* of the decision is independent of its *institutional setting.*[x]

Traditions of narrow individualism and guildism that permeate the health services have helped to perpetuate outmoded rigidities and institutional restraints. Professions and occupations that owe their content and significance to twentieth century technology still strive to operate in a context of nineteenth century legal, economic, and social organization (Somers and Somers, 401, p. 98).

The inefficiencies are for the most part by-products of the current institutional situation in medical care in which essentially public functions are being discharged by private or quasi-private groups with abundant opportunities for gratification of private group interests and with weak mechanisms for coordination and planning. At the core of this situation is the organized medical profession. . . . (Gottlieb, 169, p. 503).

While there appears no consensus, there is a strong trend: something is wrong. Precisely what and why it is "wrong" and how to "right" it is not so clear. Some suggest a "systems approach" (400; 401; 396; 397; 399; 73; 361), either via "horizontal integration" (256) or through some central clearing device (257). Some suggest "hospital complex analysis" (92, 371). But some maintain that nothing much needs be done (16, p. 81).[y]

[w]For a point of view stressing managerial inefficiency, see Kaitz (204). For some suggestions on how to attain better managerial decision making, see Jelinek (198). For an example of managerial efficiency, see Callahan and Kabat (69).

[x]Weisbrod has suggested the opposite. "The implication of the argument is that, even if the hospital industry remains essentially non-profit, economic efficiency could be increased if *hospitals would act* more frequently *as if they were profit maximizers*." (431, p. 18 emphasis added) And if whales had wings they could fly. But if they acted *as if* they had wings, they would still be nonflying frustrated whales. For other arguments for the institutionalization of the profit motive see Refs. 26 and 50.

[y]For a good review of the planning literature, see Klarman (218). A good bibliography is Ref. 89. Problems of locational efficiency are discussed in Ref. 370, and see references there. The distinction between "locality-relevance" and "functional-relevance" is discussed, with good bibliography, in Palmiere (315). For a definitive treatment of the conceptual and measurement issues in defining "service areas" see Metzner and Winter (273, chapter 5). See also Ref. 57.

Once again the basic issue is the absence of a frame of reference. Hospital costs are increasing. The number of people receiving services are increasing, and whole subgroups of the populations who previously were not within the system at all are now at least at its peripheries. Some receive services they do not medically "need" and many do not receive any care for conditions considered "in need" of care. Some services are not provided because they are too costly (dialysis), others provided are, on cost bases, questionable (heart transplants). The aged, with a short expected life-span, receive publicly subsidized services regardless of their income, but children do not. Some areas have "excess" capacities for providing services while others have no service capabilities at all. Some services that can be inexpensively provided in the doctor's office are provided during expensive inpatient stays, while in other situations where the speed of hospitalization is crucial to life-maintenance, no mechanism for it exists (heart attacks). All these conditions are "bad." Which is "worst"? If rational decisions are to be made there must exist some framework within which, based on fairly exact knowledge of the direct and indirect costs and outcomes of alternatives, the options chosen will most closely correspond to the social valuation of those costs and outcomes. The identification of precise production and cost functions, productivity and efficiency measures, as well as distributional and health indexes are necessary, but not sufficient, for rational policy formation. Rather than the slogans that either "health care is a right" or that "the Thomistic notion of a 'just' or 'fair' or 'reasonable' price has no role to play in the allocation of scarce resources" (32, p. 127), what is needed is an agreed upon social valuation system, a social welfare function.

In this chapter we have seen that while the analytic procedures and research methodologies for measuring productivity and efficiency in the hospital and over hospitals exist, little useful empirical work has been done in either area. Further, to be able to assess the indicated productivities and efficiencies of the hospital sector, there must be an answer to a previous question, in the words of Samuelson, "Efficiency in terms of what? And for whom"? The literature offers hazy answers.

Even though there is scant knowledge of productivity and of efficiency, the high and rapidly rising costs of hospital care, now on the order of $30 billion, have resulted in great concern with hospital costs. In the next chapter we consider the analysis of hospital costs.

5 The Costs of Hospital Operations

In applying our method for estimating cost functions of multi-product firms to the hospital industry, much of our investigation consisted of a search for significant variables. This search was made necessary because there is little knowledge of the functional form of the cost relationship or of which explanatory variables to include.

—Judith and Lester Lave, 232, p. 393.

Introduction

Review of the literature on definitions of output demonstrated the prevalence of multiple and sometimes conflicting conceptualizations. Costs, whether average, marginal, short-run, or long-run, direct or indirect, realized or opportunity, private or social, can only be measured for some defined set of outputs. Since no two writers employ the same definition of output, the multiplicity and disagreement found in the literature on output is necessarily present in the cost studies.[a] The indefinitiveness of the cost studies is aggravated by five additional factors.

The behavior of costs over varying output ranges, the cost function, is logically predicated upon the existence of a production function which specifies, for any level of output, the efficient combinations of relevant inputs. It is clear that no productive organization need necessarily be on its economically efficient production function: it may use a technically efficient production function with the "wrong set" of inputs or it may use a technically inefficient one (manual medical record keeping in a 1,000 bed hospital) or unnecessarily costly inputs may be used (registered nurses making up beds). Hence, even with the identical definition of output, observed interhospital cost differences will not permit the identification of the implied production functions. Therefore, observed cost differentials, as we have seen, cannot be attributed separately to technical or economic inefficiency, nor can the productivity of each of the inputs be identified.

[a]See, for example, Somers' comment that "... many measurement indices are either inaccurate or grossly misleading. The most obvious example is the traditional *per diem* ... Its drawbacks as a statistical tool for comparing the costs of different hospitals or of the same hospital over time ... seem to me overwhelming and unaccompanied by any compensatory advantages." (397, p. 355)

To assess the appropriateness of observed costs, the underlying production function should be identified. To evaluate the appropriateness of the *identified* production function, the *economically efficient* production function must be determined. That is, to assess whether or not resources are used in an economically efficient way, the economically efficient way must be known.

The second factor aggravating the difficulties of cost studies is conceptual imprecision resulting in empirical exactitude at the cost of unreality. An example is the statement: "In evaluating health services, it should be satisfactory to accept the consensus among economists on certain simplifying assumptions, such as: (1) there are no external (secondary) benefits or costs of health care. . ." (352, p. 362). The validity of this statement need not be discussed, since neither its substance nor its assertion is correct. The laxity of its implied definition of what "health services" are (presumably excluding treatment for communicable diseases and biomedical research such as that producing the vaccines against poliomyelitis), the absence of any theoretical framework to specify whether or not externalities are relevant or not, facilitate the use of those "simplifying assumptions," which then rob the results of meaning. This approach is fairly typical. Even M. Feldstein, possibly the most technically sophisticated analyst of costs, resorts to it in arguing that for health care, "appropriate standards of provision cannot be determined by reference to levels of 'need' inherent in or manifest by the community. Planning requires choice" (133, p. 201).

Economists generally tend to disparage the relevance of the concept of need. It is, however, theoretically interesting and analytically valid to distinguish between "perceived need" of the potential patient, the medically defined "need" for given conditions for the individual and for the population at risk, and the level of medical "need" society is willing to meet (see, e.g., 53; 117; 197). Exogenously determined objectives in terms of final products in health care are no more theoretically or practically invalid than those for the production, for example, of military goods. While "planning" does "require choice," neither the object nor the subject of planning is thereby predetermined.

The third factor contributing to the dubiousness of cost studies is methodological carelessness. This shall be pointed out from time to time in the discussion. One example here may suffice: use of a regression coefficient whose standard error is ten times larger than the coefficient (133, p. 34, table 2.10, item No. 25).[b]

The fourth factor is the relative absence of adequate data. In the Michigan study, for example, Foyle found that hospitals neither collect precise, accurate data nor perform any cost analysis, hence they were even unable "to relate rates to costs" (149, p. 992).

The nature of the hospital sector itself presents the fifth confounding factor. Baumol and Bowen have stated this most clearly:

[b]For an excellent review of methodologies of recent work (to early 1966) see Lave (233). See also Mann and Yett (265).

The fact that any nonprofit organization can always find uses for a temporary excess of funds—and indeed may be embarrassed to report . . . that it has some money left at the end of the year—makes it difficult to determine its cost functions. If an auto producer finds that a sudden increase in demand has swollen his receipts, he is only too happy to report higher profits; *a nonprofit enterprise, however, may well use the extra revenue in a way which, in effect, deliberately raises its costs* (41, p. 498, n. 6, emphasis added).

In assessing the cost studies these factors must be borne in mind.

In this chapter we first consider some of the major cost function investigations, emphasizing the different conceptual approaches as well as the different attempts to attain homogeneity of the "Product" whose costs are to be measured. As a result of those differences, and because the underlying production functions are not well understood, the cost function studies cannot be easily summarized nor do they yield comparable results except in one area. There is fairly general agreement among the investigators that marginal costs in the short run are a significantly large percentage of average costs, implying that short-run below capacity utilization is economically costly. After discussing major cost functions, the analytic issues in the definition of capacity, size, and economies of scale are considered and the relevant empirical findings discussed. Once again, there is little common ground among the studies, which conflict in their findings on the existence of economies of scale. The last two sections are devoted to a briefer consideration of other cost elements and to the behavior of costs over time.

Hospital cost analysis is seen to be in its infancy, but characteristic of that stage, there are signs of growth.

Estimated Cost Functions for the Hospital

Major studies of hospital costs have been done by P. Feldstein (139), Carr and P. Feldstein (74), M. Feldstein (133; 135), Cohen (84; 85; 86), Berry (46; 47), Ro (350), Ingbar and Taylor (195), Lave and Lave (231; 232; 234), and Francisco (150). These will be discussed *seriatim* generally first. In the following section, "Capacity, Size, and Economies of Scale," those relationships will be discussed in detail. This procedure is necessitated by inconsistencies in the definitions of output and of inputs.

With the objectives of determining the shapes of the short-run cost functions for a given 242 bed acute hospital and the long-run cost functions of hospitals with different sizes, P. Feldstein fits a linear regression equation to departmental data from one hospital and to aggregate data from sixty hospitals ranging in size from 48 to 453 beds (139).[c] For the single hospital, departmental costs are

[c]For other views of this study, as well as of some others, see Klarman (216, pp. 104-108), and Ingbar and Taylor (195, pp. 109-114).

estimated and then summed to arrive at the total hospital cost. The departmental dependent variables are salary expenses, supplies expenses, and all other expenses by month for a given month. The independent variable is departmental output, measured by the "single variable which best represents the output of that department," which in most cases turns out to be "adult patient-days of service" (139, p. 12). The costs of a number of departments, however, such as nursing administration, emergency room, administration, medical records, interns, and plant operation, were unrelated to patient days. This is predictable, since the operations of these departments are either independent of "patient days" or are directly a function of ambulatory services, as is seen in production function analysis.

Estimating total, average, and marginal costs, P. Feldstein finds that marginal costs are only 20-30 percent of average total costs and constant over the observed range (pp. 48-51). Realizing the tentative nature of his analysis, he warns that "it is less misleading . . . to say that the very short run marginal costs are relatively small than to say that they are a percentage of an unreliable average and to assume that this relationship is constant among different hospitals" (p. 51). Since marginal cost is constant and below average cost, average cost over the relevant range must be decreasing. This is not accountable for by the existence of significant excess capacity, since the occupancy rate was 90 percent.

Patient day as a measure of output may be appropriate for a given hospital with a short period of observation. It can be reasonably assumed that neither the facility-mix nor the service-intensity of care will vary in the span of a month. Whether it can also be assumed that patient turnover is constant is an unsolved question.

In Feldstein's study of the sixty hospitals of varying size, the output is again measured in terms of unweighted patient days. In this case all of the above assumptions become highly questionable and, in addition, the problem of case severity is also present. Hence the finding, once again, of a constant long-run marginal cost curve below the long-run average cost curve must be taken with somewhat more caution and surprise than his finding of a correlation coefficient of 0.99 between patient days and the number of beds (p. 62). The conclusion drawn by Feldstein is that since his output measure is biased downward by service-mix heterogeneity, output corrected for the number of services would demonstrate decreasing marginal costs. Demonstrating a rather strong belief in the inviolability of the law of variable proportions, he argues that even though the long-run average cost curve will probably decrease with hospital size if service complexity is allowed for, "The long run average cost curve will begin to rise when a certain size is reached" (p. 64).

The discussion of output measures in chapter 3 pointed out that there are two ways to attempt to correct for the biases introduced by variations in service intensity and service utilization. One way is to assume that hospitals with identical or very similar, service/facility mixes produce patient days homogeneous in service content. More explicitly "a group of hospitals with identical facilities would be assumed to be producing a relatively homogeneous product" (46, p. 135). The objective is to separate the effects of hospital size (measured in beds) and of service complexity on costs per patient day, the measure of output employed in the studies. This approach is tried by Carr and Feldstein (74), Berry (46; 47), and Francisco (150).

The source of data in each of the studies is the same, that reported by the American Hospital Association, although for different years. It should be noted that the A.H.A. data are based on individual hospital reports on their individual service and facility capabilities. The reports merely specify the presence or absence of services and facilities. Since neither size, complexity, nor rate of utilization by facility or service is reported (other than in gross patient days), the procedure boils down to assuming that in all these respects the reported capabilities are homogeneous over the reporting units. If that were the case, then the assumption of a "homogeneous product" would be analogous to the assumption of identical case mix and case severity, within hospitals with identical reported facilities, to whom they deliver identical, or nearly so, bundles of services. That is a rather heroic assumption.

While the econometric methods applied vary among the three studies, they each attempt to "homogenize" hospitals by stratifying them in such a way that each group contains only hospitals with the same or similar service capabilities. Carr and Feldstein analyze five groups, Francisco twenty-five, and Berry forty, each using the same definition of output, the unadjusted patient day.

Within each of their five groups, the service-facility number is multiplied by the average daily census and entered as an independent variable by Carr and Feldstein (74, p. 61). The data are then converted to patient days and linear regressions run. The results show that "economies of scale in the provision of care appear to exist over a wide range of sizes in each of the service-capability groups" (p. 61). The minimum of the estimated average cost occurs at successively larger patient days for groups with increasing services. These results are somewhat clouded not only by the autocorrelation between three of the independent variables (patient days, or PD, PD^2 and SxPD), but also by the statistical insignificance of the SxPD coefficient in three of the five service groupings. (See table 2, p. 62) Carr and Feldstein comment on their findings that the coefficient on student nurses is negative for three service groupings, and appears to be statistically significant for one, the group with the largest number of services and highest average daily census. This finding does not support their conclusion that there is "lower cost per patient day in hospitals with nursing students. . ." (p. 64). The statistical results tend to support the much narrower interpretation that in hospitals with the highest number of services and facilities *and the largest number of patients*, the presence of student nurses is associated with lower costs. Since it is not possible to "explain" this phenomenon directly in terms of services or in terms of the numbers of patients in this analysis, it can also be hypothesized that the observed effect of the presence of student nurses results not from any relationship to service complexity, but simply from the presence of a large number of patients requiring large quantities of the types of routine nursing and housekeeping chores student nurses can perform.

Berry (46; 47) is also primarily concerned with separating the effects of size and service complexity on cost. His 1967 study considers forty isoservice/facility groupings, each containing ten or more hospitals, and a linear equation in average cost and patient days is estimated for each group. The conclusion that strong economies of scale are demonstrated for thirty-six of the forty groups is based on the negative correlation coefficients for those groups, even though in ten cases the coefficients are not statistically significant. However, even where the correlation is significant, a patient day coefficient of 0.0001 with a constant term of 58.63 is less than exciting.

Francisco constructs twenty-five isoservice groupings (150). Considering patient day to be the appropriate measure of output, the question of the presence of economies of scale is addressed by fitting average and total cost as a curvilinear function of patient days. The paucity of the reported results makes evaluation of his findings, that economies of scale appear to be present in hospitals with seventy or less beds and with four or less service facilities, somewhat difficult. In most cases the regression coefficients are not reported, it is merely indicated whether they are significant or not. Where the coefficients are shown they are in the range between 0.31 and 0.49. Given that the objective is to analyze costs as a function of output, the appropriateness of the coefficient of correlation as the measure of the functional relationship is itself dubious.

An alternative method to account for service/facility variation as well as for cost variations possibly attributable to the presence of various teaching programs is to introduce them into the cost equation either as dummy variables (Berry, Francisco), directly according to the number of actual number reported (Carr and Feldstein), or as an index number (Francisco). In the latter case an index of service/facilities is constructed, thereby enabling the use of one variable instead of the large number of dummies required otherwise. Using data from 3,147 acute voluntary hospitals for the year 1963, Carr and Feldstein experiment with several approaches. (74) Output is defined in terms of average daily census, and an equation of the form

$$TC = a + b(ADC) + c(ADC)^2 + d\,(OPV)$$

is fitted, where ADC = average daily census, OPV = the number of outpatient visits, and TC = total costs (p. 53). This assumes that the "output" of a hospital can be measured in terms of the average number of patients per day and that "size" and output as measured are identical. To isolate the effect of size on cost, independently of the service-facility mix, which tends to vary with size itself, the number of facilities and services (as reported in the yearly *Guide* issue of

Hospitals, see Ref. 189), is entered as an independent variable. In an attempt to "reflect a component of long run cost associated with the provision of specialized services . . . which is relatively constant per patient day" (p. 55), the facilities and service variable, *S*, is multiplied by the average daily census and entered as an independent variable again. Additional variables to account for training and research related costs are entered as well, such as the number of student nurses and the number and types of residency and intern programs. The results indicate that "as hospital size increases, average cost declines until it reaches a minimum level at about 190 ADC and then begins to rise" (p. 60).

A number of the difficulties are realized, namely, the implicit assumption that service content and service utilization intensity are constant over all hospitals where the existence of the service capacity is reported to be present, and further, that the marginal costs of the service units are identical. The presence of multicollinearity and heteroscedasticity are also perceived, but not corrected for. Some additional biases are also present without discussion. The variables reflecting training costs, the simple counts of training programs, are at best crude measures, since they do not allow the distinction of cost differentials attributable to different levels of training. The differential patient-service benefits of the residency and intern programs may or may not be reflected in the total costs, but they are not specifically taken into consideration. The results of the analysis, therefore, are at best tentative.

Berry (47), after discussing a rather more complete model relating costs to output, quality, product mix, factor prices, and efficiency, because of data limitations, resorts to a much simpler single equation model. He measures output as average daily census, costs as per diem, and product and service-facility mix by some forty independent variables. Of these twenty-seven are dummies, representing the presence or absence of specified services or facilities, another seven are dummies representing degrees of affiliation and accreditation. In addition, the average length of stay, the proportion of outpatient activity, births, and the numbers of medical and nursing students are also included (p. 10). The data are from some 6,000 short-term general hospitals, which are then further grouped by control (governmental, voluntary, etc.) for 1965.

The resulting R^2 for all hospitals is 0.25, and for voluntaries 0.26 "explaining" 26 percent of the variation in observed per diem costs in voluntary hospitals in terms of the forty independent variables representing service-facility mix, etc., included (47, p. 13). The results are somewhat disappointing. For the voluntaries, of the forty variables included, nineteen, including some which one would expect to be important, since they are thought to reflect the intensity of service operations such X-rays, laboratories, blood bank, and radiation therapy, are not statistically significant, and sometimes the coefficients have the "wrong" sign (see 30, table 2, pp. 11-13). While this is not discussed, Berry recognizes the likely presence of multicollinearity resulting from interdependence among the independent variables. That is, the probability of observing a given service or facility is not independent of the presence of other services and facilities. The probabilities are conditional.

Trying another tack, he employs factor analysis and finds that eight common identifiable factors can be generated to explain 60 percent of the variation attributable to the original forty variables (p. 16). These range from teaching programs, through "general services," to outpatient services. The sixth factor is "identified" as "a form of routine admission program" (p. 20). But since it is composed of chest X-ray on routine admission and blood sugar test on routine admission, it could be argued that it is really a proxy variable for one aspect of the quality of care.

Berry's analysis, as well as that by Ingbar and Taylor, is typical of the use of factor analysis without a theoretic framework. The principal theoretical rule appears to be to use any and all data available, without considering their relevance or shortcomings. There is no attempt to disaggregate output beyond "patient days" on the assumption that correction for service-facility mix diversity will eliminate all of the problems resulting from variations in case mix, case severity, quality and patient characteristics. It is also taken for granted that all facilities of a given category, such as therapeutic X-rays, as reported for American Hospital Association purposes, are in all respects identical, using the same input mixes of the same quality for the same purpose at the same level of intensity. Since any analytic framework is conspicuous by its absence, there is no guide by which to assess whether the cost function to be estimated is misspecified or over identified. According to what principle, and for what purpose does one simultaneously include operating room, post-operative room, recovery and blood bank (47, p. 17)? The appropriateness of per diem costs depends not only upon the purpose of the analysis but on the crucial assumption of product homogeneity.

Francisco (150) tries both the dummy variable and the service/facility index approach with similar results. Cost is again a function of output measured in patient days, but both the nature and the value of the reported measure of association, the simple coefficient of correlation, *R*, lend little credence to the finding that, again excepting the very small hospitals with beds less than seventy, there appear to be no economies of scale. The *R*'s reported range between 0.15 and 0.49, depending on the specification of the equation.

We have pointed out above some of the difficulties engendered by the assumption that hospitals with identical service/facility capabilities produce homogeneous patient days, which is the basis of the studies we have just discussed. Lave and Lave (231) consider this hypothetical and test it.

If hospitals with the same service/facility capabilities in fact produce identical products in terms of patient days, there should be a close association between their service/facility mix and their case mix.

Recognizing that the classification of patients into isoresource categories is prohibited by the absence of available data, they carefully construct seventeen broad ICDA categories of diagnoses which are then used as the case mix measure, the dependent variable in an equation which relates case mix to bed capacity, the number of advanced services, teaching status, locational variables, and other factors such as the proportion of Medicare and Medicaid patients (231, pp. 18-32). Their procedure, a model of methodological precision and appropriateness, lends credence to their findings that "although the characteristics of size, number of advanced services, and teaching status selected as likely indicators of treatment capability did, indeed, show some correlation with case mix, they were found to explain only about one-fourth to something less than half of the variation in proportions of common surgery, common diagnoses, in surgical complexity, and in extent of surgery performed" (p. 36). The use of service/facility capability as a surrogate for case mix, and the consequent assumption of patient day homogeneity, employed in other studies, therefore seems to be unwarranted.

Using data from Massachusetts hospitals, Ingbar and Taylor undertake a series of experiments with cost models in which output is measured in patient days. The dependent variables are hospital service expenses per patient day and cost per available bed day (195, pp. 49, 53) and the independent variables included are beds, occupancy rate, weighted operations, medical and surgical expenses, and outpatient weighted radiological films. Factor analysis is employed to sort out a very large number of possible regressors (see quote on p. 85, above). Though the factors are not readily identifiable, they claim that this represents no problem since "actually identifying the factors is not central to the task" (p. 33). The approach of selecting regressors solely on the basis of factoring without any a priori criteria derived from some applicable analytic framework may be useful if the resulting factors have some independent analytic meaning. The use of unidentified factors diminishes the impact of their painstaking efforts to disaggregate data for seventy-two hospitals into a complex of some 100 service and function variables, from which then the factors are constructed.[d]

Their intent is to measure hospital costs per available bed days (and per patient day) as a function of hospital size and capacity. This intention is not realized. "None of the macro characteristics of hospitals—size-volume, utilization

[d]In chapter 3, a careful and explicit discussion of statistical and analytic methods and probably the most useful part of the book, Ingbar and Taylor discuss these issues. Their analytic techniques are justified on the grounds that "past experience, common sense, and economic theory are important aids in suggesting variables relevant to explaining costs, but they fall short of providing an exhaustive list. Given the large number of the possible explanatory variables, it would be rare indeed if the ones to use could be specified a priori" (p. 32). This assumption lies behind the use of factor analysis, which is suggested as the appropriate technique to answer two kinds of questions: "what costs should be the dependent variables in the regression equations? Which of several alternative measures of the same characteristics should be used as independent variables? The principal component solution to the factor model is an appropriate tool for finding the answers" (p. 30). It is precisely to avoid this atheoretic approach that engineering specification of the underlying production functions, statistical techniques of process analysis, and a priori conceptualization are useful.

and length of stay—are important in explaining hospital costs per ABD. . ." (p. 53). Costs per patient day do not appear to be better "explained" either. This is not particularly surprising for two reasons.

In estimating the equations for costs per available bed day as the dependent variable, and service expenses, such as medical and surgical physician expenses, radiological activity, etc., as the independent variables, they are in effect correlating different definitions of output. A more generous interpretation would hold that they are correlating different dimensions of the same output. In either case, the resulting corrected R^2's on the order of 0.5 from the various forms of the equations used can in fact be interpreted as indirect measures of heterogeneity of the service mix per available bed day. That is, to the extent that the service/facility mix variables imply a set of heterogeneous outputs while beds, available or however qualified, imply a homogeneous output, their partial incomplete correlation can be interpreted to mean that variables used to capture the product heterogeneity do not do the job.

Secondly, what appear to be significant "explainors" are essentially staff expenses: medical staff expenses, radiological and surgical activities, and medical education activities. Even where the variables are measured in "activities," it is clear that the major proportion of the costs of those activities are personnel staff costs and not expendables, such as surgical dressing and X-ray films. The dependent variable is cost per available bed day. But available beds are earlier defined (because of data limitations) as "fully staffed" (p. 32) beds. Hence it is to be expected that staff expenses will be highly correlated with "fully staffed" beds.

Analyses of department cost expenses also appear to be exercises in testing the statistical consistency of logical relationships. Departmental costs per available bed days for radiology are "explained" by the level of radiological activity, "The number of inpatient weighted operations per ABD is the most important variable in explaining operating room costs per ABD. . ." (p. 153). This, of course, argues that in "explaining" the cost of operations, the number of operations is important.

Now it is perfectly true that the cost function can, and often has been expressed as $TC = f(Q)$, where TC denotes total costs and Q the quantity of output, both per some time period. For heuristic purposes, this representation in an elementary text may be adequate to suggest that indeed total costs are somehow related to the rate of output, unless, of course, all of the costs are fixed. But the purposes of empirical research are to investigate the precise functional form and not merely to see whether costs are associated with output rates or not. As Lave and Lave stress, "estimated marginal costs tend to be sensitive to the specification of the function" even in relatively simple situations of a single output. But in the presence of multiple products, "it is essentially impossible to reflect the underlying cost structure in a single function" (232, p. 379). Ingbar and Taylor's departmental cost findings, therefore, to the extent that they do not result from autocorrelation, affirm the validity of the hypothesis that yes, costs have something to do with the rate of output.

Ro (350) undertakes a rather ambitious attempt at the economic analysis of data over an eleven year period (1952-63, excluding 1955) from sixty-eight hospitals in western Pennsylvania. Abstracting from such problems as the effects of case mix, case severity, treatment quality, or any indication of outcome, he defines output to be patient days per year. To the extent that other analysts, such as Berry, and Cohen, use the degree of affiliation as an indicator of quality, this may appear justified, since Ro excludes all affiliated hospitals. Incomparability also results.

After a thorough theoretical and methodological discussion (pp. 187-218), he specifies twenty-five independent variables to be included in one or more of the equations to be tested, which range from simple linear to a multiplicative equation with interaction terms. The variables are: patient days, beds, admissions, birth, occupancy rate, pressure index, turnover rate, average length of stay, patient days per employee, personnel per 100 beds, adjusted annual average wage rate, inpatient expenses as a ratio to inpatient operating expenses, outpatient expenses as a ratio of total expenses, dummies for nursing and medical education, percentage of urban population, and a variable measuring differences from minimum per household income in the relevant area. In addition, to account for service/facility mix, he includes five variables, in terms of "usage per 100 patient days," for anesthesia, X-ray, laboratory, operating room, and delivery room. He considers as separate variables patient care expenses as a ratio of inpatient care expenses, both of which are reflections of the previous five. The reason for the inclusion of a separate variable defined to be the number of facilities as a ratio to the maximum number listed for the year is not obvious.

The variables are then used to test a set of hypotheses about differences in interhospital unit cost relationships to turnover rate, service complexity and use intensity, technology, and so on. Some of the formulations are inventive. It is argued that "the average length of stay is chosen as the last variable to represent the scope of services. The reason for this choice is that expanded knowledge and improved methods of treatment reduce the average length of stay" (p. 204). While the formulation is interesting, the example offered, namely, reduction in stay of obstetrical patients from ten "to five days during the last two decades" (p. 204), demonstrates the tenuity of the argument. The reduction in stay for obstetrical cases certainly implies increased service intensity *per day of stay*. But the causal factor in all likelihood is medical custom, standards of "good practice," and not the increased *availability* of more complex services. Hence, variation in the length of stay, even for the same diagnosis, is not unambiguously related to the scope of existing services. Further, the hypothesis is posited in terms of "a given mix of diagnosis" (p. 204). But the measure of "output" is patient days, without any consideration of diagnostic mix.

Other hypotheses regarding size, volume, capacity, and costs are also tested, and will be discussed in the next section.

The hypotheses are tested in two stages: "First, the step-wise regression is computed with all the independent variables inserted. . . Next, covariance regression is computed with the variables thus chosen through the step-wise method" (pp. 225-56). The number of assumptions required to make this procedure valid, including normality of the distributions of the populations, is rather prohibitive for this kind of data.[e] The resulting correlation coefficients for the equations presented are in the neighborhood of 0.9, but when corrected, R_e^2 (see Ref. 203, p. 31), drop to around 0.3. Since the corrected correlation coefficients "explain" the proportion of the variation in the dependent variable attributable to the independent variables after allowances has been made for unspecified variables, this means that more of the variation is "explained" by variables *not* specified. Ro computes standardized *B*-coefficients both for the hospital constants (hospital effects) and the eleven year constants (time effects) (p. 231-32). The relative sizes of the *B*-coefficients show that all the included "independent variables combined contribute less to the explanation of variances than either the hospital effects or the year effects" (p. 232). It is in light of this fact, in addition to his use of patient days as a unit of output, that his conclusions must be interpreted:

(1) Economies of scale exist in hospital operations; (2) The higher a hospital's rate of capacity utilization, the lower its unit costs; (3) Hospitals which have a higher proportion of patient care expenses to hotel-type services expense have a higher unit cost; (4) As each hospital employee provides more days of inpatient services to more patients per year, the unit cost becomes lower; (5) Hospitals which have accredited professional nursing schools have higher unit costs; (6) There is no statistically significant difference in unit cost between hospitals with approved intern and/or residency programs and those without; (7) Hospitals in areas with higher percentages of urban population have a higher unit cost than those in areas with lower percentages of urban population; (8) Inter-hospital and inter-year differences in unit cost are better explained by a multiplicative model than by a linear model. (p. 185)

A few additional comments are in order. Regarding conclusion No. 6, the variable on which it is based is a dummy, showing the presence or absence of an approved intern and/or residency program (p. 221). A residency program with fifty residents is counted the same as one with two, or even possibly zero, for any given year. Regarding conclusion No. 7, it is assumed that "there exists a competitive labor market within the hospital industry" (p. 212), and the possibility of urban-rural wage differentials "are to be accounted for by the exogenous variables" (p. 213). Therefore, it might well be that the result

[e]For a discussion of some of the difficulties, see Christ (78, p. 146). For the most lucid and comprehensive discussion of the special difficulties in estimation procedures with medical care and hospital data, with emphasis on regression and correlation analysis, see Metzner and Winter (273, pp. 102-112, 128-33).

reflects the existence of that differential. More generally, it might also be that the urban population percentage, on which that conclusion is based, is merely a proxy for locational differentials in input as well as output and patient characteristics. Considering that in general hospitals some 60-65 percent of total expenses are payroll expenses, conclusion No. 4 is a tautology. In view of the fact that hotel-type services are not very capital-intensive and require labor inputs at the lowest skill levels, conclusion No. 3 is not very surprising at best. In sum, the conclusions must be taken with great caution.

Cohen's objectives are to isolate the effects on cost of size (84), and of the nature and quality of services performed (86). The approach in his several studies is essentially the same, with some improvements. We have discussed in chapter 3 his definition of output as the sum of cost weighted services. From a conceptual standpoint, his approach is not only interesting but promising. However, the weighting of services by their average costs, and then considering that sum as the dependent variable with the costs of services as the independent variables is, for the purposes of cost analysis, tautological. If additional difficulties were required, they may be found in the data. His cost data are for New York City hospitals, as reported by them to the United Hospital Fund of New York (86, p. 3). The hospitals report fully allocated costs. Whether costs are allocated over departments by income or by the number of services provided, they are at best rough accounting data based on full absorption cost allocation principles and hence need not reflect actual costs (149).

Cohen adjusts for quality differentials by assigning to the affiliated hospital's output, depending on its degree of affiliation, arbitrarily assigned weights of 1.1, 1.2, 1.3 relative to the output of the unaffiliated hospital (86, p. 13). He then claims that "quality, as measured by accreditations, is seen to be positively correlated with cost and to be, along with size, a significant explainor of cost variations" (86, p. 19). It must be kept in mind, however, that affiliation with a medical school is, at best, a very gross measure of quality. Further, this factor may simply isolate higher costs per unit of output, particularly in the case of his definition of output, associated with affiliation per se.

While his empirical analysis of costs is not supportable, his conceptual approach is pregnant. His view of the hospital as a set of departments producing services needs to be further specified, but is theoretically sound. His concept of output as the sum of these weighted services does not attempt to sidestep the difficulties arising from product heterogeneity, as in the studies of P. Feldstein, Berry, Francisco, and Ro, nor to "hold them constant" as these approaches would have it, but to meet them. The analytic problem arises when he considers their estimated costs as the appropriate set of weights. But in this procedure he has rather good company.

M. Feldstein, as shown in the discussion on output, defines output as the weighted number of cases where the weights are the relative average costs of each case type (133, p. 31). The case types are "specialties": general medicine, pediatrics, general surgery, ear, nose, throat, traumatic and orthopedic surgery, other surgery, gynecology, obstetrics, and other. Status upon discharge is not considered and neither are any direct or indirect measures of the quality of care.

Feldstein's data are from the British National Health Service, generally excluding both capital costs and ambulatory, or outpatient care costs (p. 61). Using an imaginative and comprehensive set of approaches, he examines different formulations of the cost functions for hospitals within the same size class (as measured by beds), and for large hospitals alone. He employs least squares estimates, principal component analysis, and a variety of other statistical techniques which will not be reproduced. Examining a wide variety of analytic and empirical questions, he considers the relationship of cost to case mix, case flow, utilization rates, as well as both short- and long-run costs and the interactions of productivity and efficiency.

Here his analysis of case mix will be considered. Case flow and utilization effects are related to scale economies and will be considered in the next section.

Working with data from 177 large non-teaching hospitals, he finds the distribution of case load over hospitals to be both skewed and bimodal (133, pp. 15-21). By regressing average (ward) costs per case on case mix, he is able to account for 27.5 percent of the interhospital variation in the average cost per case, and over 37 percent of the variation in its medical component (pp. 22-23). In this procedure he uses a linear regression equation and a multiple correlation coefficient corrected for a number of degrees of freedom.[f] However, in the estimation of the average (ward) cost per patient week, the interhospital cost variation attributable to case mix effects is reduced to 2.1 percent. This implies substantial differences in length of stay between case categories and reduces the strength of his conclusion that costs are "substantially influenced by the case mix composition" (p. 23).

Questions about the degree of homogeneity within each of the case categories in terms of the specific diagnoses, diagnostic complexity, the presence of multiple diagnoses, case severity, and patient characteristics in terms of age and sex are not reflected in case mix. For these reasons, as well as for the facilitation or the replication of his approaches on U.S. data, it would be useful to know the composition of each "case" in terms of I.C.D.A. four digit categories. It may well be that at least some of the implied heterogeneity is captured by the vastly reduced effect of case mix on costs per patient week. That this may be the case is tentatively indicated by the finding that the correlation between cost per case and cost per week is no more than 0.23 (p. 24).

That case mix may lose some of the relevant dimensions is indicated by a study of 1,707 operations in one 600 bed hospital over a period of three months in which a significant relationship between costs on the basis of patient day, or admission, and *complexity* of surgical operations was demonstrated (284). C.

---

[f]It is notable that such pedestrian methodological comments need to be made. M. Feldstein is a principal member of a very limited set of investigators whose statistical procedures are not only usually excellent, but are always made explicit.

Muller has shown that even when surgical, anesthesia, and consultant fees are excluded–since they are charged directly to the patient and hence are not "hospital" but patient costs–increasing complexity of surgery was associated with greater intensity of eight services: laboratory, X-ray, oxygen, ECG, operating room, recovery room, medical supplies, blood, and special duty nursing. Both the pre- and post-operative segments of stay had higher service intensity and higher per diem charges. For example, the average total dollar charge for major classes of service by complexity of principal surgery, classifying surgical complexity by quartiles with 1 being the highest complexity, was $2,380 in the first quartile and $846 in the fourth (284, p. 108). This seems rather convincing evidence that when case mix is composed of such broad categories as "general medicine" and "general surgery" a significant enough degree of heterogeneity is introduced to render the value of "case type" or case mix, for purposes of cost analysis, of dubious value.

Mann and Yett advocate the application of "rate-volume theory" (265). Both the volume of production and the rate of production per unit of time have an effect on cost. In the application to hospitals, they advocate "the number of beds as a proxy for the anticipated volume of output, and the number of cases per unit of time as the rate at which hospital services are produced" (p. 200). The suggestion is made that by holding constant the rate of production (cases per unit of time), the "relationship between cost and volume would yield constantly decreasing unit cost" (p. 200). Aside from the fact that "anticipated volume" is by far not the same as "volume," one may ask what must be assumed about the average length of stay, for a given hospital and between hospitals, for beds to represent the volume of output, anticipated or otherwise.

They proceed to apply this approach to M. Feldstein's equations, finding the relationship between average cost and the number of beds to reach its minimum at 438 beds (p. 200). The "average cost" is arrived at by dividing total cost by the number of cases per year.[g]

Skinner, in the Michigan studies, considers interhospital cost differentials.

[g]Mann and Yett reformulate a number of Feldstein's statements and equations. In their review of the book they criticize Feldstein for excluding capital costs by saying that he excludes "certain major capital expenditures." (265, p. 198) Feldstein in fact does not qualify his statement: "Capital costs are not included in the data." (133, p. 61) Then Mann and Yett reintroduce "beds" into Feldstein's equation "as standardizing for any capital cost variations which had not been eliminated from expense figures." (265, p. 198) Saying that by this procedure "it can be shown that each member of the family of such curves generated by changing bed capacity reaches its minimum point at a level of 32.75 cases per year . . ," they demonstrate this by reproducing their own formulations of Feldstein's equation no. 3.12 on p. 75. (265, p. 198) Feldstein, discussing his equations 5.3 and 5.4 on p. 131, says "these functions imply that the minimum cost per case would be achieved at $F = 32.7$ . . ." F is cases per bed year. This is further complicated by the fact that the only difference between Feldstein's equation 3.12 and 5.3 is that in the former the coefficients and standard errors are rounded off, in the latter they are not, but not always consistently. In equation 3.12 B has a coefficient of -3.54×10^{-2} with a standard error of 1.01. In equation 5.3 the coefficient is -3.5414×10^{-2} with a standard error that has now grown to 1.0800.

The cost measured is per diem. He uses rank correlation to conclude that there are strong, and statistically significant, relationships between per diem costs and employees per occupied bed, annual payroll per employee, scope of services, percentage of occupancy, percentage of acceptable beds, accreditation, and size. The results are tentative at best, since in rank correlation one-to-one associations are shown, but the possibility that the association is attributable to some other, intervening, variable is not measurable. Additionally, per diem costs are not meaningful (391, esp. pp. 814-17).

In an attempt to normalize for variations in the scope, quality, and intensity of services offered, differences in staff physician specialty mix as well as salary expenses, "12 distinguished hospitals," otherwise unidentified, were studied by the Panel on Hospital Care of the National Advisory Commission (340, vol. 2). These "12 distinguished hospitals" are said to be "providing unexcelled services, with the quality of staff considered almost equivalent" (vol. 2, p. 161). Costs were decomposed into general service associated costs (hotel type, housekeeping, administration, and plant), patient associated professional service costs (medical, surgical, laboratory, pharmacy, etc., except nursing), nursing costs, and training associated costs (intern, resident, and nursing education). For, presumably, the year 1966, "the average total cost per patient day is approximately $83 with the variation ranging from $54.10 to $111.53. . ." (vol. 2, p. 162). In volume 1 this is "explained" by arguing that "it is not surprising that there are wide variations in efficiency among hospitals, given the almost total absence of economic incentives for efficiency or mechanisms that would force the inefficient to improve or go out of business" (340, vol. 1, p. 55). The results cannot be independently assessed, since neither the data nor the statistical procedures are revealed. (For some further discussion, see Ref. 414.)

Capacity, Size, and Economies of Scale

What is the size of a television set? Its physical dimensions can be measured in terms of length, height, and depth: a console is "bigger" than a portable one. Its tube, or viewing surface, can be measured in terms of two dimensions, square inches, or as a representation, the length of its diagonal. A fourteen inch tube in a four foot console is not the same "size" as a twenty-one inch tube in a portable. Which is the relevant measure of size? In terms of placing the unit in an enclosed space, such as a room, the exterior physical dimensions are clearly relevant: there may be no room for a four foot console.

In terms of the size of the audience and the desired distance between it and the viewing surface, the size of the tube is relevant. The television screen in Grand Central Terminal is four feet square. Several hundred viewers can be simultaneously accommodated, but only one channel is available. The 21 inch home television screen can accommodate but eight or ten viewers, but it has the delivery capability of some 12 UHF and some 70 VHF channels. What is the relevant measure of size, and capacity? It may be argued that both audience quantity and channel capability are relevant. But the number of available channels in a community are also relevant: in a two channel rural community the set's technical capability to deliver 82 channels is irrelevant, unless the potential buyer expects the actual availability of another channel in the near future.

It can also be argued that the product of a television set is entertainment and since the programs on all channels are basically similar, channel capability is not important. It can also be assumed that all channels are received with the same clarity, visual as well as audio. Further, if it is assumed that the maximum audience is not likely to exceed six people at a time and that the maximum length of continuous viewing is eighteen hours, only its external physical dimensions and the size of the screen are the relevant dimensions. Capacity, in physical units, is then, for example, single channel entertainment for zero to six people for sixteen hours. Since the marginal cost of any additional viewer between 1 and 6 is zero, and for any length of time, constant (assuming away the problem of physical depreciation as a function of heat levels), capacity in economic units is different: it is six people for sixteen hours. An audience of four for two hours is economically "inefficient."

If the several alternative channels are considered capable of providing heterogeneous entertainment and/or other programs, channel availability becomes a relevant dimension of capacity. The famous television set of a few years ago with its three-screen reception and instant tunability demonstrates that both simultaneous as well as sequential channel capability may be relevant. Even under the assumption of program homogeneity, channel capability is relevant if the clarity of reception is heterogeneous.

The example is trivial, or should be. The output of a television set, and therefore the relevant measures of its size and capacity are quite simple problems. But the point made is crucial: no measure of size, and hence no measure of capacity, can be a priori defined without specifying the output in all its relevant dimensions. In the above simple example, it is obvious that the quantity and the time dimensionality of the audience and the channel capability of the set are aspects of quantity, and visual and audio clarity are dimensions of quality.

Figure 5-1 is drawn for an assumed cost function such that the average cost reaches a minimum at thirty units of output per time, remains at that minimum level to forty-five units of output per time period, thereafter increases, and at sixty units of output becomes infinite. That is, no more than sixty units of output per time period can be physically produced, regardless of cost. As we have discussed before, the shape of the cost function is a reflection of two sets of factors: the shape of the production function and relative input prices. The underlying production function in this instance indicates that between thirty

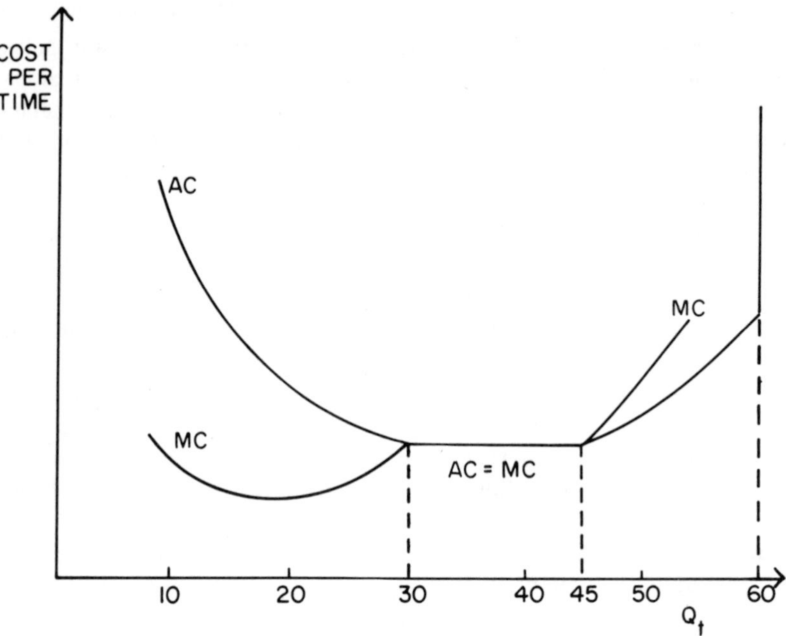

Figure 5-1. Capacity Output.

and forty-five units of output, output can be increased at constant cost, before that level costs decline as output is increased, and beyond that they increase, but no greater than sixty can be produced. This implies the presence of some indivisibilities which are fully exploited at the thirty-forty-five range, and of some fixed factor, or factors, which become limiting at $Q_t = 60$.

In this instance "absolute capacity" is 60 Q_t. "Economic capacity" is that level of Q_t for which AC is at a minimum, or where marginal cost equals average cost. In this instance $MC = AC$ for Q in the range of thirty to forty-five. Economic capacity is variable. The subtle theoretical issues need not be discussed here.[h]

Assuming still a single output, or that the output Q_t is homogeneous, the question of the *relevant* economic capacity remains if it is further assumed that (a) there can be no inventories of Q, and (b) the expected demand is stochastic. Under these assumptions, it is no longer true that "efficient" utilization of

[h]The question of whether it is the presence of indivisibilities or the desire for built-in productive flexibility, of whether absolute limits exist in the short run only or in the long run as well, are interesting issues, not directly relevant here. For a discussion of these theoretical as well as empirical issues, and for a reference to the literature, see Smith (393), as well as Schwartzman (376).

capacity occurs at, and only at, $Q_t = 45$. If demand is probabilistic, that is, only the distribution of demand in the future can be predicted, and the cost of *not* meeting peak-demand is high either in terms of the loss of future "sales," or indirectly, operating on the average at $Q_t = 40$ may be efficient. This, of course, implies a peak demand of forty-five. For purposes of cost and efficiency analysis, therefore, even in the case of a simple homogeneous output, the *relevant* economic capacity may not be the *absolute economic capacity*, and it is certainly not the absolute technical capacity. It can be argued that the relevant capacity should be defined to be forty-five, since in periods of excess demand or peak demand, an additional fifteen units of output can be produced, though on the steeply increasing portion of the cost curve. This is a question of the frequency of peaking and of the rate at which costs increase beyond $Q_t = 45$.

It is the nature of expected demand, whether predictable with certainty or stochastically, whether it is constant over time or occurs with predictable or unpredictable peaks, therefore, that determines whether $Q_t = 40$ or $Q_t = 45$ is considered "100% utilization of capacity." Simply stated, is it the absolute number of total beds or some portion of them, say 90%, that is considered "size" or "capacity"?

Consider also, as another example, that there are two outputs produced: treatment of surgical cases and treatment of medical cases. Assume that for each of these outputs only three inputs are used, beds, medical staff, and nursing staff, and that the proportions of inputs for each of the outputs, regardless of their level, are constant. Consider further that at any given time the quantities of inputs are fixed: there are a fixed number of beds, nurses, and a given medical staff.

In figure 5-2, measure on the horizontal axis the number of medical cases treated per time, say year, and on the vertical axis the number of surgical cases treated. On the assumption of given numbers of beds, nurses, and medical staff and a longer average stay for medical cases and a relatively more nurse-intensive treatment process for surgical cases, the diagram shows the following relationships. With the given number of beds, fifty medical or eighty surgical cases, or any linear combination of them, can be treated per time period. With the given number of nurses, seventy medical or fifty surgical cases per time period can be treated, or any linear combination of them. With the given medical staff, fifty-five medical and sixty surgical cases can be treated, time and linearity conditions being the same. The three inputs determine how many of each case types can be treated: consider them constraints. Therefore, only the five-sided convex area OABCD is feasible: even if only medical cases are treated, no more than fifty per period can be treated, since for any number above that there would not be sufficient beds: the bed constraint is binding. With their shorter stays, there would be enough beds to treat eighty surgical cases, but even with zero medical cases, the nurse constraint becomes binding at fifty surgical cases. When some of each patient-type are treated, all three constraints become relevant at different case proportions: on the A-B segment the nurse constraint is binding, on the B-C segment the medical constraint is binding, and on the C-D segment the bed constraint is binding. Let ABCD be called the "production possibility locus." Any combination of medical and surgical cases per period of time can be treated up to and including, but not in excess of, the possibility locus ABCD.[i] Where actual production will take place is not now the point. It is clear that since a variety of combinations are possible, some choice will have to be made. The choice to be made will be determined by how the medical and surgical cases are weighted: *how they are specified in the dominant objective function*, that function which the literature cannot specify. What is at issue here is the question: What is the relevant measure of size and capacity? Can it be beds?

We have oversimplified: there are surgical beds and medical beds, and they are not always interchangeable; and there are obstetrical beds, maternity beds, pediatric beds, intensive care beds, and none of these beds are usually substitutable for either medical or surgical beds. But on surgical cases the bed constraint is not relevant at all, and on medical cases only in the range from forty to fifty per time period. Medical staff is binding only on the segment B-C. We begin to see the rationale of measuring capacity in units of "fully staffed beds." But it should also be seen that *unless* those "beds" are multipurpose beds, they specify treatment capacity in some fixed set of case proportions. And to the extent that the demand for hospital services in terms of treatment proportions does not correspond to the case proportions implied in the "staffed bed" specification of capacity, that measure of capacity is useless. The argument can be simply restated: when more than one product is produced, with more than one input, and as long as the inputs are not fairly freely substitutable in the production of those multiple products, capacity can be meaningfully specified only in terms of the relevant binding constraints.

"Beds" do not do the job. "Bed days" do not do the job. "Bed complements" do not do the job. "Patient days" is meaningless. These are the units in which the literature "measures" size and capacity. One saving argument can be made: to the extent the heterogeneity of that gross aggregate used as the measure of output, "patient days," overlaps the heterogeneity of the gross aggregate of the measure of size, the differentials may coincide. Then we are back to the propriety of cost measures as "per diem" and to the statement, made earlier in this book, that yes, "transportation is transportation."

Even if the "measurement" of such unspecified multidimensional conglomerates were acceptable, one problem remains: ambulatory care is completely lost.

Defining output as the weighted number of cases (regardless of discharge status) and size (or scale) as the number of beds, M. Feldstein estimates the long-run average variable cost (if there were no cases treated the cost would be

[i]For a neat technical exposition of a linear programing example see M. Feldstein (133, pp. 168-82), and Dowling (120, pp. 28-74).

zero) in a number of ways. Fitting both linear and quadratic equations, when *no* allowance is made for possible interhospital differences in case mix composition, he finds that "throughout the currently observed range of hospital sizes, cost per case increases with hospital size; the quadratic cost curve does not reach its maximum until 2,580 beds" (133, p. 64). Noting the possible biases introduced by case mix heterogeneity over hospital size, he properly disregards these results as not very meaningful. It may also be noted that that may be true on purely statistical grounds: the standard errors of the coefficients on the two variables in the quadratic equation (3.2, p. 63) indicate that the coefficients are not significant, and R^2 is only 0.048.

To allow for case mix heterogeneity, he explicitly introduces into both of his equations for average long-run costs the vector of case proportions. The fit is now somewhat better, $R^2 = 0.31$ for the quadratic equation. The conclusion is that "a quadratic cost function with case mix included, implies that cost is unaffected by size. *If we disregard the standard errors*, (3.9) indicates a shallow U-shaped curve with minimum average cost at approximately 310 beds" (133, p. 66, emphasis added).[j] Since the results are not very satisfactory, Feldstein proceeds to examine the cost function in more detail, separately for large hospitals and for all hospitals within the same size class. The equations are run, plagued again by coefficients whose standard errors often exceed by several factors the coefficients themselves (see p. 72, table 3.6). From these results he draws the following conclusions:

(a) The more disaggregated models do not provide a better model of the relation between size and average cost per case than the original single equation (3.9). (p. 71)

(b) . . . All four of these models indicate a cost curve of the same general shape as that implied by the single equation: a slightly U-shaped curve with a minimum in the range of 250 to 350 beds. (p. 71)

(c) We can neither accept nor reject the theory that there are overall diseconomies of scale among the largest hospitals. What does appear most likely is that a true minimum does exist in the 250 to 300 bed range . . . Beyond 300 beds it would seem that costs do rise until about 600 beds and then probably flatten out at this higher level. In short, costs rise slightly with scale beyond the current average size but cease rising at twice that size. (p. 73)

(d) Both of these approaches support the conclusion that any tendency to increased costs in larger hospitals is of no importance. There are neither

[j]In the equation referred to the coefficients of B_1 and B_2 respectively are -0.581×10^{-2} and 0.934×10^{-5}. Their standard errors are, again, respectively, 1.728 and 1.741. This would appear to be sufficient reason to disregard the coefficients and not their standard errors. Feldstein argues, however, that "we must not disregard as 'insignificant' the possibility" that the U-shape exists. (p. 66)

substantial economies nor diseconomies of scale. The costliness index need not be adjusted for hospital size. (p. 67)

(e) The estimates of section 3.4 indicate that there are no economies of scale. (p. 73)

(f) The general empirical results presented in this chapter can be summarized briefly. The average cost function, when adjusted for casemix, is a shallow U-shaped curve with a minimum at the current average size (310 beds). Costs rise beyond this size but level off after 600 beds at about 10 percent above the minimum cost. (p. 86)

Any one conclusion, or any set of them, is acceptable—depending on whether or not "we disregard the standard errors."

As an analytic convenience, Feldstein accepts the conclusion that there is "an apparent absence of any influence on size" (p. 74).[k] Further assaying the question, he hypothesizes that the "apparent absence" may be the resultant of two counteracting factors: the "pure scale effect" and the "case-flow effect" (p. 74). Defining the number of cases treated per bed year as the case flow, he incorporates this variable into the estimating equations to reflect possible interhospital differences in patient turnover rates. The average observed case flow is 23.2 with a range of 9.4 to 40.5. His quadratic equation in case flow and beds shows an inverse relationship: case flow decreases as size increases.[l] Feldstein interprets this to show that "the pace of hospital activity may decrease with size. The inference is consistent with the more general economic argument that the specific diseconomy of large units is managerial or labor inefficiency and the increasing complexity of communications" (p. 74). This ad hoc theorizing is no more plausible than the argument that the output measure is not correctly specified.

One alternative explanation for the lower case flow, indicating a longer average stay in larger hospitals is that they treat the more complex, the more severe cases even within the same case category.[m] Within case categories as broad as his, there may well be diagnostic variation as well. Therefore, it can be maintained that if the larger hospitals treat more complex and more severe cases of increasing diagnostic and therapeutic difficulty, they are producing a *different*

[k]The synonymity of "no economies of scale," no "substantial economies of scale," and "apparent absence" of economies of scale is not obvious.

[l]In view of this result, the Mann-Yett assumption that caseflow increases as hospital size increases, is at least peculiar. (265, n. 23)

[m]The careful and detailed analysis of casemix variation by hospital characteristics carried out by Lave and Lave demonstrates that when casemix is considered in a detail greater than what is possible with Feldstein's "case proportions" approach, the hospital's size, urban vs. rural location, teaching status, are all important explainors. (231) They argue that while these hospital characteristics "cannot be considered good surrogates for casemix," (p. 37) what is relevant a propos our point here is that such "institutional characteristics as size, teaching status, and number of advanced services . . . explain only about 25 percent to 45 percent of the variation in the casemix measures constructed. . ." (Ibid.)

output. While it may appear reiterative, quality and status upon discharge must once again be mentioned, for Feldstein must assume, for example, that mortality ratios are the same for all hospitals regardless of size. That this is not the case, at least in the United States, has been shown by Roemer, Moustafa and Hopkins (357).[n] Feldstein's "inference" of the managerial inefficiency of size could be reformulated into an hypothesis to be tested by comparing case histories of patients with the same diagnosis in different size hospitals.

When the caseflow variable is incorporated in the equations estimating the average long-run cost, R^2 is increased to 0.74, a U-shape is observed, but now the minimum point, instead of being at around 300 beds, is at 900 beds (p. 75). At first Feldstein maintains that the minimum cost point at 900 beds "is an artifact of the quadratic form of the function" (p. 75). He then fits a monotonic function in log and semilog, and since the "residual sums of squares" and R^2 values are "practically equal" and there is no basis of choice between the quadratic and monotonic functions, he draws the conclusion that "if flow rates were uniform, larger hospitals would enjoy lower costs per case" (p. 75). The turning point at 900 beds, which is exceeded by only three hospitals in the sample (p. 75), now becomes accepted: "Adjustment for caseflow rate or average duration of stay shifts the minimum cost scale from the current average size (about 300 beds) to the largest sizes in the observed range" (p. 81). This conclusion is then modified by calling attention, in a footnote (p. 81, n. 22) to the fact that even though analysis by instrumental-variable-estimates shows a "smaller minimum cost size than the ordinary least squares value (738 beds instead of 903) there are too few hospitals above this size (only nine) to give much weight to this as evidence of a turning point."

A reasonable conclusion, then, at this point, would appear to be that (a) excluding case flow, if one is not willing to "disregard the standard errors" there are no apparent economies of scale; (b) if one is willing to "disregard the standard errors," rather significant economies of scale are present, with a minimum at around 300 beds; (c) if case flow is considered and the "artifact of the quadratic form" disregarded, economies of scale are even more pronounced, with the efficient scale at around 900 beds if (c.i) the case flow in larger hospitals can be reduced but if the case flow cannot be reduced then (c.ii.) the existing size of around 300 is the efficient size. Some additional questions must be raised, however.

In his discussion of the production function (see chapter 4), Feldstein concludes with a recursive model in which the *only* exogenous constraints are beds and medical staff (133, p. 120). He considers the rate of occupancy of

---

[n]This reference is also relevant with respect to Feldstein's comment that "measuring quality of medical care remains an unsolved problem" (p. 25), on the basis of which he disregards quality. Roemer, Moustafa, and Hopkins develop and test a somewhat crude but nonetheless useful and stimulating index of hospital quality by adjusting observed death rate differentials over hospitals by case severity.

existing beds to be also relevant, and hence estimates the equation for occupancy rate in beds and medical staff (p. 121, eqn. no. 4.47). Two interesting results emerge: occupancy rate is negatively related to beds (the coefficient is –0.110 and significant), and positively to medical staff (0.126 and significant).

In a study using principal component analysis on ninety-nine variables representing hospital and patient characteristics from Chicago area hospitals, Morrill and Earickson find, though using a somewhat different definition of capacity, that "personnel and payroll expenses are much better predictors of capacity than the number of beds. . ." (282, p. 231). Feldstein in his production function identifies not beds but medical staff as the constraint, and the Morrill and Earickson study substantiates this.

Utilization will be discussed below. Here it might be mentioned that Feldstein argues, in a different context, that there appears to be a positive relationship between availability of beds and their utilization (133, pp. 201-227). One of his conclusions is that "a redistribution of medical staff, rather than general funds would be necessary to reduce the effects of bed availability on the number of cases treated" (p. 215). This also clearly implies that the relevant constraint is the "medical staff."

Experimenting with a linear programing approach to the analysis of case mix specification, Feldstein shows, for other purposes, that *only* if the cases are weighted by average length of stay are *beds* the binding constraint on output, measured as weighted cases (133, p. 180). When other weighting schemes are used, beds are *not* binding: the shadow price of beds is zero.

The "shadow price" of an input is the calculated price or value which reflects how much the decision maker would be willing to pay for the quantity of that input to produce an additional unit of output. If the shadow price of an input is zero, it shows that output can be increased without any additional increase of that input. It is not a binding constraint. In figure 5-2, for example, at point B, the shadow price of beds is zero, regardless of how the relative desirabilities of treating medical and surgical cases are weighted. Beds are not a binding constraint, nurses and medical staff are.

But what is the constraint on the length of stay? Bed availablilty. If the individual components of an output bundle are weighted in terms of that dimension only which is uniquely determined by a given constraint, it logically follows that that constraint will be binding.

Ingbar and Taylor (195) use "available bed days" as their measure of capacity. The shortcomings of this concept for certain cost estimating purposes was discussed in the previous section. However, since "available bed days" is defined in terms of "fully staffed beds," it is clear that they explicitly recognize that "beds" as such may not be an adequate unit in which to measure capacity.

What is the rationale, then, for assuming that the constraint on output is the number of beds? Capacity can only be meaningfully defined in terms of the relevant constraints. *Ad extremum*, what is the capacity to deliver treatment

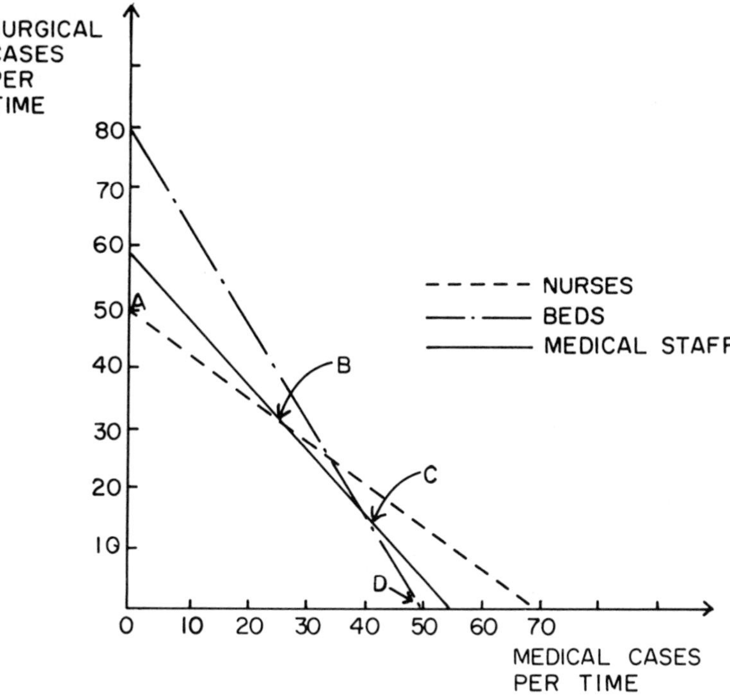

Figure 5-2. Capacity with Multiple Outputs and Inputs.

services of a 1,000 bed hospital with no medical or nursing staff? The use of "beds" as a measure of capacity is troublesome not only because of technical problems involved in measuring output-capacity relationships under that assumption. Particularly in view of his own identification of medical staff *and* beds as the relevant constraints, and an inverse relation between occupancy rate and bed size, the use of "beds" as the measure of capacity by Feldstein, as well as by others, is questionable, as shown above, on theoretical as well as empirical grounds. That this is more than simply a theoretic nicety is indicated by the current discussion of "the doctor shortage," "the nurse shortage," "the intern shortage," but not of the bed shortage.

In the analysis of short-run cost curves, the assumption that the number of beds is an appropriate measure of capacity is again made, with case flow as the unit of measure of output (133, p. 129). It will be recalled that the average case flow is found to be 23.2 cases per bed per year. The relationship between case flow (F) and cost per case shows that (a) *cost per case* would decrease with an increase in case flow, and reach a minimum at F = 32.1, (b) *cost per patient week* is at a minimum at F = 12.3 and would increase with increasing case flow beyond that (p. 130). When "capacity," as measured in beds, is introduced, (c) *cost per case* reaches a minimum at F = 32.7 and (d) *cost per patient week* at F = 18.2 (p. 131). Given the specification of output as "case treated" without any quality dimension, it is not possible to choose between "cost per case" and "cost per week." Cost per case, with or without including a "capacity" measure, would be substantially reduced by *increasing* the case flow, or patient turnover, but cost per week would be reduced by *reducing* patient turnover. In other words, increasing patient turnover would reduce cost per case, but increase cost per day (or week).

Full presentation of the sample on which the analysis is based would enable one to assess to what extent some of these results stem from data characteristics or from methodological inefficiencies. The fact that both quadratic and monotonic functions yield the same, or similar results, is not fully acceptable in terms of "but the exact general form of the function is unimportant" (p. 133). While on p. 130 Feldstein states that the observed average of *F* is 23.2 and then performs his analyses, on p. 133 it is pointed out that "only seven hospitals have *F* values exceeding the implied turning point of the short run average-cost-per-case," which has been calculated to be 32.1. Now, from tables 3.4 and 3.5 (pp. 68-70) it can be calculated that of the 53,454 beds in 177 hospitals in the sample, the seven largest ones, 3.9 percent of the total number of hospitals, have 12 percent of the beds. In the discussion of long-run cost curves, the estimated turning point of 738 or 905, depending on the functional form, is dismissed because "there are too few hospitals above this size" (p. 81, n. 22). As we have seen these "too few hospitals" contain 12 percent of the beds. In the absence of other information it can be plausibly inferred that the fit of quadratic, and monotonic functions, with direct data or data transformed into log and semilog, is partially explainable by the distortion of the distribution by the very few very large hospitals.

It is interesting to note that the relationship between case flow and cost per case appears to be the same whether size (in terms of beds) is introduced or not. The minimum point is reached at about thirty-two cases per bed per year in both formulations. It is also to be noted that the inclusion or exclusion of *case mix* is also without effect on the estimated case flow effect on cost per case (pp. 131-32). Feldstein's analysis of the effect of case mix was discussed above. Case mix is considered crucial because of very substantial interhospital variation in case proportions (133, p. 15); the distributions of cases in each category are bimodal and highly skewed over hospitals (Ibid.), that is, "many hospitals do little or no work in a particular category and . . . a few hospitals concentrate a much higher than average proportion of their work in these areas" (Ibid.); because "there is a high degree of interhospital variation" (p. 21); because "the proportional casemix specification effectively removes the problem of multicollinearity in the workload specification that would be present in severe form if the actual numbers of cases were used" (p. 63); because "omitting casemix may substantially bias the cost-curve estimates" (p. 66). Yet, when the relation between average cost per case and the number of cases per bed year is estimated it matters not whether case mix is included or not.

The explanation may be quite simple: the effect of case mix variation is reflected both in case flow and in average cost per case. This is recognized by Felstein explicitly (p. 131). Then, however, what is the merit of the argument that "substantial savings in cost per case could be achieved by increasing case-flow rates" (p. 134)? If the case mix is variable, bimodal, and skewed, *and* reflected in case flow, case flow can be increased only by changing the distribution of case mix.

Further, if case mix basically reflects length of stay effects and if length of stay variation in turn is the reflection of differences in case severity and diagnostic heterogeneity within the case category, case flow rates are not subject to much manipulation. There is some indirect evidence of this in Feldstein's table 5.2 (p. 135), where the results of the calculations of separate cost functions by hospital size groups are presented. The average cost per case equation in beds, case flow, and case mix is estimated for groups of hospitals:

Bed (Size) Range	Value of Case Flow at Which Cost per Case is Minimum	Elasticity of Cost per Case with Respect to Case Flow
72-117	44.4	−1.11
118-302	30.9	−0.90
303-488	29.9	−0.85
489-1,064	27.6	−0.88

Cost is most responsive to case flow, and reaches its minimum at the highest case flow in the small hospitals. The cost effect of case flow is less pronounced, and cost reaches its minimum at the lowest case flow in the largest hospitals. If (a) the larger hospitals get the more complex and more severe cases—as Feldstein's own discussion indicates—and (b) the length of stay is related to case complexity and case severity, the case flow variation by size reflects differential length of stay resulting from variations in treatment patterns by disease stage and severity. This further diminishes the power of the conclusion that "substantial savings in cost per case could be achieved by increasing case-flow rates" (133, p. 134).

The nature of the binding constraint is also crucial in the discussion of the relationship between costliness and the length of stay. Per diem costs between hospitals can be easily distorted by "deliberately holding patients a day or two longer than medically necessary" (397, p. 239). The argument is that since the ancillary services are concentrated in the first few days of stay, by extending the length of stay the per diem cost per admission, or the cost of stay, to the hospital, can be reduced this way. If the binding constraint on output is "beds," as is generally assumed, this implies that during those "extra" days of stay ancillary equipment and personnel are idle. In real, or opportunity terms, the cost is therefore increased, not decreased. For the same per diem charges hospital revenues could be increased by an increased patient turnover and an increased intensity of service utilization. If the binding constraint is medical staff, or service capability, the cost of those "extra days" is the cost of hotel services only: the shadow price of beds is zero.[o]

The most inventive and exhaustive analysis in the literature, that by M. Feldstein, therefore, yields contradictory tentative conclusions. The reasons are to be found not in methodological errors, but rather in the absence of a comprehensive analytic framework, inadequate specification of variables and parameters, and shortcomings of data. Other analysts have not been able to overcome these difficulties.

Klarman (216), Lave and Lave (232 and 234), Long (256), Mann and Yett (265), Ro (350), and Stevens (407) use as their measure of "size" the number of beds. Ro recognizes that the absolute number of beds should be deflated to represent that proportion of beds not in use for extended periods, and hence considers "bed compliment" (350, p. 193). Stevens considers beds and patient days to be interchangeable. Carr and Feldstein, in a careful discussion, realize the shortcomings of "beds" as a measure of size and consider that the ideal measure would be the "average number of patients for whom care can be provided in an optimal manner" (74, p. 52). Since the total number of beds may or may not represent this capacity, they evaluate two alternative measures (a) the reported number of beds less the average daily unoccupied beds, an "adjusted bed" concept, and (b) the average daily census. The latter is then used in their analysis as the measure of size. Ingbar and Taylor, as has been already discussed, take "patient days" and "available bed days" as measures of size and capacity (195). Cohen (e.g., 86) considers the weighted average of services, but then translates them into "patient days" and "beds." The various investigators also employ differing definitions of output. It is not surprising, therefore, that there is no agreement on whether economies of scale exist, and if so, whether they are significant.

Ro, after stating that "in the regressions calculated but not included here, the number of beds are sometimes found to be related positively to the cost per stay and sometimes negatively" (350, p. 243), concludes that economies of scale exist. His estimated long-run cost curve decreases over the entire range of his sample, varying in size from 36 to 794 beds. This would imply a downward sloping long-run supply curve which, in the absence of externalities, either internal or external to the industry, is a theoretically, as well as empirically, thorny question. His faith in traditional economic theorizing comes to the

[o]For a thorough discussion of the differences, and their implications, between "output" and "capacity," see Metzner and Winter (273, pp. 16-18).

rescue: "This is not to rule out a U-shaped cost curve for hospitals of all sizes. As size increases beyond *800* beds, managerial diseconomies and decreasing labor efficiency will *sooner or later* outweight the economies of further specialization and efficient techniques" (350, p. 245, emphasis added). The maximum "size" in his sample is 794. This is, of course, convenient, but not proven. Among other things, it confuses size of *plant* with size of *firm.*[p] Many large hospitals tend to have separate units in separate wings or separate buildings, specialized by function: maternity units and pediatric units, for example, tend to be physically separate. Aside from the difficulties of measuring the "size" of the entire hospital in units of aggregate if unsubstitutable beds, to what extent do these individual units represent separate "plants" of the same "firm"? There is no discussion of this in the literature at all. The hypothesis that *plant* diseconomies will be present in possibly multiplant hospitals cannot be offered as a conclusion.

M. Feldstein, as has been shown, concludes that economies of scale are present, with the turning point at 300 or 900 beds depending on how the statistical results are interpreted. The tenuity of this set of conclusions has been discussed extensively.

P. Feldstein (139) concludes that economies of scale do exist, and Carr and Feldstein (140) find a shallow U-shaped curve with a minimum at around 190 average daily census, which implies that beyond that rather small "size" diseconomies exist.

Ingbar and Taylor (195) not only find that economies of scale do not exist, they find an *inverted* U-shaped cost curve, with a maximum at around 150 beds, or 200 beds, depending on the year of the data (pp. 105-107). Their "least efficient hospital" (p. 107) is almost exactly that found to be "most efficient" by Carr and Feldstein. They reasonably conclude that "whatever its exact shape—the average cost curve does not fall monotonically, at least in the 30-330 bed range of hospital size. . ." (p. 107).

Berry (46), on the other hand, finds economies of scale to exist over the entire range (p. 138).

Cohen finds economies of scale to exist, with the minimum of a U-shaped curve at around 160-170 beds in one sample, and a minimum at around 290-295 in another sample, and hence concludes that ". . . hospitals between 150 and 350 beds are most efficient for ordinary patient care" (84, p. 20). When allowance is made for the "more output" of affiliated hospitals, however, the economies are even more pronounced and now the minimum cost is reached at 540-575 beds with "unweighted" output (p. 15), and at either 640, 700, or 790 beds, depending on how the affiliated output is weighted (p. 16). When inpatient days are used as the measure of output, he finds the minimum cost at either 240 or 320 beds, depending on the presence of the quality variable (pp. 17-18).

[p]For an excellent yet uncomplicated discussion of the relationships between economies of scale in plants and multiplant firms, see Bain (31, esp. pp. 146-69).

The Panel on Hospital Care, in its analysis of data from the "12 distinguished hospitals" ranging in "size" from 300 to 1,500 beds concludes that there are no economies of scale (340, vol. 2, p. 161).

Klarman, after a review of the literature up to 1964 (216, pp. 104-108), concludes that "a U-shaped curve for the long run is plausible" (p. 107). The "plausibility" is posited on the theoretical arguments of a basic textbook in economics and a complete misspecification of the measure of output: "as the size of the hospital increases, cost tends to be raised by the provision of a wider range of services. . ." (p. 107). This of course assumes that output as measured by "patient days" or "average daily census" is precisely the same regardless of variations in case complexity, case severity, and service intensity. The untenability of the last is precisely the question to which P. Feldstein, M. Feldstein, Carr and Feldstein, Berry, and Cohen address themselves, albeit without much success. The fallaciousness of this argument is recognized by Lave and Lave, who conclude that *because* neither economies nor diseconomies are demonstrated the assumption that economies of scale *do* exist is likely to be correct (234). To the extent that service-facility complexity is positively associated with size, and positively associated with a more complex output in treatment terms, the fact that diseconomies are not observed implies that economies of scale are present. The output measure, in other words, is assumed to be symmetrically biased downward: the larger the "size" (in beds) of the hospital, the more its output is biased downward when measured in patient days, or other gross aggregates. The argument is theoretically appealing, but not proven. In a later and much more careful work with better data, Lave and Lave conclude that "our results indicate that if economies of scale exist in the hospital industry, they are not very strong" (232, p. 394).

The strong hold of theoretical assumptions, particularly in the light of contradictory empirical evidence, is demonstrated by Morrill and Earickson, who maintain that "a more complex output is, of course, one explanation for apparent diseconomies of scale . . . Returns to scale probably obtain for hospitals within a similar group."(282, p. 225) To demonstrate the relation between "size" and "a more complex output," they assume, probably correctly, a strong relationship between that and facilities-service complexity. If that does not work, perhaps economies of scale can be identified by studying the hospital at the departmental level (Kushner, 227). In any case, economies of scale probably exist and they can be "captured" either by mergers (179) or at least by the sharing of some services (95).

We may summarize the findings on the existence of economies of scale in table 5-1.

That average per diem costs and the number of services offered by the hospital are strongly positively correlated is shown in a number of studies (14; 182; 391). The single largest component of costs, however, is shown to be that of the nursing service, which, unless further specified, is itself an aggregate and probably a function of the length of stay (4; 139, p. 9; 216, pp. 108-111).

Table 5-1
The Existence of Scale Economies: Summary of Findings

Investigator	Existence of Economies of Scale	Minimum Long Run Average Cost Point in Terms of Beds
Cohen (84)	Yes, strong	150-350 depending on output definition
Cohen (85; 86)	Yes, strong	540-790 depending on quality measure
Ingbar and Taylor (195)	No	
Lave and Lave (234)	Probably yes	?
Lave and Lave (232)	Probably no, and if so very weak	?
Francisco (150)	No	
Klarman (216)	Yes	?
P. Feldstein and Carr (74)	Yes	190
Ro (350)	Yes	900
M. Feldstein (133)	Yes	300-900 depending on equation specification
Panel on Hospital Care (340)	No	

In summary, then, the question can be posed: What are the shapes of the short-run and long-run cost functions of hospitals? Are there economies of scale? The answer from the literature is clear: "The exact general form of the function is unimportant" (133, p. 133), but "whatever its exact shape" (195, p. 107), and depending on the methodologies and definitions used, economies of scale exist, may exist, may not exist, or do not exist, but in any case, according to theory, they ought to exist.

Other Cost Elements

P. Feldstein, M. Feldstein, and Ingbar and Taylor, in the studies previously discussed, also consider departmental costs in detail. The large proportion of costs generated by what may be called "fixed labor factors," nursing and administration (30-37 percent and 12-14 percent, respectively) seems to be a consistent finding. There is no agreement on the cost implications of a nurse training program. P. Feldstein finds that the net benefit to a hospital of having a nurse training program is negative: it implies a positive cost, if a low one. He finds that the presence of student nurses accounts for something less than 1 percent of operating expenses. Carr and Feldstein present similar findings with somewhat more strength (74, pp. 56-62).[q] Ro, on the other hand, shows that,

[q]But see references at pp. 56-62 in Carr and Feldstein for contradictory evidence. See also, Butter (38), for an excellent recent survey.

according to his definition of output, the presence of nursing training programs increases unit costs by some 10 percent (350, p. 235). Ro also maintains that costs are uninfluenced by the presence of intern and/or residency programs (350, p. 235), while Lave and Lave indicate the opposite (232). P. Feldstein shows that the presence of interns is correlated with the intensity of service-facility use. Uses of laboratory, radiology, and central service departments appear to be positively correlated with the presence of interns. Further, the variable that best "explains" the differences in interhospital monthly drug expenses is also the presence of interns. "The drug prescribing activity of interns is an interesting and anomalous factor which affects hospital costs during any period" (139, p. 53). This would clearly imply that in analyzing the costs of intern and/or residency programs, the indirect costs generated by their impact on the activity levels of service departments should be examined.

That teaching hospitals, at least in New York City, tend to have per diem costs some 21 percent higher than that in non-teaching hospitals has been demonstrated (e.g., 87, p. 103). This has been attributed to a variety of factors, including higher quality of care and the continuing education they offer the attending physicians (324). However, no precise studies of the cost effects of intern/residency programs have been published. Two beginnings are represented by Campbell and by Carroll (70; 75).[r]

It is notable that no detailed analysis of the costs of providing outpatient services have been done.[s] Nor are there any detailed studies relating the costs of community services to the costs of hospital operations. Some of these questions are considered under costs of care under differing practice settings, such as prepaid group vs. solo fee for practice, and under different insurance coverages. It will be briefly reviewed in chapter 6 on Demand and Utilization.

One of the characteristics of the studies so far discussed is their exclusion of indirect costs borne by the patient, such as time costs.[t] This has been explicitly considered by Long and P. Feldstein. Since their purpose was to incorporate a measure of time-cost and inconvenience-cost into planning for hospital bed distribution, the study, while demonstrating the inefficiency of facility fragmentation without any coordinating mechanism, is not directly relevant (257).[u]

Cost Behavior Over Time

Given the diversity of views about the shapes of cost functions, and even questions about their identifiability, there is good reason to expect that while

[r]For a general discussion of the special problems of teaching programs, see Somers and Somers, Ref. 401, pp. 108-113, and research costs, Wing and Blumberg, Ref. 439.

[s]But see, Roemer and DuBois (356).

[t]For some recent economic studies of the money costs of time in traveling, see, e.g., Beesley (43), and Mohring (277).

[u]For critical evaluation of this study, see "Discussion," Ibid.

consensus would obtain that costs have gone up, no agreement exists on the causes. Views range all the way from the assertion that in a "land of plenty" resource constraints are no longer binding and the problem is really that insufficient resources are devoted to medical care: "We must marshall the resources of the country in a semi-military, although democratic, manner to keep pace with, if not to exceed, the growth of the population and the endless proliferation of medical discoveries and technology" (16, pp. 77-78). Some suggest that while costs have gone up, perhaps one ought not to worry about it too much:

It is a bitter irony that the nightclub dancer earns more than the medical technologist . . . Americans have unobtrusively adopted a convenient system of double values under which they are cheerfully willing to pay for life's pleasures and patently reluctant to shell out for life itself. (206, p. 495)

Some view costs increases of huge proportions as endemic to all developed industrial societies: "It may well be that rapidly rising hospital costs are 'inherent' in a modern industrialized society" (12, p. 198). This is seen as taking place in the United States at a rate below that of other similar countries, such as the U.K. and Sweden.[v] (12; 17) No "causes" are advanced, but the assertion is made that neither the existence nor the nature of controls inhibits cost increases (Ibid.).[w] Not only absolute but proportional cost increases are seen:

. . . In all high income countries there has been a secular trend for expenditure on health services to increase as a proportion of national income or national product . . . Moreover, it appears that in *all* countries for which data are available, an increasing proportion of total health expenditures has been devoted to hospitals. (7, p. 92, emphasis added)

A.R. Somers maintains that cost increases, as measured by per diem units, are perhaps the necessary corollaries of the increased quality of care resulting from the use of the products of medical knowledge and technology. The improved care was facilitated by the institution of third parties:

It is because–and only because–most Americans now have substantial portions of their hospital bills, even part of their doctor bills, paid by such third parties that the progress in medical science and technology could be translated into

[v]For an excellent and detailed international comparison of cost trends, see Abel-Smith (6 and especially 7 with which it is often confused). For an interesting comparative analysis of public health care costs, see also Pryor (332, esp. pp. 151-81, 416-19, and Appendix E).

[w]In the Netherlands, for example, between 1958 and 1968, hospital costs increased by 339 percent (395, p. 51).

actual health services and the rising demand inherent in recent demographic and sociocultural changes could be met even on an approximate basis. (397, p. 349)

The cost increases, further, as measured, are *overstated* by the use of per diem (397, p. 348). Not quite, says Reder, the opposite is true: at least in some dimensions quality has been decreased, hence cost increases are understated.

Since professional standards and public surveillance both limit deterioration in the quality of medical care per se, the pressure of cost increases is deflected, at least partially, from raising product prices to lowering the amenity aspects of quality. (337, p. 127)

Using time series data from seventy-four hospitals for the period 1961-67, Lave and Lave construct and test two models. In one the "relation between average cost, utilization, size, and time" is first estimated for each hospital and then the "causes of the variation in the estimated parameters among hospitals" is investigated (232, p. 380). The second procedure assumes that there is no interhospital cost function variation and a single cost function is estimated from pooled data. They find that the relative rate of cost increases among hospitals is positively related to the initial cost level and to size, and that location, urban-rural, has no effect. The size effect is speculated to be a reflection of the presence or absence of teaching programs and location, since location and the presence of a teaching program are not independent of size. This is tested, and they find that while the presence of teaching programs is a significant factor in the hospital's rate of cost increase (those with teaching programs had cost increases 1.3 percent greater per year than those without), urban-rural location is not significant (232, p. 386).

However, when the second approach is tried, the utilization variable becomes insignificant, and so does the size variable. The role of the level of initial cost is also changed: "hospitals with high initial costs had a much larger than normal cost increase in 1961, but a much smaller than normal cost increase in 1967" (p. 392).

Many causal factors have been mentioned: the "overexpansion" of facilities (H. Somers, 400, p. 707), "unnecessary and uncoordinated facilities" (A. Somers and H. Somers, 401, p. 220), increased costs of technological change, lack of increase in labor productivity, increased numbers of functions, third party cost "pass-through," physician income maximization, "catching up" by hospital employees combined with the effect of almost universal reimbursement which makes hospitals more willing to grant pay increases (211, p. 35), general pressures on administrators to engage in more costly hospital activities (135, p. 5), increased financial charges stemming from increased commercial borrowing, changes in medical education, increases in the general standard of living, the absorption of functions previously performed by physicians, the pricing of functions previously performed free, the absence of incentives for productivity and efficiency (199; 217; 271; are representative).[x]

These causal factors will not be examined in detail. But an understanding of their roles can perhaps be learned from our discussion of Productivity and Efficiency in chapter 4.

Two thoughts may be kept in mind, one from the Gorham Report, and a statement by Piel:

A major obstacle to the analysis of changes in the amount of care received per dollar of expenditure is that there are no generally accepted measures of output, input, and productivity of the hospital sector. (271, pp. 31-32)

. . . Most of the cost increases reflect the waste of resources that are encouraged by the present modes of delivery of health care that lay the emphasis on episodic and acute treatment. In a structured regional system it would become possible to establish physical and social incentives for more efficient use of resources. (327, p. 348)

Summary

In this chapter we have discussed the nature of hospital costs and the empirical investigations of their behavior. We have shown that given the differences in conceptualization, the various measures of output, the multiplicity of size, capacity, and quality variables employed, it is of little surprise that there appears no consensually held view on either the short-run or the long-run cost behavior in hospitals. In general, marginal costs are thought to be a very significant percentage of average costs in the short run but there is no agreement on whether economies of scale exist, and if they do, at what size.

It is quite likely that more reliable and repeatable studies will be forthcoming in the not too distant future. The approach of disaggregating case categories into well-defined case mix to reflect output differentials and constructing individual hospital cost functions as pioneered by Lave and Lave appears promising. The paucity of useful data is also likely to be remedied, to some extent, by the increasing enforcement of comparable, and fairly detailed, record keeping which appears to be a concommitant of the increasing role of federal programs, such as Medicare, in the financing of hospital costs.

Though there is scant empirical or theoretical understanding of how hospital costs behave, which is quite understandable in view of the analytic difficulties and the lack of work on production functions, there is a general belief that

[x]For an interesting and useful decomposition of medical care cost increases for the period 1929-69 in the United States into factors related to increases in per capita utilization, changes in population composition, and inflationary trends, see Ref. 213.

increases in demand pressures facing hospitals are important factors in their increasing costs.

We may not know what it is exactly, or how its production and distribution are brought about, but at the yearly cost of some $70 billion, of which the largest single component, about $30 billion, is hospital cost, something called medical care is produced and distributed. There certainly appears to be a demand for it.

6 Demand and Utilization

"Only the slave has needs; the free man has demands."

—Kenneth Boulding

"My name is Alice, but—"
"It's a stupid name enough!" Humpty Dumpty interrupted impatiently. "What does it mean?"
"*Must* a name mean something?" Alice asked doubtfully.
"Of course it must," Humpty Dumpty said with a short laugh: "*my* name means the shape I am . . . With a name like yours, you might be any shape, almost."

—Lewis Carroll

Review of the extensive literature on the nature of demand, utilization, and "need" however defined, and of their interdependence, is not our purpose here. Since, however, the interaction of the conditions under which services are produced, of the nature of supply, and of the demands for those services is assumed to be relevant for price determination, and since, according to our discussion in chapter 1, the demands for hospital services are interactive and complex, we now consider briefly some of the relevant aspects of demand and utilization.

In the first section we present the outline of a demand model for medical care and for hospital services. We show that unlike the demand for the usual consumption goods, the demand in this case is not for specific goods but for good health, or more specifically, for the remission of disease states. We consider that each individual has some expected health status and some perceived one. When a negative difference between the expected and perceived health levels exist, when there is a health status disequilibrium, the initial decision process begins. In the formulation we stress that different levels of health status disequilibrium lead to different kinds of patient originated demands. Further, that a large segment of the demands for health services, and particularly those for hospital inpatient services, are physician legitimated or physician originated. Hence we show that much of the demands are not exogenous, but are generated within the medical care system. Thus we establish that there may exist minimally four types of demands, each resulting from varying sets of demand determinants. Further, since the conditions under which felt needs for medical care services may exist are at best probabilistic for the individual, there may exist option or contingency demands.

Next we consider the empirical studies of demand behavior to find that most of the formulations are either fragmentary, stressing only the demands for inpatient care, or incorrectly formulated by disregarding the endogenous nature of some demands. The studies on price and income elasticities are on the whole faulty, since the elasticities are measured not in relation to quantities of services, but in relation to a proxy, the expenditures for the services. Thus, while the conclusion from the empirical studies that price and income elasticities have been decreasing since insurance has largely replaced income and prices as the principal demand determinants may be instructive, the absolute values found are tenuous at best. This is supported by the pathbreaking analysis of Andersen and Benham. Observed demands are intersection points between demand and supply schedules, or utilization. So we consider the studies on utilization and utilization variations.

Utilization variations are differently attributed to socioeconomic variables and are seen to be influenced by supply conditions as well as by the nature of incentives facing physicians. This part of the literature lends support to our formulation of the four demand model, stressing the role of physicians and the availability of alternative supply sources.

All the demand studies and most of the utilization studies define outputs in narrow terms, disregarding the dimension of quality. To the extent that quality is discussed at all, some economic analysts maintain that we already have too high a standard of quality and not enough variation within it, certainly less than would obtain under conditions of economic Utopia, perfectly competitive equilibrium. We then demonstrate the meaning of quality variation by citing some case reports of poor quality of care.

Attempts to maintain high quality care while encouraging the choice of economically efficient treatment processes where alternatives exist are incorporated into experiments with different practice settings, particularly prepaid comprehensive group practice. We consider some of the findings from studies on prepaid group practices for the light they may shed on their impact on utilization to find that in fact inpatient processes, particularly admissions and patient days per population aggregates, have been significantly reduced by them.

The conclusions in this chapter are similar to our findings in the previous chapters. While some innovative work is now being done, most of the demand studies and utilization analyses suffer from weak conceptualization and imprecise definition of the relevant variables. Further research studies in terms of demands for specific kinds of services, for specified diagnoses, are required to enable us to isolate the role of economic variables. Further, the role of the provider, the physician, in the decision-making process that leads to the generation of demands ought to be explicitly incorporated in the demand constructs.

A Demand Model for Medical Care and Hospital Services

Consider that the medical care process may be initiated by (1) the potential patient voluntarily; (2) the potential patient involuntarily; (3) a social mechanism directly; and (4) the potential provider of services. For our present purposes there are no significant analytic difficulties in cases (2) and (3). While there are substantial ethical issues present in determining the relevance of patient preferences when he is unable to indicate them (as in a severe cerebral accident) or when social preferences override them (as in involuntary confinement, or until recently, abortions), the initiation of the care process is not within his domain and hence his preferences need not be examined to predict utilization behavior. Rather, it is when either the patient or the provider is the initiator of the care process that we must consider the mechanism, and the possible role of economic variables within it, by which that process is initiated.

While the complex subjects of perception and felt need are properly within the domains of psychology, sociology, and anthropology, it seems reasonable to assume that, at any given time, an individual has some expectations regarding the appropriate level of his or her health status. When the individual perceives his actual health status to be less than his expected health status, there is a *perceived disequilibrium* in his state of health. The perceived disequilibrium leads to a perception of felt need and initiates a sequential decision process to identify actions conceived to be appropriate to the degree of felt need.

An individual's desired health status is some function of a multitude of objective and subjective factors such as economic and family status, education, role expectations, degree of socialization, geographic location, work experience, age, past health experience, and societal norms. We are assuming here that these and perhaps other considerations will result in the individual's estimation of the health status appropriate to his age, social position, and role within a given societal structure; and, that the expected health status is in fact the desired health status. A degree of functional impairment, for example, which would be considered a sufficient deviation from expected health status by a 30 year-old male to lead to the presence of felt need for some action by him might well be consistent with the expected health status of a 65-year-old male. Needless to say, whether the 30 year old is a ski instructor or a file clerk may make a difference; as might, in the case of the 65 year old, whether the individual is a retired postal clerk or an active conductor. Felt need for some action, however, is not uniquely a function of disequilibrium in the state of health. It may also be present when desired health status is prospectively defined, that is, when in the individual's estimation some present action would yield a higher expectation of attaining desired health status in the future. Felt need for preventive care is of this nature. Felt need for preventive care may also result from the potential patient's reluctance to rely on his own perceptions of his state of actual health. Thus it is likely that the more knowledgeable he is about disease history prior to the symptomatic stage, the less likely he is to trust his own perceptions.

The argument so far can be summarized symbolically. The individual at any given time t has a desired health status which is his *expected health status* H_t^*. The expected health status is a function of a set of situational variables.

$$H_t^* = f(A,E,R,S,N,H_{t-1}) \qquad 6.1$$

Where *A* is age, *E* education, *R* role expectation, *S* societal and family status, *N* cultural norms, and H_{t-1} the individual's previous health status experience.

At any given time the individual has a *perceived health status*, H_t. The relation between the expected and perceived health status is expressed by the relation

$$H_t^* \gtreqless H_t \,. \qquad 6.2$$

If, and only if the perceived health status is below the expected one is there a health status disequilibrium, H^d.

$$H_t^* - H_t > O{:}Hd \qquad 6.3$$

When H_d exists, the motivation for some action exists.[a]

Given the perception of some signs, symptoms, disabilities, or discontinuities in his experienced health level that signal, as it were, the presence of health status disequilibrium and thus generate a degree of felt need for some action, a decision process to select the action perceived to be appropriate is initiated. At this stage of the decision process the potential patient is faced with four options: (1) Do nothing, but wait for the disequilibrium to correct itself; (2) Undertake self-medication (lots of orange juice and a day in bed, say); (3) Seek information and advice from informal, non-scientific, non-medical sources, such as family members or friends; or (4) Initiate contact with a medical care provider. Note that while both options (2) and (3) may be properly defined as "seeking care," we shall consider only option (4), entry into the medical care system, as initiating the medical care process, since it is only then, with the exception of over-the-counter, self-administered medications, that the resources of scientific medicine are called into action. The decision process is an iterative one. For a given perceived level of disequilibrium the decision in period 1 may be to do nothing, in period 2, to self-medicate, and if still "nothing happens," in period 3, to seek care. We have consciously used "period" without further definition, for what is an appropriate "period" is itself a matter of perception of both time and

[a]For a similar conceptual framework which considers the demand to exist for good health and within which good health is a depreciating stock which may be increased by investment, including the purchase of medical care, see Grossman (174).

of the nature of the signs, symptoms, etc. Thus the length of the period for which the "do nothing" option is thought to be appropriate will differ depending on whether a pain of similar intensity is perceived in the stomach or in the chest.

Consider now that the action of choice is option (4), entry into the medical care system. At this point the potential patient has presented himself to a medical care provider and by that action has translated his felt need into effective demand. Let us now consider the mechanism by which felt need becomes demand, the point at which medical care utilization begins.

In received economic analysis we assume the existence of some preference function which is an ordered set of the individual's felt needs for commodities and services purchasable on the market. Whether, and to the extent, the so-ordered felt needs are translated into effective demands depends, among other factors, on the relative prices of goods and services and the potential consumer's income, or budget constraint. The preference function is assumed to be a priori given and there is assumed to be one complete ordering at a time. Given the rather continuous, repetitive, and predictable nature of general consumption activities, it appears both reasonable and fruitful to assume that an individual can rank quite well his preferences today for steak, hamburgers, and chewing tobacco tomorrow. He is not only likely to have experienced each at some past point on his consumption path, but can be reasonably sure that hunger will strike again tomorrow. Further, his previous experience with the three commodities had enabled him to associate with each the presence or absence of hunger satisfaction, as well as other properties such as taste, texture, smell, color, etc. Since the consumption experience is repetitive, he has had an opportunity to learn their properties as well as his satisfaction with them and thus rank in his preference ordering each of the commodities. In cumulative consumption behavior information is ipso facto generated without engaging in any specifically information generating activity. The preference function, in this sense, can be reasonably said to represent the consumer's informed tastes. Note that this is not an argument for "consumer sovereignty." External influences, advertising, or taste creation of any nature are fully consistent with the assumption that the consumption itself is an information generating action as conceived in all learning paradigms.

Given the informed preference function, the budget constraint, the alternatives, and their prices, the consumer is assumed to translate his "preferences" into effective demand. We need not inquire into how that preference function had been shaped, how felt needs are perceived and under what conditions, or with what level of intensity they enter the preference function. We do not generally consider whether the potential consumer is in fact hungry now, or whether he has eaten in the last three days, or whether the contemplated purchase is for a dinner party tomorrow. His preferences are informed, they exist a priori, and they are independent of his circumstances. His predicted consumption choice is presumed to result from his equating at the margin the known prices and the expected satisfactions attached to each of the options.

The fundamental but unstated assumptions embedded in this model of consumption behavior are that the potential consumer has subjectively predicted his contingent states of felt need, that he has ranked them, and that, consequently, he is in command of a completely ordered set of contingency needs. The consumer, in other words, is assumed to have contemplated a set of all possible future states of the world, to have evaluated the expected outcomes under all possible strategies open to him, and to have selected a strategy for all possible future events. Even if we allow for "impulsive" or other "irrational" consumption behavior from time to time, these strong assumptions may be quite sufficient for the analysis of repetitive, continuous, learned, and information generating consumption behaviors. The states of the world, the analogues of felt needs, in terms of the need or relative preference for means of shelter, items of food, commodities and services of recreation do not radically change over relatively short periods of time. Given a reasonably long time horizon, the consumer can probably fairly reasonably predict his future hence expected felt needs in these areas; he has learned which goods and services he perceives to be the best satisfiers, or choice objects, of those felt needs; thus he can be said to come fully equipped with a preference ordering over all possible events which, in conjunction with the constraints and parameters of the choice situation (in the consumption case, prices and income), enable him to make rational choices. A rational choice is one which, subject to the constraints, is expected to result in the maximization of his preferences. Consider now the case of health status disequilibrium.

Recall that health status disequilibrium results from the perception of signs, symptoms, and disturbances, and leads to the presence of felt need for some action. Here we must consider a dichotomy between recurrent or chronic symptomatology on the one hand, and episodic, nonrecurrent, new to the person, on the other. In the case of recurrent disturbances the assumptions of learned behavior, predicted states of felt need, identified choice objects, and rational choice embedded in the theory of consumer choice are likely to be met. The chronically ill have learned to interpret the signs, evaluate to some extent their severity, develop a concept of duration and severity, and have had the previous stream of experience as a guide in the choice of the appropriate action. A patient with angina pectoris can generally recognize the onset of an attack by the site and intensity of pain; knows when to take nitroglycerin; and generally knows the length of duration of the symptoms after medication that indicates the probable need for further medical intervention. The chronic patient is also likely to have experienced the familiar disturbance in a variety of situational contexts, hence the situational factors probably wash out. The experienced patient, therefore, both as a result of his familiarity with his own conditions and as a result of his familiarity with alternative medical care interventions and their prices to him, can be expected to behave according to the predictions of the theory of informed consumer choice. This does not imply that the action chosen is in fact the action which under the same circumstances would have been chosen by a medical care provider. The interpretation of signs, symptoms, etc., is probabilistic, their perception over time may be dulled or intensified, and they may signal the presence of a different, new condition or a different stage in the history of the old one. The action learned to be appropriate to perceived situations and hence chosen may be clinically the wrong action.

For now we conclude that in the case of recurrent or chronic illness, patient decision making is amenable to the analysis embedded in the theory of consumer choice with the roles of prices and income in their accustomed places. Let us consider the choice situation in the case of nonrecurrent, episodic, new to the person signs and symptoms.

Implied in our argument so far is the postulate that the perception of state of health disequilibrium and the resultant felt need for intervention which occurs under unanticipated situations, unforeseen states of the world, unconceptualized conditions, lead to choice behavior characterized not by learning but by ignorance.

Here we must distinguish between the perceived severity and implications of the perceived signs and symptoms. It is not merely an unnecessary complication to suggest that while different individuals may perceive the same signs, they may, resulting from purely personally different thresholds, perceive different degrees of severity and, as a function of disparate levels of knowledge, cultural norms, and socialization, draw different inferences. Surely there is an element of overstatement here, since all social beings have learned at least some appropriate behavioral norms; peer group behavior, family behavior, behavior norms communicated by social means as well as expectations of normal body functions provide both enforcement to the conception and perception of abnormality and some guides to the action appropriate to it.

It appears reasonable to assume that there exists a set of signs and disturbances which, within a given cultural system, always and without exception result in a level of felt need resolvable only by seeking care from a clinical provider without delay. That is, for some H^d option (4) will be chosen: enter the formal system. It appears both trivial and grotesque to suggest that in urban America of the 1970s anyone with a compound fracture of the ulna, with bone protruding from the torn tissues, would willingly choose to wait for it to go away, or attempt to set it himself, or ask a friend for advice on the best medication.

In general, we can identify a set of signs and disturbances consensually perceived to be of such severity that it results in an extreme degree of felt need and consequently in the initiation of utilization. When the perceived disequilibrium in the state of health exceeds some level, when, in other words, direct intervention by a provider is perceived to be life critical, the economic choice algorithm is irrelevant. "Money is no object." But note three points: (a) we are talking about making initial contact with a provider, and *not* the management of the process of care; (b) we are referring to an individual's own choice; and (c) we are saying that the individual would not willingly choose otherwise. These three points merit emphasis.

While we are suggesting that some set of signs will always result in the speediest feasible contact with a clinical provider without prior calculations of personal economic costs, we are not suggesting that the clinically determined appropriate therapy will similarly be undertaken in all cases without an economic calculation. While it could be agreed that certain signs of heart failure will send just about anyone to see a physician without first calculating the cost of the visit, it appears less reasonable to suggest that surgical intervention or placement of a pacer, if that be the appropriate therapy, will inevitably and automatically follow in all cases without prior economic calculations. Regarding our second point, the condition giving rise to the perceived signs may incapacitate the patient in which case, of course, his preferences become inoperative, inexpressible, or dysfunctional (as in some extreme mental disorders). In this case the potential patient falls into either categories 2 or 3; initiation of care is either involuntary or is by some social mechanism directly.

The third point stresses "willingly," namely that given a set of signs, an individual would not *willingly* choose actions other than immmediate initiation. For the choice to be operational, a potential provider must not only be physically available and attainable, but must be accessible to the potential patient. Institutional, racial, or economic barriers to access are neither unknown nor uncommon. While the refusal to treat patients, even in urgent conditions, stemming from racial discrimination is now prohibited in most states, there are few if any legal constraints on the refusal by private providers to treat patients whose ability to pay for services is in question.

On the whole, however, we conclude that there exists some set of signs and symptoms of severity sufficient to induce a degree of felt need which can be assuaged only by immediate initiation of care without prior economic calculations. An indication, or proxy, of the magnitude of demand for initial care in this category is the percentage of emergency room contacts adjudged to be urgent.

At this point the potential patient enters the medical decision process. Now the initial professional decision takes place. The professional medical decision maker, the physician for short, evaluates the presenting patient and may arrive at one of two alternative decisions: professional H^d exists, or professional H^d does not exist. The physician, that is, using professional medical standards, may concur that health status disequilibrium exists or he may not, for two reasons. First of all, the physician's evaluation may lead to the conclusion that the signs and symptoms do not indicate the presence of a condition of sufficient nature, degree, or severity to infer the existence of a disequilibrium. Secondly, the physician may conclude that while the signs and symptoms reveal a state of health *different* from H^*_t, the patient's expected health status, medical intervention is unwarranted and likely to be of little effect. Hence the patient may have to readjust his expected health status, to a now lower level, thereby eliminating the perceived disequilibrium.

If the patient agrees with the professional evaluation, the medical process terminates with either his acceptance that the perceived condition does not imply divergence from his expected health status, or that his expected health status has to be scaled down to the perceived level. If the patient does not agree, the process begins again by his seeking a different professional to reenter the system.

Alternatively, the physician may agree that in fact H^d exists, that there is a probable diagnosis indicating the appropriateness of clinical intervention. Of course the patient may not agree, but assuming his perceived H^d presupposes his willingness to comply, a sequence of decisions now leads to the generation of demands for medical services. At this point the factors we indicated in chapter 1, and particularly in figure 1-1, p. 3, come into play. The alternative supplies of services and their prices and payoffs to both the patient and the physician, as well as the patient's socioeconomic characteristics and the physician's preferences interact to determine the specific quantities of derived demands for services and their locations.

Prior to proceeding with the discussion of health status disequilibria of lower values or of smaller perceived degree, we should consider the question of whether the felt needs for some action arising from such perceived disequilibria are in the same category as the felt needs for food, shelter, etc., as they appear ordered and ranked, and expressed in terms of goods, in the hypothesized preference function. To engage the discussion of "basic" and "created" or "cultural" needs, or preferences, is to enter a psychological-philosophical morass. Avoiding the quicksand, we might note, however, that values other than the mere ability to assuage hunger are generally attached to most items of food: values other than the sole function of keeping out the cold and rain are attached to most varieties of shelter; and the essential function of wine is other than the satiation of thirst.

We might here consider that goods whose fundamental attributes inhere in their ability to satisfy biologically originated felt needs have as yet other attributes or abilities to satisfy additional personal or cultural values as reflected in some felt needs. It is perhaps more fruitful to consider that felt needs originating in biological stimuli, such as hunger, have historically, and differently in different cultures, become encrusted with other felt needs of social, cultural, religious, and other origins. Goods with the attributes thought suitable to satisfy these latter perceived needs thus become valued for more than their ability to eliminate the biological stimulus of the basic felt need; they are valued for their symbolic, ritualistic, conspicuous, or hedonistic attributes. Both filet mignon and hot dogs have the attributes to satisfy hunger, both margarine and "the high price spread" provide the same nutrients, yet there is little question which is preferred and which is the "inferior good." While one may observe great diversity in personal "tastes," within the same cultural context there is generally consensus on which members of the set of substitutes are preferred. And note that they are preferred not for superior abilities to satisfy stimuli but for their ability to satisfy a more diverse set of stimuli: they are multi-purpose goods.

It is significant that the services and commodities over which the consumer is assumed to have preferences are called "goods." There is surely a degree of circularity in the argument which maintains that a consumer selects from among a bundle of goods and that they are "goods" because they are within the choice set.

Consider the obverse: consider that a consumer is forced to play a game in which he dislikes all possible proximate outcomes. Assume that all proximate outcomes and their associated probabilities are known to him and that he must make a choice. The notion is neither bizarre nor unrealistic.

Suppose a traveler with rather well-developed culinary tastes is stuck at dinner time in a seedy diner where his choices are ham and eggs, chili, hamburgers, and for some strange reason, pompano amandine. The stimulus whose satiation is the ultimate outcome is hunger. The proximate outcomes are those associated with the menu choices each of which, as we shall see, he may dislike to differing degrees. He prefers the pompano, when well made, only lightly broiled and juicy yet firm, and dislikes it intensely when not properly prepared. But he also dislikes, even when well made, ham and eggs, chili, and hamburgers, in that order, for dinner. Now suppose that he dislikes ruined pompano even more than he dislikes well made ham and eggs and in his estimation the chances of getting a well-prepared pompano amandine in the dumpy diner are close to zero, while the chances of getting the ham and eggs well prepared are about half and half. Though he dislikes all his options, or in other words, would prefer a different game, he must nonetheless choose the alternative which he dislikes the least. He chooses the ham and eggs. Now this conceptualization of "the only game in town" is not original and neither is the strategy which in the vast literature of game theory has the name of "minimize regret."

Conceiving medical care to be intervention to correct a perceived health status disequilibrium, it seems plausible to suggest that the decision process which might result in the initiation of care is, similarly, a game played not to maximize outcomes, but to reduce losses and to minimize regret. It is the only game in town.

Let us consider another example. Suppose our reluctant consumer observes that his kitchen drain is clogged. He of course might wait awhile, hoping that it will clear by itself, taking a chance that the cause of the original obstruction will further impact. Next he might try a home remedy in the form of lye, or caustic soda, depending on his awareness that he might thereby damage his dishwasher. Finally, he might call a plumber. Now needless to say, the price he expects to pay the plumber is relevant and if his friendly plumber made house calls free of charge our reluctant consumer might well call him sooner, perhaps at the first sign of sluggish discharge. Yet it is equally plausible that unless he enjoys friendly chats with the plumber and a messy kitchen, he would rather not engage in this activity. There are few felt needs involved other than to have a functioning kitchen. And the plumber is the only game in town. The reluctant consumer must choose among "bads."

We have introduced these considerations into the discussions of choice making when a state of health disequilibrium is perceived to suggest that to consider the "preference for medical care" to be a member of the set of usual consumption goods is misleading. With the exception, perhaps, of preventive care, and in the pathological case of hypochondria, for the patient to initiate medical care utilization is to enter reluctantly into an unwanted game. Medical care is not a good; it is a least "bad."

This is not to argue that in some cases and in certain situations the choice field is not broad enough to include some positive attributes of the sick role. To go on sick call may not be "good," but it is certainly much better than to go on K.P. Here again, cultural norms, social expectations, peer standards, may encrust or endow, depending on one's perspective, the process of initiation of care with positive values even in the absence of perceived disequilibrium. In certain subcultures and at certain times, not to see your analyst once a week is to be out in the cold; in others, to see one is to be in hot water.

To recapitulate, we have said that if there exists a health status disequilibrium, H^d, of sufficient degree, patient contact with the formal medical care process is initiated resulting in some level of patient originated demand for services, D_{IF}. (See chapter 1, pp. 1-3) D_{IF} is composed essentially of initial contacts: office visits, emergency room and clinic visits, and so on. But perceived health status disequilibrium varies in perceived severity, seriousness, immediacy, and implications.

Consider, for ease of exposition, that there exist only two different levels of health status disequilibrium as perceived by the potential patient: H^d_e, a level of disequilibrium conceived to be emergent, and H^d_n, a level *not* considered to be emergent. What is considered to be emergent by the patient will no doubt be influenced by all of the factors (see 6.1 above) which enter into his expectational state and, in addition, whatever level of medical knowledge the potential patient commands. Psychological and situational variables also, no doubt, play a role. "Emergent" is here broadly used to mean perceived conditions which require immediate medical consultation since they are seen by the potential patient as either gross divergence from his expected state, such as trauma (e.g., broken limbs), or because they are thought to be life threatening (e.g., suspected cancer, heart attacks, etc.). We consider that while in the second case the economic algorithm is probably valid, in the first it is not. That is,

$$D_{IF_1} = f(H^d_e),$$

$$D_{IF_2} = f(H^d_n, P_m, Y). \qquad 6.4$$

In perceived emergent cases, the disequilibrium state is directly translated into patient originated demand, with the prices of medical services, P_m, and the patient's income, *Y*, playing no role in the decision. When the disequilibrium is not perceived to be emergent, both the potential patient's income and the prices of medical services are relevant demand determinants. Patient originated demands, therefore, have these two elements.

$$D_{IF} = D_{IF_1} + D_{IF_2}. \qquad 6.5$$

But now consider that after initial contact has been made, there is professional evaluation of the health status disequilibrium presented by the patient. As we have suggested earlier, the physician may or may not agree with the patient's estimate of his own state. Let us focus attention now only on those cases in which the physician considers that medical intervention is appropriate and again consider that there are two polar alternatives: the health status disequilibrium in the *physician's* estimation is emergent, H^d_{em}, or it is not, H^d_{nm}.

We make the reasonable assumption that when a condition in both the patient's and physician's estimation is emergent in the sense of being traumatic or life threatening, the physician's medical decision is strictly condition (or patient) focused and hence the economic algorithm is not applicable. The consequent physician originated demand for services is determined by his estimation of medical appropriateness and the physical availability of resources, or service capabilities. That is,

$$D_{M_1} = f(H^d_{em}). \qquad 6.6$$

When in the physician's estimation the disequilibrium is not emergent, the physician originated demands for services, D_{M_2}, are determined by his characteristics, C_M, subsuming under that his objectives in terms of physician relevant outcomes, the prices of services, and the patient's income, *Y*, again considering insurance coverage as an element of income. That is,

$$D_{M_1} = f(H^d_{nm}, C_M, P_m, Y) \qquad 6.7$$

The observed demand, D_o, or total utilization, is the equivalent of total demand, D_T. But that is now seen to be composed of four elements.

$$D_o = D_T = D_{IF_1} + D_{IF_2} + D_{M_1} + D_{M_2} \qquad 6.8$$

Needless to say, all of the four demand elements may to some extent overlap. What the patient considers to be emergent the physician may or may not; what the patient considers to be nonemergent the physician also may, or he may consider it to be emergent. There are other complexities, such as the possible outcomes of preventive care or routine examinations and the possible interactions between patient income and expected prices on the one hand and on the other, what the patient perceives to be a disequilibrium level requiring immediate medical attention. Nonetheless, if this formulation is correct, some immediate conclusions can be drawn.

It is obvious that price and incomes are relevant demand determinants in only a subset of observed demand, in D_{IF_2} and D_{M_2}. Studies, therefore, of price and income elasticities which do not consider this four-tuple of demands will probably underestimate both, since in the observed quantity relationship there are included demand components which are price and income inelastic. It is also obvious that the observed demands are outcomes of interacting decisions by patients and by physicians.

The constraints facing each of the two participants in the decision are not the same. Their preference functions by definition cannot be the same. While it is true that the patient's ultimate objective may coincide with at least some, or even a large part, of the physician's ultimate objectives in terms of health outcomes, or as we have stated in health status disequilibrium correction, the physician will have objectives (or preferences over outcomes) that are strictly physician focused, or physician specific in terms of income, leisure, status, professional esteem, etc. This means that the analysis of observed demand as a function of patient preferences, the prices facing patients, and the constraints, particularly income, acting upon patients, is deficient.

This is one reason why demand studies ought to be in terms of well-defined products and services, or outputs, for given diagnostic categories. We have seen that the conceptualization of the hospital's output as the "patient day" presents as a heterogeneous aggregate a set of decomposable specific outputs. The same is true of demand or utilization studies in terms of "admissions" of "office visits." Hence both for the purposes of meaningful productivity and cost studies as well as for the purposes of meaningful demand studies, the outputs of providers (whether they be considered final or intermediate outputs is here irrelevant) ought to be defined in homogeneous service units flowing to specified diagnostic categories, ideally incorporating a measure of severity and of quality. Then at least some of the demand components could be separated, since standards of the medical appropriateness of services in terms of diagnoses either exist or could be constructed.

Is the existence of health status disequilibrium predictable? The incidence in a population of conditions requiring medical intervention is predictable with a fairly high degree of accuracy. Further, since various medical pathologies are related to age, sex, occupation, and environmental conditions, the population subgroups among which the incidence of given conditions is suspected to be present at one time or another can be identified. Such subgroups are called "populations at risk." The populations at risk for cancer of the cervix and cancer of the prostrate, to use an obvious example, can easily be identified by sex, and for carcinoma of the prostrate, further defined by age since its prevalence among men over sixty is significantly greater than among men in lower age groups. There is now sufficient evidence to identify fairly well the populations at risk for a large set of seriously disabling diseases, such as arteriosclerotic disease, emphysema, cancer of the respiratory system, congestive heart disease, among others. The population at risk for other conditions, such as upper respiratory infections, urinary tract infections, and a host of other infectious diseases is more generalized, or, in other words, less well predictable. Just as with continuous throws of a fair coin it is possible to predict with a high degree of accuracy the probability of "heads" and "tails" frequencies, while whether on one given throw the coin will fall "head" or "tail" is less predictable, so with the predictability of the occurrence of medical conditions in populations at risk and in specified individuals within it.

The occurrence for any specific individual of conditions requiring medical attention is but poorly predictable. Since the conditions under which need is perceived cannot be predicted with certainty, demand is said to be probabilistic. It is possible, therefore, that any group of consumers and/or physicians will have some level of conditional demand for hospital services on the expectation that within some calculable period they will in fact experience those conditions under which need will be perceived and effective demand demonstrated: option demand may exist.

Option demand, or contingency demand, has at least two implications relevant to demand analysis.

The prevalence of private health insurance is an indication that many, if not most, individuals recognize its existence. Health insurance, in principle, is a risk transfer mechanism: the risk of incurring expenses resulting from the occurrence of certain medical conditions is transferred from the insur*ed* to the insur*er*, in more general terms, from the individual to the collection of individuals who are members of the insured pool. This is a mechanism for transferring financial risks only.

The existence of insurance in no way guarantees the availability of facilities, physicians, or other providers. Hence the other relevant implication of contingency demand is that groups of individuals, or communities, may wish to maintain and be willing to pay for, the service capabilities, or potential supplies, required to satisfy them. Less than full occupancy, the maintenance of service facilities though infrequently used, and other examples of "under-utilization" may well be examples of the presence of option demands. They are the precise analogues of provision for peak demand. To the extent that "under-utilization" of facilities is attributable to duplication of facilities we have an example of the consequences of organizational fragmentation. If in electricity generation each generating plant had to make provision for demand peaks occurring in its own area without a connecting network that facilitates power exchanges among areas with differently timed peaks, we would have excess capacity in each. In the hospital sector, we have an absence of such networks. Since, on the whole, each hospital is seen by the community, and is conceived by itself, to be an independent unit without relation to the other facilities that exist within the relevant medical catchment area; since there are no provisions for organized exchanges of unused capacity; since facility sharing is neither provided for nor encouraged; since there is no mechanism for central allocation of admissions on the basis of capacity constraints, unnecessary duplication may result. The duplication results, in part, from individual, uncoordinated attempts to provide for contingency demands.

In addition, therefore, to the four-element demand structure that we have posited, there exists another element, contingency demand.

Needless to say, the simultaneous existence of such multiple demand elements and their correspondingly different demand determinants complicates demand analysis. But not only the analysis of demands facing the hospital is made more complex and difficult, the questions of pricing strategies and of efficiency pricing are also seen in a different light. For if "the" demand is recognized to be composed of multiple elements, each with its own differential price sensitivity, it may well be that no one homogeneous pricing policy may be appropriate. This issue will be considered in chapter 7.

The conclusion of the demand model here presented is that a multiplicity of demands exist. Some elements are clearly exogenously determined, as in traditional analysis, while other elements are endogenously determined by the medical decision makers themselves. And in all cases, the demands presuppose the existence of some level of health status disequilibrium which leads to their formation. Analysis in terms of the usually assumed well-behaved preference function in which one element is the "preference" for medical services and commodities is likely to be inappropriate and misleading.

Let us consider the empirical analyses of demand.

Empirical Demand Studies–General Considerations

> With the arrogance that characterizes our profession it is customary to refer to a set of moderately dull exercises on some constructs arising from mediocre, casual utilitarian psychological theorizing as "the theory of consumer choice."
>
> –Martin Shubik (387, p. 410)

Consider now how traditional demand analysis approaches the issues of the demands for hospital care.

For economic analytic purposes "demand" is conceived to be a relationship in quantities of goods and services, prices, and incomes. The "demand for" a commodity is a specified relationship: the quantities of the commodity, or service, that would be demanded for *any* given value of its price, assuming the prices of substitute and of complementary commodities to remain constant, as well as the incomes and tastes of consumers. The "quantity demanded" at a given price, which may also be called the "effective demand," is the amounts that are actually purchased in some specified time period at that price. It may also be called "observed demand." In this fundamental sense "effective demand" or "quantity demanded" or "observed demand" are all identical with "utilization": the observed utilization of hospital services at a period of time is the quantity demanded of those services, at the extant prices of those services and of their substitutes, incomes (of which insurance is one aspect), tastes, attitudes, and health beliefs (preferences), states of knowledge, and levels of expectation. Should the prices of services the demands for which we are investigating change, there might or might not be a change in the quantity demanded. The price-quantity relationship, assuming all other demand determinants to remain constant, the price elasticity, is one aspect of demand behavior that has received extensive attention. The relationship between quantity demanded and income, assuming all other demand determinants to remain the same, the income elasticity, is the other major dimension of demand which is present in the empirical studies.

It is generally assumed that some preferences for hospital services exist and that these preferences are translated into effective demand, or utilization. We have pointed out that the analysis is complicated by the possibility that the preferences that are translated into effective demand are those of consumers *and of* physicians, and, that, with the exception of that segment of demand which the consumer can himself express, demands for the services of hospitals are expressed, or translated, by those who can legally "order" the services: physicians. Additionally, the relationship between quantity demanded and the price is not independent of the strength of perceived need, which in turn is likely to be a function of the emergent versus non-emergent nature of the perceived medical condition giving rise to perceived need, and through it, to demand: the price elasticity of demand for care is likely to be a function of the nature of medical conditions leading to the existence of demand.

Whether consumers have preferences, or demands, for the individual components of the medical care package, among them "hospital services," or whether such preferences and hence demands are conceived of in terms of end results, health status, or in terms of processes leading to expected changes in health status, the specification of preferences has not been much discussed theoretically, except by Grossman (174), and no attempt at empirical analysis has been made. Discussion of differential utilization patterns under prepaid group practice has implicit in it the assumption that the demands are expressed either for health status or for processes and hence the relative prices of alternative processes expected to lead to the same end results help determine relative demands for them. Changes in own and in other prices have been tentatively studied.[b]

There has been considerable discussion of the relation of "need" to demand. Economists tend to disparage the concept of "need," however defined (27, p. 3; 53; 133, p. 201). The most extended discussion of the relationship, and the most comprehensive survey of the literature, is available in Donabedian (119, see also 117). The distinctions between "professional need," "detectable need," and "effective demand" are best discussed in Metzner and Winter (273). The applicability of demand analysis in the prediction of hospital utilization is clearly explained and demonstrated in P. Feldstein and German (141). The results of confusion between "need," "demand," and what the observed data actually represent (known to econometricians as the "identification problem") is demonstrated in Stevens (407).

Some recent economic analyses do explicitly consider the possible presence of need.[c] There appears to be no agreement, however, on *how* it is to be defined and by *whom*. Jeffers et al. (197), for example, in a useful if elementary discussion of the relationships among the concepts of need, want, and demand, define need narrowly as a function of "biological and psychological health states as *perceived by expert medical opinion*" (p. 57, emphasis in original). This assumes that only those conditions evaluated by medical experts as warranting medical intervention correspond to needs, thereby disregarding patient felt needs as well as social definitions of need. In most states, until very recently in all states, a potential patient could have all the "need" for abortion she pleased, but societal definitions of what needs will be met, in the sense of being legitimately translatable into demand, prevented both patients and "expert medical opinion," even where willing, from actualizing such felt need.

An even narrower definition of need maintains that it exists only when the conditions for which care is appropriate are either emergent or urgent. This is

---

[b]For a good but methodologically conservative discussion of the concepts of demand, as well as of need, see Pauly (319), as well as Bailey (27), and P. Feldstein (138). Some interesting and inventive analysis is presented by Anderson (10). The most detailed examination of hospital expenditures as related to general consumption expenditures is Newman (309, chapter 4). Detailed studies are those of Anderson and Sheatsley (18), Fitzpatrick, Riedel, and Payne (147), Riedel and Fitzpatrick (347). For a very recent and up to date study and survey, see Anderson and Hull (12). Auster, Leveson, and Sarachek (25), present an ambitious but conceptually unclear and statistically insignificant general model. Barzel (35), discusses some aspects of demand formation in advanced analytic terms, which then he proceeds to disregard. An interesting and stimulating discussion is found in Boulding (53). An excellent critique of demand studies, based particularly on their exclusion of health states as demand determinants, and an argument for their inclusion is Leveson (246). The best general discussion and data on demand is Andersen and Anderson (13).

[c]An attempt to develop an econometric model is made by Larmore (230). The level of analysis is indicated by the conclusions: "Doctors tend to prescribe hospitalization or bed rest which constitute bed disability, but which prolong life. Persons whose lives are extended by medical treatment may experience disability associated with convalescence or terminal illness (p. 58)

implicit in P. Feldstein's statement that "it is important to be able to estimate what amount of medical care is need alone, i.e., emergent or urgent care" (136, p. 10). This presumably means that the amount of services delivered to patients in emergent or urgent conditions, and that amount alone, corresponds to "needed services," while all other levels of services are discretionary. A need for services, as opposed to merely a demand for them, exists in emergent or urgent cases only. While this concept of need is surely much too narrow, it is consistent with our formulation (relations 6.4 and 6.6, above) of demands in which the demand for care for conditions seen as emergent is not influenced by the price of services, or by patient incomes.

A more general, if also more tenuous, concept of need would define it in terms of high and increasing standards of care. Presumably both patient felt needs and professionally defined needs are relevant. The difficulties of arriving at consensually accepted standards by which to evaluate the presence of need are well illustrated by Rafferty's statement: "This is not to deny that some patients in the hospital do not 'need' to be there, but what is the relevant criterion? Many, perhaps most, of the autos on the Long Island Expressway in the five o'clock rush do not have to be there either" (333, p. 163).

Hospital services for which "demand" is expressed, and in terms of which the demand relationships are studied, are usually expressed as "beds" (339). The variability of demand along a continuum of illness severity is generally not recognized, although a few attempts have been made, in conceptual and/or descriptive approaches, to make that distinction (27). There is no general agreed upon framework for the analysis of demand and hence the specific model developed and tested tends to vary with the analyst. The dependent variable tends to be beds, or "hospital day," a weighted measure (Andersen, 10, Appendix B, p. 87), or sometimes length of stay considered explicitly (359). The independent variables usually included are traditional economic variables, such as price (both the out-of-pocket price and insurance) and the consumer's income, demographic variables in terms of age, sex, family status, and education, and whatever other sociological or other data the analyst has at hand or is concerned with. No agreement exists on the weight of any of the variables, with perhaps two exceptions: the consumer's income and the supply of beds.

When the demand analysis is concerned with a community's demand, or need, for hospital facilities, the "population-bed ratio" is the usual measure, without any further consideration of the availability and non-substitutability of different types of beds. Among other factors, this is implicitly recognized by Somers and Somers, who contend that there is no optimal population-bed ratio (401, p. 57). They suggest "occupancy" as the best measure which also disregards any existing differentiation by (a) the nature of beds, (b) the nature of the hospital, and (c) the relevant service area.

That the demands for hospital services are probabilistic is sometimes recognized by considering the demand for inpatient services to take the shape of the Poisson distribution, which we shall discuss below.

As in production and cost analyses, the focus of attention is inpatient care. While some scant attention has been paid to the demand for outpatient services, the models and analyses do not consider inpatient and ambulatory services to be interdependent, and hence demand analysis proceeds as if each were an island.

The possible existence of demands endogenously generated is implicitly recognized, though poorly conceptualized, in the discussion of what has come to be known as "Say's Law of hospital beds," namely, that it is available supply of beds which partially determines the demand for them. For hospital administrators, and for some economists as we have seen in the discussion of efficiency, this has been translated into a rule of thumb efficiency criterion: "a filled bed is a billed bed."

Let us now consider in detail three basic issues: the economic and socio-demographic determinants of demand; utilization variations and appropriateness; and demand and utilization patterns in various practice settings.

The Nature of Demand: Economic and Socio-Demographic Variables

Rosenthal develops a demand model to estimate bed requirements by "a process that relates the specific characteristics of each area to its utilization of hospital facilities" (360, p. 19). The "relevant areas" are defined in terms of political boundaries, that is, states. This immediately raises the question of whether it is meaningful to consider a state, e.g., such as New York or Michigan, to be the relevant area for purposes of analysis. The implication is that the state can be considered to be fairly homogeneous in terms of those characteristics which are then related to the demand for, or utilization of beds: the intra-class differences are assumed to be unimportant. It would appear intuitively obvious that, for example, New York City and Wayne and Washtenaw counties (including Detroit) on the one hand, and Upstate New York and the Upper Peninsula of Michigan on the other, are more "like" each other in terms of income and other socioeconomic as well as racial characteristics than New York City and Upstate New York.

The model is to include "taste and preferences as well as price and income" (p. 20). Since it is difficult at best to get such data on an aggregate state-by-state basis, Rosenthal assumes that "the socio-demographic characteristics of an area reflect most of these tastes and preferences in some systematic way" (p. 20). The same doubts about the relevance of state-wide data are again applicable. Considering the dependent variable to be utilization in a given state, measured in (a) patient days, (b) admissions (both per population), and (c) average length of stay, he estimates the equations in 12 independent variables by using least-squares multiple regressions.[d] The tenuous nature of underlying theory is

[d]For a discussion of the appropriateness of the procedure, which is questionable, see Christ (78, p. 146). A generally excellent discussion of the conceptual and methodological issues in utilization studies is found in Bice and White (48).

indicated by the selection process which resulted in the list of variables used: ". . . The particular variables were selected on the basis of their popularity in the literature" (p. 23). The "economic variables" are per diem charges, two variables regarding income distribution (families with under $2,000 and those with over $5,999 yearly income), and the percentage of the population in the state with hospital insurance coverage. The socio-demographic variables run the usual gamut from age (percent under 15, and over 64) to race. The results show respectably high corrected correlation coefficients while the regression coefficients tend to be statistically insignificant.[e] Rosenthal concludes that the price elasticity of demand for beds is high. This conclusion is again suggested, based on a different study by Rosenthal (359). The methodological difficulties of both studies would suggest that the conclusions be received with great caution. (For an incisive critique, see Fuchs, 156.)

Reder has argued that while there may be some price elasticity in the aggregate, the demand for beds in any given hospital is likely to be very price inelastic since the decision to enter is largely that of the physician. "As a first approximation, I venture to guess that demand for beds in a given hospital is independent of their prices relative to those of other hospitals in the same area" (339, p. 477).[f] This formulation implies the assumption that price competition between hospitals is completely absent. Newhouse has suggested that while, in general, there is little price competition, since consumers are ignorant of price and quality differentials (a propos physician services), when prices are known they are likely to be misused, since consumers associate price differentials with quality differentials (303, p. 175). Whether the association is valid or not, he does not test.[g]

In several studies P. Feldstein has suggested that the price elasticity of demand is not significant. There are a number of difficulties in evaluating the validity of both the price elasticity and income elasticity studies.

Price elasticity is a relationship in prices and quantities of services. The measurement of both prices and of the quantities of services therefore becomes crucial. Consider first the question of price.

In a study of "Hospital Cost Inflation" (135), M. Feldstein considers the relevant concept of price to the consumer, or patient, to be the cost of hospital services net of insurance "relative to the price of other consumer goods and

[e]Whether the correlation coefficients are "meaningful" is debatable in light of the untenable necessary assumption of the normality of the distributions sampled.

[f]The relevance of the lack of consumer information and information search activity for market organization is shown by Nelson, who demonstrates the existence of much higher rates of concentration in markets where purchases are made in relative ignorance of quality variation and on the bases of past purchases rather than search (299).

[g]While making an argument that efficiency as such need not attract demand, Rothenberg cogently argues that if perceived quality differentials exist in an equilibrium situation, where patients have distributed themselves among hospitals of varying quality under conditions of own payment, they may shift if third party payment is introduced. With the introduction of insurance payments, substantial portions of potential patients will shift to the higher quality hospital, even if it is less efficient. He calls this "demand bunching" (361, p. 226).

services" (p. 3). We have suggested previously the error of introducing in such manner the assumption that consumer "preferences" for hospital services are neatly lined up with preferences for all other goods and services in some hypothesized global preference function. But quite aside from the faulty theoretic formulation, in the theoretic discussion which follows that statement, gross price is taken to be the *average cost per patient day*, on a state basis (p. 12). To arrive at the net price, the gross price is adjusted by an estimated insurance variable which measured the proportion of the state population covered by insurance (p. 14). While some of the needed assumptions may be troublesome (such that the ratio of utilization by the insured and uninsured is constant), the difficulties are compounded in the estimation of the insurance variable, INS. It is estimated in the following way:

$$\text{INS} = \frac{\text{CONS}}{\text{TEXP}}$$

where CONS = "aggregate net expenditures on short-term hospital services by consumers,"

TEXP = "aggregate total expenditures on short-term hospital services including net payments by consumers, insurance companies and the government." (both on p. 13)

Since TEXP includes all payments to the hospital by consumers, carriers, and government, it is clear that it includes payment for services other than patient services. Teaching, research, and community services are included in the output spectrum for which total payments are made. Since TEXP includes payments for services other than patient services, INS, the insurance variable is biased downward, and hence the INS adjusted net price to consumers is biased upward, for patient services. Perhaps none of this makes any difference, since in the empirical work testing the price adjustment model the relative price variable becomes the gross price deflated by a "CPI index variable" (p. 28, where CPI is the Consumer Price Index, not further specified as to component). But the gross price has been previously defined as the "average cost per patient day" on a statewide basis (p. 12). Since the average cost per patient day, just as TEXP, includes the costs, allocated according to different principles in different hospitals, of outpatient services, some teaching and research activities and possibly other output, it might be some reflection of the prices *faced* by patients for inpatient care but not the prices *received* by hospitals for such services. This is simply one example of the difficulty of properly identifying and then measuring the relevant measure of price. Similar difficulties arise in the appropriate identification of the quantities of services.

Price elasticity, as we have mentioned earlier, is a relationship in terms of prices and quantities of services. Since it is difficult to obtain data on quantities of services in terms of physical entities, a proxy is usually employed. The proxy is expenditures for specific services. Whether the relationship be between office visits and prices or between "hospital care" and its prices, the observed prices are related to *expenditures* for those categories of services. In a system of multiple pricing, by income, race, location, etc., given expenditures need not correspond to the same set of services, either in terms of quantity or in terms of quality. That this is so is recognized by Fein (130) and demonstrated by Andersen and Benham, who show that the computed (income) elasticities measured in terms of services are about half of those when measured in terms of expenditures (11, p. 90). Future price elasticity studies, therefore, would be more revealing if both the price and quantity variables were more precisely identified: net out-of-pocket prices to consumers and quantities of services. A further refinement of distinguishing between demands corresponding to different levels of perceived health status disequilibrium would also be useful in identifying price and income elasticities useful for generating accurate utilization predictions.

The price and income elasticity characteristics of demands for medical care are useful in predicting future rates of utilization under different assumptions about price and income changes. Thus, high income elasticity would imply that as incomes increase, utilization will more than proportionately increase. A high price elasticity would imply that under a kind of national health insurance scheme that requires little or no out-of-pocket payment at the time services are received (such as the Kennedy Bill), the demand for services would very significantly increase. Note, however, that the predictions are based on traditional demand theory. If our suggested demand model is appropriate, only that proportion of demands that correspond to patient generated, and only in non-"emergent" cases, is price sensitive.

The literature on income elasticities exhibits shortcomings similar to that on price elasticities.

Silver finds very high income elasticities, 1.8 for hospital expense and 2.2 for medical expenses, for example (388). There are at least two reasons why his results may be biased: the price variables employed represent third party payments as well as out-of-pocket expenses, hence they are not net price, and second, the use of "expenses" to measure the quantity of services consumed, as has been pointed out by Fein, and Andersen and Benham, among others, introduced a strong bias. One's confidence in his results is further reduced by Silver's discussion of them:

> The coefficient of the percentage Negro (X_{11}) is negative, which might mean that, other things equal, Negroes are healthier than whites and therefore require less medical care but is more likely to mean that cultural and other factors result in Negroes' receiving less medical care for a given problem. However, these speculations should not be emphasized, since the coefficient of X_{11} is not statistically significant. (p. 132)

P. Feldstein, on the other hand, finds that the usually important economic variable, income, tends not to be of significant explanatory value here. Though his statistical procedures, and data, are subject to serious doubt, he shows that the income elasticity, while it may have been as high as 1.5 before World War II (140, table 14), is now below 1 for all medical care expenditures, and hence even lower than that for hospital admissions (p. 12). This is further demonstrated, along with evidence that the role of income in the past has been replaced by that of the presence or absence of insurance coverage, by P. Feldstein and German (141, esp. pp. 29-30). Andersen and Benham substantiate this point in the so far most detailed and careful analysis of income elasticity. They find, among other things, that since insurance reduces the out-of-pocket price, it "diminishes the importance of income as a determinant of the consumption of medical care" (11, p. 92).

The contrary evidence, that there is a very strong relationship between health status, the utilization of all kinds of services, including that of hospitals, and income, is demonstrated in several places, the most comprehensive of which is *Delivery of Health Services for the Poor* (107, esp. pp. 9-36). Somers and Somers have argued that increasing income and education levels tend to reduce the demand for inpatient care (401, p. 62). Even though there is little evidence on the independent effect of each, there may be good reason to assume that since the correlation between them tends to be very high, income will generally capture the education effects as well.

The mechanism by which higher income levels translate into the reduced demand for inpatient and increased demand for office visit care is not clear. "Accessibility" and "amenity" differentials between publicly supported hospitals and private physician offices may be one factor. This effect may be observable if those with low incomes who find private office visits unattainable and hence demand care at hospital facilities on an ambulatory or inpatient basis, switch to office care when increasing income levels permit. Additionally, it may also be, that, even if the poor have lower health levels (see e.g., 107), hospital based care is viewed as an undesirable substitute.

It has also been suggested that economic variables are of little or no "explanatory" value. Coe and Friedman, for example, have suggested that the sociological "variables" of educational level, social class, ethnicity, etc., are the relevant factors to consider (83, esp. pp. 42-44). This disregards the fact that in the United States at least, the usual non-economic measures of social class, and of ethnicity, are very highly correlated with income. Other studies go to other extremes, such as excluding variables on family size, education, and occupation on the basis of data unavailability, while including "color" because "by color we wish to measure any genetic differences between the races which might reflect on health" (*sic*) (230, p. 35). This was written in 1967.

An analysis of hospital use in defined diagnostic categories was not able to identify any demographic or socioeconomic patient characteristics systematically related to utilization differentials (347, esp. pp. 165-71). M. Feldstein, however, in his detailed study of maternity care in the United Kingdom, shows a very strong relationship between hospital utilization and social class (133, chap. 8).[h]

The analyses tend to be tenuous for a variety of reasons. Perhaps the major reason is inadequate development of a theoretical framework incorporating those "special" characteristics of the nature of demand which are in several places discussed and then assumed away. That the demand is stochastic, that there is no possibility of consumers' carrying excess stocks, that the observed demand is the resultant of some as yet unspecified interplay between consumer and physician preferences (or decisions), that we might well be dealing with commodities and services which, in Lancaster's words, form "an intrinsic commodity group" with the special aspect that "substitution effects will occur only for relative price changes within the group and will be unaffected by changes in the prices of other goods" (229, p. 144), is not incorporated into any model that has been empirically tested. Neither do the analysts of demand consider the complexities engendered by consumer ignorance and by the multiple availability of services at differential prices; nor the fact that one of the peculiarities of the demand for inpatient care is that, in the absence of income maintenance programs, this is one of the few commodities along with leisure, whose consumption ipso facto absolutely reduces income. In technical terms, the consumer does not choose between various commodities along the same budget constraint. The decision to "purchase" inpatient care simultaneously *shifts* the budget constraint down: unless income maintenance is assured, the decision to enter the hospital is also the decision to give up earned income for the period of hospitalization. The choice, therefore, is not to change consumption patterns with a given income level such that real income is maintained, but to shift consumption which directly *reduces* real income: "more" inpatient care at the same time means "less" of *every other* commodity, less of income. The "intrinsic commodity group" approach appears to be doubly relevant, but has not been adopted.

In summary, the evidence on price and income elasticity, the two basic measures of the role of economic demand determinants, appears to be that insurance, where it exists, has become the most important demand determinant, when the analytic formulation is one of exogenous demand. The role of price elasticity is reduced both by the potential patient's ignorance of available alternatives and their prices and by the reduction in out-of-pocket prices stemming from generalized inpatient care coverage by health insurance. In-

[h]An interesting argument that seeks to explain the relationship between demand levels and economic status in terms of disaffection is presented by Hyman (193). He maintains that low economic status tends to lead to generalized "discontent with the system," which in turn leads to lower utilization.

surance, however, may have lead to estimated reduced price and income elasticities, and hence to increased demands for inpatient services, by quite another route. To the extent that insurance reduces the out-of-pocket cost to the patient, it also reduces possible patient reluctance to comply with medical regimens requiring inpatient care, thereby facilitating increases in physician originated demands. We shall consider this question in the context of utilization variations, and appropriateness, to which we turn next.

Utilization Variations and Appropriateness

"But I don't want to go among mad people," Alice remarked.
"Oh, you can't help that," said the Cat: "we're all mad here. I'm mad. You're mad."
"How do you know I'm mad?" said Alice.
"You must be," said the Cat, "or you wouldn't have come here."

–Lewis Carroll

That variation in utilization, measured as admissions or length of stay, exists, is well documented (308; 133; 354; 146; 90). The analysis of the differences has followed two basically dissimilar approaches: (a) physicians and medically-oriented analysts have tended to investigate the extent to which differential utilization patterns are medically "justified" or "unjustified"; (b) economists and other social science analysts have attempted to relate the observed differentials to a variety of factors, largely disregarding the quality of care, or medical "justification." One result: the studies are not comparable.

If a "built bed is a filled bed," a "filled bed is a billed bed," or in a somewhat more elegant formulation: "demand is not an independent variable but a function of the supply and the length of the queue" (133, p. 193). The existence of a positive correlation between bed availability and bed use was found by Roemer and Shain, and since 1959 hardly a year goes by without someone else also commenting on the issue (e.g., 397). There is much literature on the proof of the hypothesis that availability has a positive effect on use (353; 355; 391; 349; 308; 271; 401, pp. 57 and 64). The nature and shape of the functional relationship escapes specification. Newell suggests that ". . . the supply of beds itself modifies demand. In an area with few beds, the patients, practitioners, and consultants are accustomed to few admissions, and short durations of stay. In an area with many beds, the 'threshold of admission' may be lower, and cases who have passed over that threshold may be retained for longer than necessary" (308, p. 756). Others have argued that the private preferences of physicians and the differential financial payoffs associated with ambulatory versus inpatient care

are the causal factors (401, pp. 62-63).[i] The most extensive analysis has been undertaken by M. Feldstein (132; 133, pp. 193-222).

Again using data from the N.H.S., he finds that the correlation between bed-days per 1000 population and bed availability is 0.838. That is, over 70 percent of the British interregional variation in bed usage can be attributed to variations in bed availability (p. 196). Computing the elasticity of utilization in terms of admissions and length of stay, he develops what is called the "responsiveness index" (132, p. 562), to disaggregate the separate effects of differences in length of stay and rate of admissions. Feldstein finds it both "surprising and somewhat discomforting" that the elasticity of the average length of stay, with respect to total beds, is only 0.35, while that of admissions is 0.65. That is, the responsiveness of admissions to changes in bed availability is about twice as large as that of the length of stay. The finding is interesting, but tractable to different interpretations.

The notion that regardless of bed availability, "the number of cases requiring treatment should be less variable" (p. 204) and that the observed constancy of length of stay results from "playing safe" (p. 216) by both physicians and nurses constitute merely one set of hypotheses. An alternative set would be that while it is correct that "the number of cases requiring treatment should be less variable," the treatment is not correctly specified. Consider that there are possible a number of types of admissions, for example, elective, emergent, and diagnostic. Consider further that for elective and diagnostic admissions substitute treatment processes exist on an ambulatory basis. Variations in admissions, therefore, may indicate no variations whatever in "treatment," but variations in the chosen treatment process: the "output" of the various possible production methods is precisely the same, the difference is one of choosing more or less input-intensive processes. American experience with differential utilization rates under different practice settings tends to imply this. And there is some indirect evidence of this in Feldstein's own data.

In his table of "Elasticities by Diagnostic Category" (table 7.10, p. 219), the coefficients are statistically insignificant from zero (the standard error is more than twice the coefficient) for acute appendicitis, peptic ulcer, hemorrhoids, tonsils and adenoids, and varicose veins in females. One would expect no significant difference from zero for acute appendicitis, as well as for the stage of peptic ulcer at which it becomes hospitalized. This leaves upper respiratory infection (URI), female abdominal hernia, arteriosclerotic heart disease, and malignant neoplasms to explain. Medical practice, at least in the United States, indicates a substantial degree of treatment process (or treatment setting)

[i]Based on his analysis of case mix variation as a function of the occupancy rate, Rafferty argues that the observation of a higher proportion of discretionary cases during periods of low occupancy "should not be regarded with alarm . . . Supply does not create demand, but increased supply does permit the satisfaction of existing, through previously unfulfilled wants. The problem is less a question of who should not be in the hospital than a question of how high a standard of care we really want to provide" (333, p. 163).

substitutability—certainly within such broad and otherwise undefined categories as URI and arteriosclerotic heart disease—between ambulatory, home, and inpatient care. The elasticities for these categories are the highest, 1.53 and 1.14, respectively. The broad category of "malignant neoplasm" is subject to the same argument.

The fact that nearly a third of arteriosclerotic cases admitted die in the hospital (p. 220) is not relevant for this purpose. (It is quite relevant considering Feldstein's definition of output.) To test the hypothesis that the differential responsiveness of admissions of arteriosclerotic patients indicates that the physician for "unconscious reasons . . . is making a choice that he might not find acceptable if it were made explicit" (p. 217), one would have to identify the responsiveness of mortality within hospitals from arteriosclerotic heart diseases to admissions. If Feldstein's implied hypothesis were correct, one would expect to find no responsiveness in the mortality rate. A finding that the death rate from arteriosclerotic heart diseases *in* hospitals responds negatively to admissions would tend to show that alternative treatment processes influence admissions for elective patients.

Some evidence for the hypothesis that the elasticity of admissions is influenced by the availability of alternative treatment processes is presented in an excellent and careful study by Rafferty (333).

Short-run case mix variation in two general community hospitals totalling some 320 beds in a given community was analyzed by using patient records in thirty-seven diagnostic categories accounting for "the most frequent causes of hospital admission" (p. 156). Rafferty finds that there was no relationship between the rate of admission and occupancy rate for patients in twenty-four of the diagnoses, while there was a strong direct relationship in seven diagnoses, and an inverse one in six. Unfortunately, his categories seldom coincide with those used by M. Feldstein, but his computed admission elasticities tend to substantiate the argument that we may be observing treatment process substitution. Rafferty finds high negative elasticities of admission (ranging from −1.20 to −3.27) for precisely those diagnoses which are not urgent and are amenable to ambulatory treatment, such as stomach ulcer without ulceration or hemorrhage, intermenstrual bleeding, cystitis etc. Further, among his twenty-four diagnoses for which admissions do not appear to be related to occupancy rate are the ones that one would not expect to be so related, such as acute coronary occlusion, concussion, cerebral hemorrhage, etc. Further, two of the diagnoses for which Feldstein's reported results show admissions elasticities not significantly different from zero, acute appendicitices and hemmorhoids, are also shown to have zero elasticities.

He also offers the intriguing and plausible hypothesis that there may be strong two-way interaction between occupancy rate and length of stay (LOS). LOS may contribute to increasing occupancy rate, the higher occupancy rate may result in the admission of a larger proportion of admissions with relatively more serious diagnoses requiring longer stay. Thus "both mean stay and the rate of occupancy could continue to rise, without any change in either the total number of admissions or the discharge policies of the staff" (p. 161).

Regarding the lower responsiveness of the length of stay, Feldstein may be misled by his earlier assumption that quality cannot be measured, or that at least, standards do not exist. Along with other analysts of the length of stay variation (359; 379; 407; 295; 308), no attempt is made to consider whether applicable utilization criteria exist.

Those who have considered the quality question in demand and utilization analysis sometimes conclude that in fact there is "too much" of it, at any rate the quality of care is higher than it would be "in full competitive equilibrium" (305, p. 452, n. 2). While the total demand for inpatient care may be price inelastic, the argument continues, the demand for quality is price elastic. Insurance programs that provide total coverage would result in higher quality standards than would obtain under conditions of the economist's Utopia, "full competitive equilibrium," and hence result in the misallocation of resources, allocative inefficiency (p. 453), since patients will choose too much quality, more, that is, than they would be willing to pay for out-of-pocket if they had to. If this hypothesis were correct, one would expect negative correlations between occupancy rates and average costs to the patients in hospitals. That is, patients would be expected to "choose" the lower priced, to them, hospitals, and hence price and occupancy rate ought to be negatively correlated. The opposite in fact, is the case. And the higher the cost, the faster the hospitals tend to grow in size (232, p. 381).[j]

The issue of quality is not quite as unexplored in the medical literature as the economic analysts would have it. In fact quality criteria, including standards specifying optimal length of stay ("justified" or not "justified" in the medical literature) not only exist but have been applied (90; 146; 237; 322; 321; 384; 382; 363; 267; 226; 104). The observed relative constancy of length of stay may indeed be "playing safe": adhering to quality standards. One could even posit that the observed unresponsiveness of the length of stay to bed availability is an indicator of the *absence* of organizational slack: there is no "overuse." Unless there exists some model which incorporates the degree of substitutability between inpatient and ambulatory processes for diagnostic and elective categories, and availabilities of therapeutic and diagnostic facilities on an ambulatory basis, and their relative resource costs, we are not able to interpret unequivocally differential admissions rates as either "efficient" or "inefficient."[k]

---

[j]The absence of a quality factor in demand analysis is not unique to the hospital or health care field. Indeed it is common in all demand analyses, on the assumption of product homogeneity. For a discussion of this problem and an imaginative analysis of the demand for tractors as characteristic bundles of differential quality, see Cowling and Rayner (93).

[k]For an outline of such a model, see Navarro, Parker, and White, 298. A study of utilization patterns by diagnostic categories also concludes that there appears to be significant and unexplained variation (Lerner, 240). For an excellent discussion of the interrelations between theory, methodology, and utilization studies, see Glasser (167). For examples of the use of pre-admission screening to reduce utilization, see 267 and 363.

Perhaps the attitude that "criteria" are not applicable is justified in view of the opinion of one of the most respected students:

> The present patterns of use of hospital care in North America and Europe make no sense, i.e., they show no association with any given set of circumstances. The obvious conclusion is that the volume of "proper" hospital care is highly elastic, so elastic that I feel I can generalize there is no "proper" level of use of hospital care than can be established as a standard. (15, p. 728)

That this is a somewhat difficult position to maintain is shown by a number of studies in the United States. It has been shown, for example, that when judged by criteria established by panels of practitioners specializing in diagnostic categories within which medical records were examined, there is both detectable *under*utilization and *over*utilization. In one study it was found that 9.6 percent and 6.8 percent of the cases studied were respectively "overstays" and "understays" (146, p. 474). Admission rate differentials may also be systematically related to poor quality of care either because of "overstays," or because of "understays" during which inadequate treatment is rendered, followed by repeated readmissions. Both the arguments that "quality cannot be measured" and that "quality is too high," that we have "Cadillac only," disregard the variation around some optimum, in both directions. Granted, such optima are possibly neither ubiquitously applicable nor timeless, but then very few criteria of any kind are. It may also be that the concern with what some take to be "too much quality" and the attitude that it can't be measured anyway, results, at least in part, from insufficient appreciation of what "poor quality" means medically. We reproduce below some examples of what is considered "poor quality" by peer evaluation in a recent year in perhaps the world's foremost medical center, New York City. All of the patients were covered by comprehensive hospital insurance.

1. No. 107. 52-year-old female hospitalized fifteen days. Cholecystectomy: not indicated on basis of history, physical findings, or diagnostic findings. p. 85
2. No. 357. 59-year-old male hospitalized twenty-four days. Operation for duodenal ulcer. Expired fifteen days postoperative. History and previous treatment minimal. Longer period of ambulatory treatment indicated. Technique of removal of impacted ulcer questioned. Inadequate followup of dehydration post-operatively. Only one hematocrit and total white count on day of death. p. 72
3. No. 261. 35-year-old male hospitalized fifteen days. Laparotomy with negative findings. Vagectomy. Jejunostomy. Discharge diagnosis afferent loop syndrome. (Note: patient also carried with diagnosis of lymphosarcoma from prior gastric resection, although pathology report failed to confirm this.) Indications for surgery not present; procedure not justified. p. 70
4. No. 250. 22-year-old female hospitalized twenty-seven days. Apparent re-

action to propylthiouracil for hyperthyroidism. Dosages of thyroid medication grossly inadequate, and poorly spaced. Modern therapy (surgery or RAI13) not discussed. Number and variety of medications other than those indicated bewildering. p. 62

5. No. 223. 45-year-old male hospitalized five days. First episode of precordial pain, mild diabetic. Completely inadequate cardiac appraisal. No serial electrocardiograms or transaminase. No repeat sedimentation rate or blood count. Discharged without clarification. p. 61
6. The following refers to the *same* patient over a period of four years:

   250-7.
   57-year-old male hospitalized fifteen days. Diabetic with ulceration of great toe. Superficial evaluation. No complete urinalysis. No check of elevated urea nitrogen. No electrocardiogram. Discharged with ulceration still present.

   Six weeks later
   57-year-old male hospitalized fifteen days. Diabetic with ulceration of great toe. Superficial evaluation and management.

   Two years later
   59-year-old male hospitalized nineteen days. Diabetic with acidosis, mid-thigh abcess, X-ray evidence of pneumonitis. Handling of acidosis inadequate. Discharged with a temperature of 101.

   Six months later
   Diabetic with congestive heart failure and severe anemia (6.1 grams hemoglobin). Cardiac status not fully explored. Etiology of anemia not determined. Discharged without cardiac drugs.

   Four months later
   60-year-old male hospitalized eight days. Diabetic with effusion of knee. Handled on orthopedic service for degenerative arthritis. Medical status not evaluated. Episodes of syncope not investigated.

   One year later
   61-year-old male hospitalized eight days. Diabetic with rectal hemorrhage and anemia. Although ulcerated hemorrhoids found, no treatment instituted. No further search for anemia. No overall medical evaluation. No chest film.

   One month later
   61-year-old male hospitalized eleven days. Diabetic with severe cachexia. Chest tap revealed 3500 cc of body fluid. Malignant cells found. Attending's admission note discusses "alveolar capillary block" and then no note for nine days, when patient expired. Signed out as carcinoma of the lung. No chest film. (All of the above on p. 61, all page numbers in 416.)

It is notable that these horror stories exemplify both underutilization and overutilization, sometimes in the same case. It is also notable that no evidence on the ambulatory histories of these patients is known. All of the cases may also satisfy one criterion of utilization: "In a short run, an optimal level of utilization is that which leads to the lowest possible unit cost with the given capacity" (350, p. 247).[l]

In addition to the failure of utilization studies in terms of bed availability to include any indicators of the appropriateness (medically) of what they are "measuring," it has also been shown that their predictive value is no better than that of the simple extrapolation of the five year trend of the patient-day-population ratio, and significantly worse than a general demand model with a lag variable (P. Feldstein and German, 141). Development of the "Pressure Index" by Rosenthal is another attempt to analyze utilization. In this case, the previously hypothesized causal relationship is reversed: it is the "pressure" on existing facilities, in terms of utilization intensity related to existing capacity, that is seen as the causal factor in the increase in the number of beds, which then is utilized. Stevens also takes the same tack: ". . . Increases in supply are seen as a function of the degree of demand pressure on capacity," which is then said to be measurable by the ratio of the "required" occupancy rate to the "maximum" occupancy rate (407, p. 27). The problem of interpreting the results arises even before they are reached, since the "required" occupancy rate is then "measured" as the *observed* occupancy rate (table 1, note 3), and the "maximum" occupancy rate is taken to be that rate of occupancy which "given the frequency distribution of the daily census by size, would be consistent with some probability of space shortage criterion, that is, the hospital being full to capacity, say, on the average 1 day in 100 days" (p. 27). Both of these, as well as other attempts at this kind of "bed requirement" analysis, are based on the assumption that the daily census in any given hospital is Poisson distributed.[m] It must be assumed that admissions are randomly distributed, and further, that the standard error of the mean is a decreasing function of the mean itself. Hence, as the size of the hospital, measured in *beds*, increases, deviations around the mean of admissions are reduced, thereby yielding higher occupancy rates.

There is substantial evidence in the literature that this assumption is not tenable for a given hospital: admissions and discharges are systematically related to the day of the week (248; 254; 313; 406), with admissions peaking on Sunday and lowest on Friday; admissions to different types of services, i.e., medical-surgical, pediatric, obstetrical, have differential distributions and peaks (256; pp. 218-21), and both the daily census and the occupancy rate are partially determined by the bed distribution within a given institution over various service units (51). Nevertheless, the assumption of the applicability of

[l]In addition to those already cited, criteria of optimal care for specific diagnoses during the entire illness episode have been developed by Schonfeld et al. (128; 372; 373); and Gold and Stone (168). In general, for references to this literature, see Donabedian (116 and 119).

[m]For the most extended discussion of the application of the Poisson distribution to admission patterns, see Rosenthal (360, pp. 46-52).

the Poisson distribution continues to be made.[n] Fruitful efforts in the direction of using a more plausible distribution have been made by P. Feldstein and Long (257), where a shift parameter is introduced to take into account seasonal and daily patterns, and Long (256), where the argument is clearly made that while the Poisson is inapplicable to any given hospital, it may be so for an entire community. The "Pressure Index," therefore, rests on rather dubious theoretical grounds.

Alternative explanations of demand, or utilization rates have been offered in terms of, for example, the "adequacy" of physicians, as "measured" by physician-population ratios. Roemer has argued that ". . . when the supply of physicians becomes critically limited (about 110 per 100,000 persons or less) the rate of hospital admissions tends to go upward" (354, p. 128). Stevens has also argued that "the crucial link between the hospitals as suppliers and the market is to be found in the staffing policies of hospitals" (407, p. 17). The argument is in terms of the "Physician workshop," which has the opposite set of implications: the more physicians the greater the number of admissions. Somers and Somers come to somewhat conflicting conclusions. One argument is that the private financial incentives of physicians are reflected in high rates of admissions (401, pp. 62-63). Another argument is that the very substantial increases in the last decade in the use of hospital outpatient facilities is attributable to the fact that "this is the one type of hospital service that the public can get without the assistance of professional 'gatekeepers' who guard the doors against 'improper use of all other services' " (401, p. 73). This either means that the "gatekeepers" are inefficient when it comes to guarding the gates against inpatient care, or that potential patient demands for services are in fact greater than observed levels of demand, after they have been filtered through the professional judgment of admitting physicians. The general argument that the observed national average occupancy rate of 75-76 percent indicates no shortage of beds in view of the fact that some large hospitals continually operate at 90 percent, is also questionable (401, pp. 57-58). Since this "measure" does not consider either bed unsubstitutability or locational variation, the assumption must be that (a) all beds, whatever ward they happen to be in, are substitutes for each other, and (b) there is a sufficient degree of geographic mobility. Otherwise, the empty hospital bed on the maternity ward in Saginaw, Michigan, will be of little potential benefit to the inadmissible patient to the crowded hospital in the Bedford-Stuyvesant section of Brooklyn, New York. That the example is made extreme only by the use of the geographic concept of distance is demonstrated for New York City itself by Klarman, in his excellent study of New York hospitals (219). The further atomization of the bed distribution by type of accommodation, type of hospital, and ethnicity is clear. The Chicago study shows similar results, and

[n]For a critical discussion of the applicability of the Poisson distribution, see Young (445), and Long and Feldstein (257). For a different evaluation of both the Poisson distribution's applicability and the relevance of the "pressure Index," see Klarman (216, pp. 107, 140-42).

discrimination in addition (71). In some relevant sense, the "distance" between Harlem and Saginaw, Michigan, may not exceed the "distance" between Harlem and Long Island.[o] Recognition of some of the "fragmentation factors" has, in part, lead to the incorporation of the concept of "option demand."

Both Reder (337, p. 152) and M. Feldstein (134, p. 145) have suggested that all of the traditional, and even the innovative definitions of output, have neglected to take into account the reduction in uncertainty yielded by the existence of some excess or standby capacity. A given community may be quite willing to pay a price for attainment of some probability greater than zero that "effective care will be available when requested . . . " (134, p. 145). Reder expanded on this, by pointing out what should have been obvious before, that since "an increase in reserve productive capacity . . . involves pecuniary outlay (which is recorded) while its yield (delivery convenience) goes unmeasured" it is not included in output and hence measures of output and of productivity will be biased downward. He did not point out the corollary: measures of existing capacity will be biased upward.[p] A somewhat similar argument is advanced by P. Feldstein, who maintains that since it is the "rest of society" which essentially "purchase" the "probability of being able to use these services when needed" (139, p. 74), its costs ought to be borne not by the sick, but by society. In an elegant formulation, Weisbrod terms this the "collective-consumption" component of personal consumption. If, as he correctly argues, the hospital "provides a valuable stand-by service . . . its value cannot be measured by the number of its users or the fees collectable from them alone . . . (The) option will have value for persons who never become patients" (432, p. 474).[q] But, again, the assumption of option demand is not developed and not incorporated into the models.[r]

While it appears obvious that hospitals provide other services in addition to inpatient care, the utilization studies do not take cognizance of them. The few

---

[o]For an interesting comparison of international differences in bed-population ratios, see, again, Abel-Smith (6 and 7). The United States in 1959, for example, had a lower bed-population ratio than Sweden, or Czechoslovakia (6, p. 39). The U.S. physician-population ratio was also lower than that in Israel, or Czechoslovakia. But U.S. per capita total expenditures for medical care were 2.7 times that in Israel, and twice as great as in Sweden. In 1961, Australia, Canada, Czechoslovakia, France, Iceland, Norway, Sweden, Denmark, and the U.K. had more beds per population than the U.S. (7, p. 18). See also Mobry (261), and Weinerman (427).

[p]Recall our earlier discussion of the relevant measure of capacity under stochastic demand and "penalty payments" assumptions. What is the acceptable probability that a patient will not be able to "be accommodated" on the day the admitting physician considers it desirable? Once again, the question is unanswerable in the absence of relevant value judgments. That decision must be made in the absence of theoretically refined decision rules does not mean that the value judgments underlying and implied by existing rules of thumb ought not to be made explicit and clear.

[q]Long (255), by conveniently assuming that uncertainty does not exist, disagrees with Weisbrod. The error of this argument is then shown by Lindsay (250).

[r]For a brief but comprehensive survey, and guide to the literature, of factors that are held to be responsible for current increases in the demand for hospital care, and medical care in general, see, A.R. Somers (398).

studies that have addressed themselves to outpatient services show that since 1953 the utilization of outpatient facilities has increased about five times more than the utilization of inpatient care, as measured by admissions (367, p. 1). In a time series analysis of the data for 1963-69, Russell and Davis show that the huge increases in outpatient visits appear to have been generated by two sets of factors: the decrease in the price of outpatient visits relative to the prices of inpatient care and of physician office visits; and increases in the rate of occupancy. In an argument which realizes the interconnections between inpatient and ambulatory care, they suggest that the provision of subsidies for increased outpatient care facilities and the simultaneous restriction of bed availabilities would bring about a shift from inpatient to ambulatory care (367). The same argument and additional empirical analysis is presented by Davis and Russell in several other papers (102, 103). While the arguments and the analyses are persuasive, they are robbed of the force of conviction by the use of gross prices, without netting out insurance payments, and by the definition of "ambulatory care" so as to indiscriminately include emergency room visits, outpatient clinic visits, diagnostic visits to laboratories within hospitals, referred visits, visits to specialists, etc. The demand determinants influencing the various types of visits tend to be different and hence their price elasticities cannot be assumed to be the same.

To recapitulate, our tour through the literature has demonstrated another agreement to disagree. Variations in utilization are seen to be related to the availability of alternative sources of care, but we are not quite sure how. Nonetheless, there appears to be sufficient evidence to maintain the hypothesis that there are different demand elements differentially affected by price and income variables. Utilization is observed demand (in actuality the points of intersection between demand and supply functions), hence utilization studies would yield greater results if they were more acutely focused on the demand elements, considering explicitly the quality dimension of care.

We have demonstrated that the disregard of the quality dimension of care is partly attributable to the absence of data, the difficulty in incorporating into economic analysis a dimension which is but hazily understood, and a rather cavalier disregard both of what medical literature there exists on the question and what "quality variations" in actuality really mean.

One of the important aspects of experimentation with different practice settings for the provision of care is the attempt to bring about more medically appropriate and economically efficient patterns of utilization. Next we examine this attempt.

Demand and Utilization Patterns in Different Practice Settings

> Alice laughed. "There's no use trying," she said. "One can't believe impossible things."

> "I daresay you haven't had much practice," said the Queen.
> "When I was your age, I always did it for half-an-hour a day. Why, sometimes I've believed as many as six impossible things before breakfast."
>
> —Lewis Carroll

Analysis of the differential demand and rates of utilization in different practice settings and/or under differing financial arrangements proceeds under three generally, but not unanimously, held assumptions: (a) the price elasticity of the demand for medical care is significant and hence changes in the relative prices of services will lead to changes in their utilization; (b) group-practice, by facilitating specialization and the increased use of ancillary personnel will benefit from economies in scale in the quantity of output, and from the increased likelihood of peer review, in its quality; and (c) changes in the financial incentive systems facing providers will elicit changes in their medical behavior. For the analytic purpose here, namely, as an example of what the rest of the literature neglects, the interaction of the supply and demands for hospital provided services, inpatient and/or ambulatory, with the sources and prices of alternative service providers, it is useful to consider that insurance of varying breadth of coverage and prepaid group practices are basically similar in one sense, and fundamentally different in another.

From the standpoint of attempts of various kinds to deal with the problem engendered by the probabilistic nature of demand, "insurance" and prepayment are both basically risk-transfer mechanisms: the individual who purchases insurance or enrolls in a prepaid plan transfers his risk to the insurance company or to the prepaid group. This can be seen as an exclusively financial arrangement. In another sense, however, they are very different indeed: for while insurance is a transfer of risk, spread over, so to speak, the dominant institutional form of medical practice, "the mainstream," in the prepaid group not only risk is transferred by the enrollee, but he also agrees to receive a different pattern of care within a different institutional context.

Consider, for the moment, that two types of fire insurance exist: In the traditional one, the insured agrees to receive a sum of money in case his house burns down. He will then have to depend on the existing real estate and construction industry to repair and/or build anew. In the other form of insurance, the insured agrees that in case of fire, the insurer, according to *his* specifications, standards, and practices, and by the use of *his* employees, will repair and/or build anew, in one of some alternative locations of *his* choice. To reduce the probability of serious fires occurring, the insurer makes available monthly or yearly fire-hazard inspections by his own inspectors, and the inspection of the garage is "thrown in" because of the likelihood of fire spreading from there to the main house. Now two things should be clear, two aspects which the proponents of group-practice ceaselessly emphasize: in the traditional form of insurance the major way of reducing the insurer's probability of having to pay out the principal is *not* to insure the "bad" risks; in the other form of insurance, to maintain the house hazard free: the self-interest of the insurer is to have continuous "care."

Continuous and comprehensive family care of high quality produced at economically efficient scales within an institutional framework that removes the distortions of financial barriers and/or incentives to deviate from it, is the major objective, if not claim, of prepaid group practice.

Insurance can be viewed as a risk-transfer mechanism. When the insured-for event occurs, the benefits may take the form of a lump-sum payment, the amount of which is a function of the event, specified in the insurance contract. Benefits may also take the form of payments in specified amounts for specific services, to be paid directly to the beneficiary or to the provider of the service. Co-insurance or a deductible portion may or may not be present. The services covered may vary in scope from very limited to unlimited.

It can be suggested that "unlimited" insurance does not exist in the United States. That, in part, depends on what is meant by "unlimited." Commercially sold insurance, as well as Titles 18 and 19, is very limited, generally excluding dental, opthalmic, psychiatric, and pharmaceutical care, and in addition, usually incorporates a limit on the length of time during which payments will be made. The "insurance" provided members of the Armed Forces does not incorporate any limits on time or scope of services: it is total, "unlimited," insurance, for total unlimited care. Professionals are eligible for total care even after retirement.

For the purpose of analyzing utilization patterns, insurance can also be considered a mechanism which systematically alters the relative prices of some or all services to the insured, to the beneficiary, and, to some extent, to the seller of the services. The more limited the scope of coverage, the fewer relative prices will be affected. When insurance is "complete," *no* relative prices will be changed. Lancaster's concept of the "intrinsic commodity group" is once again relevant (229, p. 144).

Some special sets of commodities, or services, can be considered to comprise "bundles" such that substitutions among the various components of the bundle will be affected *only* by changes in the relative prices of those components, and completely *unaffected* by changes in the prices of commodities or services not members of the bundle. Such a special set is termed the "intrinsic commodity group"; members of such set are said to be "intrinsically related." Changes in the relative prices of intrinsically related commodities are likely to induce substitutions, *within the set*, when substitutes exist. Changes in the relative prices of intrinsically related commodities will affect the purchase pattern of other, not so related commodities, only through the income effect. That is, to the extent the prices of purchased members of the intrinsic set are reduced, the consumer's ability to purchase more of other, not so related goods, is increased. Large price changes in the intrinsic groups, or small price changes for large groups, will have substantial income effects. Changes in the prices of commodities not belonging to the intrinsic group will have no effect on the purchase patterns of members of the intrinsic group. Hence the theoretical expectation that if the price of some service within the intrinsic group is reduced, such as the price of diagnostic services on an inpatient basis, while the price of a substitute (yielding the same objectively determined characteristics) is not, such as diagnostic services on an ambulatory basis, there will be an increase in the quantity demanded of the first in favor of the second. Selective insurance coverage is said to have this effect.

It is unfortunate that the extended discussion of "moral hazard" has not considered this point. Although Lancaster published his fundamental reformulation of consumer theory in April, 1966, it seems not yet to have struck a responsive chord. In addition to the unarguable fact that consumer demand for many, if not most, components of the intrinsic set composed of medical care commodities and services is effected only through physician legitimation, which the "moral hazard" argument does not fully consider, two other factors mitigate against its existence: (a) substitution in favor of an intrinsic group induced by a decrease in the prices of all its components is likely to be small, hence the price elasticity is likely to be small; (b) even in a system where out-of-pocket prices (direct money prices) are reduced to zero, indirect prices may remain positive. The indirect price of medical care services is minimally in terms of time, in addition to transportation costs, inconvenience costs, as well as fear. If our previous argument is correct, that medical care services are special in the sense that an increase in the purchase of hospitalization from zero to any positive amount simultaneously reduces income, then, especially for those who are gainfully employed, but for all others as well, except when indirect prices are also zero or the consumer is pathological (a hypochondriac may enjoy a weekend on the medical ward and prefer it to one in Aspen), the assumed large price elasticity as price approaches zero, resulting in the "moral hazard," is not likely. As the Duchess said: "Tut, tut, child! Everything's got a moral, if only you can find it." Increased utilization, at least initially, may have several morals, of course. One may be the existence of previously unmet medical need. On the "moral hazard" argument, see Arrow (22), Pauly (319), and Arrow (24).

That the "moral hazard" argument is theoretically unsound might be further indicated by a study of the effects of multiple insurance coverage on patterns of hospital care. A sample of hospitalized patients in the Pittsburgh area shows that 34.4 percent had *no* insurance, 54.1 percent had *one*, and 11.4 percent had multiple (two or more) insurance coverages. Those with no insurance had the significantly longer stays and larger number of services. There was only one area where those with multiple insurance appear to have received more, or better, care, that is, demanded more insured services: accommodations. Those with multiple insurance had, on the average, more frequently private or semi-private accommodations, (Ferber, 144). For an argument against multiple coverage, see Luck (259).

Increased hospital admissions, in the recent past, accompanied by reductions in the length of stay, have been attributed to two factors, both of which are attributable to the changes in the relative prices of services induced by selective insurance coverage. The Gorham Report concludes that these factors are: "... More patients have hospitalization insurance than have coverage for other types of medical care," and therefore the physician may place "his patient in the hospital rather than treat him at home or in the office since the patient's insurance company will pay the bill" (271, p. 33). The other factor is that "hospitals may be overutilized to suit the convenience of physicians. A busy doctor may put a patient in a hospital to conserve his own time" (Ibid.). The first factor may be called the direct effect, the second the indirect. It can be argued that if the physician admits patients for his own practice conveniences, such elective admissions would be, at least to some extent, reduced if the patient had to pay out-of-pocket for such admissions, both by patient resistance and possibly because physicians might be less likely to choose the relatively more expensive of the available treatment patterns.[s] The indirect effect may also be seen to be a function of the physician's objective to maximize his income. The second vice-president of the Equitable Life Assurance Society of the United States has said:

> We have put the onus of controlling costs on the individual, through deductibles and coinsurance. We speak of over-utilization, and we penalize the patient for what the professional does: the professional, the physician, controls whether or not the patient is in the hospital and how long he stays there. But we penalize the patient for something he does not control. In light of today's hospital charges, that is indeed a $100-a-day misunderstanding (125, p. 114).

In situations when alternative treatment or diagnostic processes are available, the alternatives have different resource-intensities and hence costs. The monetary costs, however, are borne not by the physician, but by the patient, directly, or indirectly when one or more of the alternatives is covered by insurance. Even if the absolute payoff to the physician is identical from each treatment process, to maximize his income he will choose the one process which minimizes *his* input in terms of time. This is an almost pure case of externalities in production: the private and social costs and returns from alternative treatment processes, leading to the same end results, are not the same. To the extent that the physician is able to increase his private productivity, and hence income, with the use of more capital-intensive processes, the direct benefits accrue to the physician, and the costs both to the insurer and, ultimately through premium increases, to the insured: in the private accounting system of the physician, the benefits are recorded, but costs are not. This is analogous to other negative

---

[s]For the most complete summary and critical analysis of the large literature on the impact of insurance and prepayment on utilization, see Donabedian (115; 118; 119).

externalities in production. The dumping of wastes in public waters by industrial plants is another example of the simultaneous generation of private benefits and social costs.

The physician externality argument, however, is not quite that straightforward. It can also be argued that if the binding constraint on the supply of medical care services, inpatient and/or ambulatory, is in fact the physician input, then there may be indirect benefits to the process that are also not accounted for. If, resulting from his increased private productivity, the physician is enabled to treat more patients, patients who otherwise could not have been treated, or would have had to wait longer for treatment, are the indirect beneficiaries of increased hospitalization. Whether this is accounted for or not is partly determined by whether or not the physician charges in such a way as to "capture" these indirect benefits. Even though there may be some doubt, given current levels of physician income, about whether there is any benefit not captured by the physician, some evidence exists to indicate that not all benefits to patients may be reflected in charges. While the time-intensity of physician services is price rationed, the time-spacing of it, with some exceptions, is not: queuing is the ordinarily used mechanism. Jumping ahead in the queue is at the physician's option and in terms, usually, of his evaluation of the importance of the time dimension of treatment. Also, presumably, some patients would prefer to pay higher prices for more prompt treatment, or for other differentiations by a given physician. There is evidence, however, that the famous "sliding-scale," which is one reflection of this, among other things, is not as prevalent as in the past, if prevalent at all. See, e.g., Scitovsky (377).

While not formulated in these terms, the studies of utilization differentials attributable to financial arrangement and/or practice setting differentials are concerned with these issues. The questions usually put are: Are there different patterns of utilization within similar population groups? If there are, what are the effects of the nature of the insurance plan or of the organizational aspects of practice?

There is some considerable evidence that hospital utilization, or the demand for hospital services, is significantly *reduced* by prepaid group practice.[t] A study of the utilization rates within the Health Insurance Plan of Greater New York (HIP) and Group Health Insurance (GHI), which provides coverage of the same scope, but on a reimbursable basis to fee-for-service physicians in solo practice, has shown that, for the age and sex adjusted populations of the two plans, admissions per 1,000 were 70.2 for HIP and 88.3 for GHI (110, p. 1712, table 1). Hospital days per 100 population were 74.4 and 95.5, respectively, for HIP and GHI (110, p. 1723, table 9). There was no attempt to analyze the factors to which such substantial differentials may be attributable, but the hypotheses were posited that it is the absence of diagnostic facilities in GHI physician

[t]The most up-to-date and detailed discussion of the economics of group practice is found in P. Feldstein (136). See also 123, 171, and 214.

offices and the form of payment mechanism under HIP that might account for the observed differentials. Since HIP pays the physician on a capitation basis, the financial incentive to hospitalize is assumed to be reduced.

The interaction between ambulatory and inpatient treatment patterns is given added emphasis in a study of utilization pattern changes attendant upon the introduction of ambulatory facilities into a community where previously such ambulatory services were not available. The experience in Boston's Columbia Point shows that the introduction of ambulatory services, in the form of a neighborhood health center, has significantly reduced admissions (44).

An extensive study by Perrott and Chase (reproduced in 340, vol. 1, p. 66, ff), shows very significant inpatient utilization variation. For the period 1960-65, the utilization patterns of Blue Cross-Blue Shield and indemnity benefit plans were compared with those of group practice plans. Hospital days per 1,000 covered persons ranged between 407 and 415 for groups, 672 and 924 for the Blues, and 657 and 945 for indemnity plans. Further, the increase in utilization between 1960 and 1965 was negligible for the groups, 37 percent for the Blue plans, and 43 percent for the indemnity plans. The National Advisory Commission on Health Manpower interprets the results the following way:

> Almost none of the factors that encourage excessive hospitalization exist in the plans providing comprehensive care. The patient's medical expenses are covered whether incurred inside or outside the hospital; extensive out-patient facilities are available to the physician; the physician is paid on a salary or per capita basis, so that unnecessary hospitalization does not add to his income; in fact, under some plans unnecessary hospitalization may actually decrease his income. Not only are hospitalization rates significantly lower in prepaid comprehensive care plans but, perhaps even more important, such plans appear to have avoided the sharp increase in hospital use that has occurred with regular hospital insurance. (340, vol. 1, p. 66)

It has also been suggested that even in the absence of group practice "a highly disciplined fee-for-service program administered by a union health and welfare fund may have an important influence on hospitalization . . . This factor may be responsible for bringing the hospital rate down to at least the comparatively low level consistently shown in the past for HIP covered groups" (Densen, et al., 111).

Extensive studies of the best known prepaid group plans, the Kaiser Permanente groups, have shown consistently lower inpatient utilization for the enrollees. Kaiser of Northern California, for example, in comparison with California as a whole, has only 51 percent as many beds per 1,000 population, 59 percent on an age adjusted basis. On an age adjusted basis, the number of hospital days per 1,000 population for Kaiser is only 69 percent of that for the whole state. And though the average length of stay is somewhat higher (102 percent), the average daily cost is lower (88 percent) (340, vol. 2, pp. 209-11). Total expenses, per capita, for Kaiser members are also significantly lower than for non-members. The cost implications are also interesting. In the period 1960-65 total hospital costs for the United States increased by 43 percent, for Kaiser California regions, 11.3 percent (340, p. 212). The basic reason adduced is that "Kaiser has been able to achieve substantial savings because it has been able to get individual physicians to control the costs of providing medical care" (340, p. 216).[u]

Kaiser has also been compared with Blue Cross-Blue Shield and comprehensive plans (such as that provided by General Electric) with somewhat conflicting results. Lower costs for Kaiser are found once again, but this time both ambulatory and inpatient utilization for Kaiser is found to exceed that of the other two plans (420). Both results may be interpreted somewhat differently from that of the authors'. Since no evaluation of the observed differentials was made by the use of any medical criteria, any concept of medical "justification," it is as likely as the opposite conclusion that the higher levels of utilization for Kaiser constitute a higher level of care, better care. Further, in view of the fact that Kaiser members received more care at a lower cost, only minimal assumptions are required to conclude that Kaiser members were better off. (For a critical review of this study, see Lerner et al., 241.)

Unfortunately, all of these studies are subject to some serious criticisms, the most damaging of which may be the question of population comparability. While age adjustment is a necessary first step in the correct direction, income, education, occupation, and race are generally not standardized for in these studies. The results may further be biased by the exclusion of services received, or purchased, outside the plans. This is not to argue that the much lower levels of hospitalization shown for Kaiser North California may, nevertheless, be significant, truly reflective, that is, of the phenomena.

An extensive study of medical groups in the San Francisco area by Bailey seems to demonstrate that if there are any economies of scale to be achieved, they are meager indeed (28; 29; 30). Comparability with other studies, and the evaluation of the findings, is made difficult if not impossible by Bailey's definition of "group." He is concerned with internists in private practice in groups of one to five. Hence these are neither multispecialty groups, nor comprehensive, nor prepaid, the three distinguishing characteristics of groups such as Kaiser and HIP. He does find that physicians in groups work fewer hours per month. Feldstein points to this finding to infer that if physicians work less but earn the same or more than physicians in solo practice, "they must be more productive" (136, p. 33). Bailey, however, in his findings attributes part of the physicians' earnings to their excessive use of laboratory facilities, which they own themselves. Reder maintains that the separation of group practice produc-

[u]For the further development of this idea, and additional analyses, see "Report of the Panel on Hospital Care," pp. 129-164, 340, Vol. 2.

tion into physician generated and laboratory generated is not legitimate since the laboratory generated outputs should be considered as inputs into the physician generated outputs. He also makes the point that the reduced transaction costs of laboratory use and referral within large groups may lead to higher quality care and that "part of the economies of scale *may* lie in superior quality of care at a constant deflated dollar cost to the patient" (336, p. 277, emphasis in original).

In a paper entitled "The Economics of Group Practice" (301), Newhouse presents a critical economic evaluation of group efficiency. His evidence is difficult to interpret since his sample of private practitioners is composed of twenty "groups," eleven of which are solo and only two have five physicians, the largest "group." Results from the "sample" are compared with data from three clinics, one in a medical school, one in a teaching hospital, and an independent one. Each of the first two clinics is reported to have had "more than 100,000 visits per year," while the third had only 15,000 (p. 5). The data for these three clinics are averaged. The paper's title, to say the least, is less than apt.

There is some contradictory evidence. A study of Blue Cross experience with the inclusion of outpatient diagnostic service benefits in Wisconsin concludes that "inclusion of outpatient diagnostic benefits does not have a reducing effect upon the frequency of inpatient admissions and total costs" (404, p. 12). The study's methodological poverty reduces the strength of its conclusions. Nevertheless, there is some supporting evidence from the other end of the treatment spectrum. It has been often suggested that the absence of appropriate alternative long-term care facilities increases the average length of stay and hence the cost of the illness episode. Hurtado et al., present evidence that the availability of extended care facilities reduces hospital utilization indeed, but with no change in the total cost of care (192, esp. table 10).

It has also been argued that while extension of insurance coverage to ambulatory services might reduce the rate of hospital utilization, total costs, contrary to the previous findings, may be increased as a result of the identification of previously undiscovered pathologies (397). But contrary is the argument that the availability of the "fire inspectors," i.e., "preventive care," would reduce overall utilization and hence costs (52, pp. 33-35). Here, as in the rest of the literature, "preventive care" is ill- or not defined. What is usually meant, it appears, is a pattern of care within which the diagnosis of a pathology requiring treatment is made at an early stage of history. Early diagnosis, then, is defined as preventive care. This must be recalled, since other patterns, such as the private and social consumption of pollutants, nutritional deficiency, among others, which might also be "prevented" and which are known to contribute to lowered health levels, are not included in "preventive care."

Donabedian, after an exhaustive critical review of the literature on prepaid groups, concludes:

> The available data on hospital utilization are consistent with the notion that prepaid group practice through changing the nature of the incentives to the

physicians and introducing professional controls, lowers the hospital utilization rates for many surgical and nonsurgical conditions. (115, pp. 15-16)

Layton, at the end of his international comparative study of utilization rates, concludes in a similar vein. He maintains that since in countries with social insurance schemes the coverage is broad, inclusive of care provided in settings alternative to the hospital,

> . . . The overuse of hospital facilities . . . is considerably less likely . . . since neither the doctor nor the patient has anything to gain in the countries being studied by seeking or recommending hospital care when less costly alternatives are also provided in the programs. (235, p. 166)

Recall that our purpose here was not to consider the literature on practice setting, or group plans, as such.[v] It was to demonstrate that, in fact, the demand for hospital facilities is not independent of the demand for and prices of substitutes, and that at least some of the literature demonstrates this. With some exceptions, the evidence is persuasive that at least for some conditions, and possibly for many, substitutability between ambulatory and inpatient care exists. There is also some evidence that inpatient utilization can be substantially reduced by appropriate ambulatory care not only because of the substitutability of services, but also because some patterns of ambulatory care are more likely to facilitate treatment at the earlier stages of disease history, thereby obviating the necessity of admission, than are other patterns. Physician relevant outcomes of different treatment processes can also be altered. While it can be argued that, at least to some extent, physician originated demands for services are a function of the marginal revenues, in terms of income, the provision of those services yields to the physician in solo practice (278), when renumeration is divorced from physician originated demands that link is broken. That such patterns of care are most likely to occur in the institutional setting of the prepaid group is one of its major claimed advantages.

At least one thing seems clear: demands for, and costs and prices of, hospital operations are not independent of substitutes. The analysis of demand and costs on the assumption that the "hospital" is an isolated activity center focusing, for the most part, exclusively on inpatient care, is likely, therefore, to be either partial or incorrect.[w]

---

[v]A late, and very interesting analysis of the impact of practice setting on surgical procedure rates is presented by Bunker (64). A good survey of the literature on ambulatory care is that by Roemer and DuBois (356). A good analysis of ambulatory care related to income and insurance differentials is presented by Kovner, Browne, and Kisch (224).

[w]According to American Hospital Association data, about 36% of X-ray and 11% of laboratory services are performed on an ambulatory basis. The existence of alternative treatment processes is also explicit in the literature on PPC (Progressive Patient Care). See, e.g., Gee (162), and Griffith et al. (173). Cost reductions in the neighborhood of some 40-50 percent are reported by Patierno (316), and Stiefel (409).

Summary

In this chapter we have presented an approach to demand analysis which stresses the multiple nature of demands for medical care. While the ultimate demand may well be for good health, the formulation here presented of the demand for services emphasizes that the underlying states of felt need, represented as different levels of health status disequilibrium, differentiate between kinds of patient originated demands. The special role of the physician in legitimating and initiating the provision of services is incorporated by considering a significant demand element to be physician originated. That the provider himself, in some analogue of the "dependence effect," satisfies objectives of his own by the treatment choices that he prescribes for the patient implies that at least some demands are endogenously generated.

We have seen that while there is some direct and some implicit realization of the patient-physician interaction and the consequent complex nature of demand formation in the literature under the rubric of demand-supply interactions, for the most part the demands are assumed to be exogenously determined. Hence the price and income elasticity studies, which show both to have been decreasing at least since World War II, are of dubious value, particularly for policy analysis purposes. We have also seen that the utilization studies tend to disregard the relevance of medical criteria in terms of quality and appropriateness.

As in our discussions of outputs, productivity, and costs, we must once again plead for some specific and meaningful conceptualizations and definitions of what is to be measured and evaluated. The recent studies on case mix by Rafferty and on demand by Andersen and Benham are moves in that direction, the one by analyzing utilization in terms of diagnostic categories and the other by measuring income elasticities in terms of quantities of services.

Studies of utilization patterns under different practice settings, particularly in comprehensive, prepaid group practices, tend to demonstrate that treatment substitutes exist and that the choice of the economically more rational alternatives may be enhanced by organizational factors and by changing the nature of financial incentives facing physicians. It is safe to say, however, that all the answers are not yet in. None of the comparative studies have included quality as a dimension of the different care patterns, hence little is known of quality differentials, if any. While it can be expected on a priori grounds that internal audits and peer review as organizational components of prepaid group practices lead to a better quality of care, there is no evidence to support it.

Our emphasis on the quality of care may seem excessive to some. We have given some examples of just what "lower quality" or possibly "Volkswagen" medicine might mean. The analysis of pricing is also complicated by the investigators' inability to incorporate quality as a dimension of care. It might be argued that increasing the quality of care would be expensive in resources and may lead to inefficiency in resource allocation by providing a level higher than what people would be willing to pay for. It would fail the welfare test. Since we prefaced the previous chapter with a quotation from Sidney Alexander, it may be appropriate to use another to end this one.

A conceptually simple test for both justice and happiness together can be based on a fundamental principle of morality expressed in the question "how would you feel if you were in his shoes?" If we have to make sense of saying that one state of the world is better than another, we can, I submit, do it in the following way. If a reasonable man completely knowledgeable of the conditions in both states is given the choice of taking a chance with equal probability of being anyone concerned in either state A or B and he chooses state A, we can say that state A is better than state B. Sidney Alexander, "Comment," in J. Margolis (ed.), *The Analysis of Public Output* (New York, 1970) p. 26.

If we were to apply this "place-taking" test, most of us, presumably, would not opt for lower quality.

7 Pricing and Reimbursement Strategies for Hospitals

> But at the fundamental level of discourse . . . we cannot regard the price system as a datum. On the contrary, it is to be thought of as one of the instrumentalities, possibly the major one, by which whatever social value system there may be is realized.
>
> –Kenneth Arrow, 1967

> . . . The price system is intrinsically limited in scope by our inability to make factual distinctions needed for optimal pricing under uncertainty. Nonmarket controls, whether internalized as moral principle or externally imposed, are to some extent essential for efficiency.
>
> –Kenneth Arrow, 1968

> None of this matters for positive economics. The terms can be defined for each problem in the manner appropriate to the matter to be discussed and need be given no more precision than the question requires.
>
> –Joan Robinson

Few of the students of hospital pricing would accept "the price system as a datum." Most, however, would argue that it is "one of the instrumentalities . . . by which whatever value system there may be is realized." None, it appears, has taken seriously Arrow's 1968 recognition of the possibly limited scope of the pricing system in attaining private and social objectives. Hence most of the discussions proceed in a manner inappropriate to the matter by disregarding that the medical care sector, and within it the hospital sector, presents not a single one of the many conditions under which simple incremental pricing rules can theoretically be shown to lead to economic efficiency.

In the first section of this chapter we consider in some detail the necessary and sufficient conditions under which marginal cost pricing not only corresponds to but actually leads toward the economist's Nirvana: Pareto Optimality where allocative and distributive efficiency are simultaneously attained. We then proceed to show that since the necessary conditions in terms of price competition, free entry, resource mobility, informed preferences, etc., do not obtain, marginal cost pricing may not be a panacea but a further distortion.

After considering incremental and peak load pricing proposals, we turn to some of the possibly promising suggestions of one or another form of fixed price contracting, exemplified by capitation prepayment and prospective budgeting.

The chapter stresses the need for precise a priori specification of objectives for the operationally meaningful description of production processes, and an understanding of the relation of hospital outputs to those of the rest of the system, before efficiency pricing rules can be devised.

Theoretical Difficulties in Efficiency Pricing

The theoretical discussion of efficient pricing policies generally proceeds under a number of strong assumptions. The assumptions specify those *necessary conditions*, in structural, behavioral, and value terms, under which certain pricing behaviors constitute both the *necessary and sufficient* conditions for the efficient allocation and distribution of resources. We shall briefly discuss some of these of particular relevance to hospital services pricing.[a]

Necessary Conditions: Structural. The first necessary structural condition S_1, specifies that markets exist. There must be organized markets in which exchange between buyers and sellers takes place, generally in money terms. The second necessary structural condition S_2, specifies that the markets must be perfectly competitive. That is, there must be a large enough number of buyers and of sellers for each commodity and service which is sold through the market, such that each of the buyers and sellers are price-takers. No single buyer or seller, or any group of them jointly, can determine the price at which the transaction takes place: there are no price-makers. S_2 may not hold for every time period, some deviations may occur. However, S_3 specifies that there must be free entry to each of the markets and hence short, temporary deviations in S_2 may be self-corrective if S_3 is met. The free entry condition is important in terms of guaranteeing that the atomistic markets assumed under S_2 will be competitive both in the short run and the long run. "Free entry" refers not only to firms, but to factors of production as well, so that it may be termed "the perfect resource mobility" condition. When free entry does not obtain, "barriers to entry" are said to exist. Barriers may be financial, technological, legal, or other, such as racial discrimination. The fourth condition, S_4, specifies that there exist perfect states of information. This does not imply that information *qua* information cannot have a positive price. It does mean the total absence of unpredictability. The condition can be relaxed and uncertainty entered. However, each buyer and seller must have either perfect information, if free, or access to information at the same price, if not free. For example, this means, among other things, that the technically efficient production functions, if they exist, are known to all who might possibly wish to use them. It can be readily seen that a violation of S_4 may also be a violation of S_3, but need not be: "technical production secrets" violate S_4 and are likely to prevent entry to the

[a] A full treatment will be found in Graff (170), or Baumol (38). For a brief but both simple and exhaustive treatment, see Bator (36).

production process which is secret, hence will be a barrier and thus violate S_3. Patents, on the other hand, violate S_3 but not S_4. It is further assumed, S_5, that there exist no technical externalities in production. The interaction between the production processes of honey (by bees) and apples (by trees with the aid of pollinating bees) raises this problem. The production of patient care (by residents and interns) and of medical knowledge and/or training (of residents and interns and their professors) is of this nature: joint production or externality.

Necessary conditions: Behavioral. The first necessary behavioral condition B_1, specifies that each consumer has a utility or preference function, expressed directly in terms of commodities and services. That is, consumers have self-known preferences directly for commodities: in their preference functions the prices of those commodities, or any other factors, do not appear. We need not be concerned here with further assumptions on the shapes of the preference functions, although certain shapes, said to be "not well-behaved," will lead to some difficulties.

The second condition, B_2, specifies that consumers will attempt to maximize their preference function: they will so allocate their given income that further reshuffling of the commodity bundle that they purchase at the existing prices in the markets will not yield any increase in satisfaction. B_3 specifies that producers, or entrepreneurs, will have the unique objective of profit maximization. The seller of commodities and services in the markets, given some other assumptions about technology, factor prices, etc., will always act in such a way that his profits will be maximized. The fourth, B_4, specifies that there exist no externalities in consumption. That is, the preference function of no consumer is influenced either directly by what some other consumer purchases, or does not purchase, or indirectly, by including in his own preference function the satisfaction level of some other consumer: Mr. Smith, who has a wife just beginning her first trimester and a six-year-old son in school is not made either better or worse off by whether or not his son's classmates purchase, or otherwise acquire, Rubella vaccinations (the direct interdependence through consumption). Mr. Smith is also utterly nonchalant about the "health and happiness" levels of his neighbors, as well as his son's classmates, independently of their consumption patterns (the indirect interdepence through "other's" welfare level). If neither condition be met, severe difficulties arise.

Necessary conditions: Value Terms. Here we merely discuss two, the first V_1, specifies that the income distribution, both at the start and at the end of the "game," is optimal, socially approved. This is of crucial importance for, as we shall see, under certain additional pricing conditions it can then be said that resources are efficiently allocated according to the signals generated in the market. It will be said that the "dollar votes" determine the allocation process.

The distribution of the "dollar votes" among the "voters" is the question of income distribution. The difficulty arises from the fact that while we may all vote with our "dollar votes" in the market, unlike in the political process, from which this analogy was drawn by some economist ages ago, the principle of "one man, one vote" does not apply: some can vote early and often, and others not at all.

The second basic value assumption, V_2, is seldom presented explicitly as a statement of values, but rather either as a dominant principle or as a deduction from the other assumptions. This is the principle of "consumer sovereignty." Consumer sovereignty means more than just that consumers are sovereign; it requires the normative judgment that individual preferences count and that no single individual's, or no group of individuals' preferences dominate. Since it has been already assumed that externalities, or neighborhood effects in consumption are absent, individual preferences and their expression through consumption behavior are considered inviolate and inviolable. Given the economist's penchant for simplifying assumptions, this principle is most easily demonstrated in a Robinson Crusoe economy–prior to the appearance of Friday.

The general principle is somewhat modified by the specification of those preferences which are translatable through consumption behavior, since once the income distribution is given, of two sets of equally inviolable preferences only those backed up by the "dollar votes" will actually count. While the principle of equal preferences thus becomes modified into "equal dollar weighted preferences," this assumption is the foundation on which the arguments for "free consumer choice" are built. It is often suggested that this is a statement of the "ideal state." But that statement itself is a value judgment on the role of individual preferences; for in other "ideal states," not unconstrained individual preferences, but modified collective preferences may be accorded the status of dominance.

As with other often reaffirmed general principles, reaffirmation is a recognition of its breach. General principles can either be operationalized, in which case they are reaffirmed by actions, or they can be violated in action, but repostulated, as in preambles to congressional bills or in the opening paragraph of learned articles.

While more often observed in the breach than in action, the general acceptance of the concept of consumer sovereignty, at least in principle, attains great importance in theoretical and practical discussion, for it places the burden of proof on those who question its operational meaning or applicability. This becomes manifestly clear when we consider the concept of marginal cost pricing, for if there is any other principle which among economists competes with consumer sovereignty for the first price of being on the ultimate rung in the hierarchy of values, it is none other than the principle of marginal cost pricing.

If, and only if, all the above conditions are met (S_1 through S_5, B_1 through B_4, and V_1 and V_2), the conditions *necessary but not sufficient* for efficient resource allocation exist. The additional conditions can be generally expressed in prices: the earnings of all productive factors must equal the marginal value of their contribution to production (wages equal marginal revenue products, and the same for all other factors), and the prices of commodities and services must equal the marginal costs of their production. These so-called marginal equivalency conditions can be derived from atomistic markets and free resource mobility only if it is assumed that there are no economic rents.

The observable reality of these conditions is not at issue here. Not even Adam Smith could argue that they reflect empirical reality. But the assumptions are important, for once the assumptions are made then it can be proved that in equilibrium, the consumer's marginal rates of substitution will be exactly equal to the marginal rates of transformation in production, and, therefore, there will be no possible way to reallocate resources such as to make any *one* person better off without making at least one *other* person worse off. We have Pareto Optimality. That is, if all necessary structural, behavioral, and value conditions are met, marginal cost pricing of all factors and commodities is both a *necessary and sufficient* condition to attain Pareto Optimality, the efficient allocation *and* distribution of resources.

The unfortunate theoretical moral of the story is this: If *any single* necessary condition is violated, marginal cost pricing is *neither a necessary nor a sufficient* condition to attain "efficiency." And efficiency itself can not be defined in the absence of a social welfare function. That, perhaps, accounts for Mishan's famous dictum: "The fashion remains to court disillusion at the static level in a formal manner, and pessimism informally at the dynamic level" (275, p. 249).

We have discussed the conditions in the most adumbrated manner, but we have discussed them because in economic theory it is no longer arguable that *any* system of pricing will lead to "efficient" solutions *unless* all the conditions are met. Neither is it very strongly arguable that when several of the conditions are violated, any interference to remove one of the violations may move the system *even further* away from the "efficient" point (actually surface) than it was to begin with.[b]

This can be seen easily in mathematical terms. Assume a function with several hills and valleys, and one large mountain: several local maxima and minima and one maximum maximorum. The function is not well known over its entire range, not all the second derivatives are known. If a local maximum is attained, any movement away from that local maximum may be toward a local minimum, and in any case, either toward or further away from the maximum maximorum: if the topography is not well known and it is dark, movement from a hillock may mean moving towards a valley, and further away from the mountain. A fixed rule, such as marginal cost pricing, or "go West, young man," is only good if in fact it will lead us West, and if we want to go there. The theoretical argument is most elegantly presented in a recent paper by Baumol and Bradford (42). They

[b]On this point see Lipsey and Lancaster (251).

prove that in second best situations marginal cost pricing is inappropriate. Further, that in the real world we are always in a second best situation. "In a world in which marginal cost pricing without excise or income taxes is normally not feasible, the solution we have usually considered to characterize the 'best' is none too good, because it is simply unattainable" (p. 280).

Detailed documentation of most, if not all, of the necessary conditions is not required here. Some of the structural conditions were discussed in the sections on the objective function. We have shown, for example, that the literature generally agrees that there are barriers to entry in the hospital "market," and that price competition between hospitals does not exist. S_2 and S_3, in other words, do not obtain.[c] Whether "markets" as such exist is itself debatable. Certainly, it is clear that for some services markets *do not* exist: the markets for psychiatric insurance, particularly long-term care, do not exist.[d] It is likely that S_1 is itself violated. Neither the presence of perfect information states (S_4) nor the absence of significant technical externalities in production (S_5) can be seriously advocated. In fact, one aspect on which all students generally agree is the heavy dose of consumer ignorance in terms of disease states, alternative suppliers (source of care), and of course, the future, which for any one individual is largely unpredictable, except at its terminus. The structural conditions which are required for marginal cost pricing to lead to an efficient allocation of resources are absent.

Most of the behavioral conditions are also subject to question. Even assuming that consumers do have well-defined preference functions, it is unlikely that they are expressed in the required terms of commodities and services, such as tetracycline, chlortetracycline, oxytetracycline, or dihydrochlortetracycline. Lancaster's reformulation, which we have referred to several times, would certainly substantiate this. The additional complicating fact that consumers may simply be purchasing technical information, which in turn determines what they will pay for, but not legally purchase, has also been discussed. If S_4 is violated and consumers don't know the alternatives, in, for example, treatment processes, their preference functions in terms of commodities and services may be empty: if I have never been to Nepal, but want to go from there to Bhutan without knowing what means of transportation may exist, my preferences may be expressed in some characteristics of transportation such as speed, comfort, and conviviality, and not in units of packhorses, donkeys, Jeeps, and Sherpas.

That "hospitals" are profit-maximizers is at times offered as a tentative hypothesis, but the consensus is that they are not (e.g., 431). Hence B_3 can

[c]For a discussion of the theoretical difficulties in the analysis of firm behavior under the assumption of no price competition see, e.g., Archibald (20). This literature is extensive.

[d]There are additional indications that markets for at least some services consumers would be willing to purchase do not exist, or do not exist legally. Euthansia is not purchasable. An obvious service for which an illegal market has long existed, and for which now a legal market may be in the making, but does not completely exist, is abortion.

safely be said to be violated. The absence of externalities in consumption is an extreme assumption for medical services in general. There can be real questions of their extent, applicability, and effects. But that such interdependencies exist, minimally for communicable diseases and environmental factors, is not debatable. Hence condition B_4 is not observed: only the extent of violation is in question. Indirect interdependence, as we have defined interaction not through actual consumption but via satisfaction levels, is minimally indicated by the argument, and public policy statements, that "medical care is a right." In fact, it may fit the category of "merit good."[e]

That the existing income distribution, for medical care purposes, is not considered "optimal" is evidenced by public programs which differentiate the price to the potential patient based on his income: Medicaid. Categorical programs, in terms of population subgroups and of special disease categories, offer further evidence that the incomes of some population subsets are not considered optimal for any kind of medical purchase patterns, and that the incomes of *no* member of the population may be considered optimal for certain types of care required by specific diseases. It also seems obvious that the existence of "poverty programs," of O.E.O., of aid to the cities, and other public programs at nearly all levels of government, and also of non-public aid programs, would indicate that, at least in some sense, the income distribution is not considered optimal either by society as a whole, or certainly by those elected to make social decisions. It can also be argued that for the purposes of analysis, some amalgam of public programs and of dominant party platforms represent, if imperfectly, a revealed social welfare function. That revealed social welfare function does not appear to indicate that the income distribution is optimal without interference.

The *necessary and sufficient conditions* in terms of pricing do not exist. That hospitals do not set the price of each of their products equal to its marginal cost, or any approximation thereof, is a logical deduction from the previous discussion of outputs and costs: there *are* no economically meaningful operating definitions of output to which the unknown marginal prices could be equated, even if they were known. We have shown that cost components are not known. Not even charges are known on a national basis. A pilot study by National Center for Health Services Research in 1968 showed that charge statistics for selected services *could* be collected, but they are not (328). Those most closely concerned and connected with hospitals advocate what might be called "compensatory full cost" pricing: "They should be designed to recover full cost of

[e]Merit goods are commodities or services which satisfy "merit wants." Merit wants are preferences or wants "considered so meritorious that their satisfaction is provided for through the public budget, over and above what is provided for through the market and paid for by private buyers . . . The satisfaction of merit wants, by its very nature, involves interference with customer preferences" (Musgrave, 288, p. 13. See Musgrave for a full discussion). Newhouse reformulates and discusses merit wants as applicable to medical care (304). See also Pauly, 319.

services used and to provide a margin of return to offset losses in departments which are in the nature of a community service, such as emergency departments and clinics for indigents" (149, p. 997). This is representative. "There is no need to recapitulate in detail the economist's objection to 'full-cost pricing'–its arbitrary allocation of joint costs, the likelihood that it will yield results deleterious to the general welfare by discouraging the consumption of decreasing-cost output, etc." (Baumol, 40, p. 119).

Whether the other necessary and sufficient condition, namely that returns to factors be equal to their marginal value productivities, is absent or present is open to question. In our discussion of productivity we have briefly discussed the "lag theory of wages." If indeed there is a "lag," or was one, it would indicate that the condition is violated. But whether it is or not, it can be shown that it should be. For if S_2 is violated, that is, at least some of the buyers and sellers of factors are pricemakers, monopolistic or monopsonistic, the simple rule of marginal equivalence no longer applies.[f]

Both the theoretical and empirical questions of efficient pricing rules (but not for medical care) have been very extensively discussed by economists. We need not reproduce it here. It is true that no overwhelmingly accepted conclusions have been derived. However, it is also true that the presence of the predicates, the necessary conditions, is generally considered sine qua non. The major topics of theoretical debate revolve not around whether or not marginal cost pricing is always both a necessary and sufficient condition. The major question is quite different: Under what conditions do what kinds of pricing policies lead us to specified objectives? One overriding objective may well be, for a number of economists, to "let the market do it." But even those economists would tend to agree that "marginal cost = price" is not the Golden Rule, except in a Golden World.

> . . . Price making is surely of importance subordinate to such matters as economic efficiency and equity. . . (Williamson, 434, p. 30)

> . . . Since the distribution of income must be taken into account, there is no general pricing system which will be more efficient than all others for all sectors of the economy. Different pricing principles are economic tools which find applicability in different circumstances . . . Marginal cost pricing may very well increase welfare in certain specific situations. The fact that it is not applicable as a general system does not mean that it should be disregarded altogether . . . But one statement can be made: the search for a panacea, for a single simple rule . . . is, because of the technological requirements of the different parts of the economy and because of the problems of redistribution, a vain search and even a foolish one. (N. Ruggles, 364, p. 125-26)

As I see it, the argument for marginal cost pricing, like many propositions in modern welfare economics, is more concerned with diagrams on the blackboard

[f]For an elegant proof of this point, see Hirshleifer (188).

than with the real effects of such policies on the working of the economic system. (Coase, 81, p. 119)

. . . [T]he principle of marginal cost pricing is not in practice to be followed absolutely and at all events but is a principle that is to be followed insofar as this is compatible with other desirable objectives and from which deviations of greater and less magnitude are to be desired when conflicting objectives are considered. (Vickrey, 423, p. 605)

The crucial importance of explicit and precise assumptions and of their evaluation in normative analysis, when policy recommendations are sought, has been emphasized before. The emphasis may not have to be restated in the discussion of alternative pricing policies proposed by some students of the field if their assumptions were a bit more tangentially related to real phenomena. A somewhat extreme but typical example is the following: ". . . We treat prices as basically determined by competitive forces . . . Throughout the analysis we assume the absence of uncertainty" (Ruffin and Leigh, 365, pp. 2-3). It is in this light that Koopmans' warning must be viewed:

In normative analysis, the purposes of the analysis are not limited to the empirical testing of the set of postulates, and need not even include the latter objective. The new purpose is that of recommending, to one or more persons or organizations represented in the analysis, a choice or course of action which can be expected to serve his or their objectives better than or at least as well as, alternative actions open to them . . . In such cases, the recommendation is as good as the postulates from which it is correctly derived. . . (222, p. 134)

An additional fundamental problem for efficiency pricing is this: for all insured services a dual-price system obtains. The prices paid by the consumer, beneficiary, of the services are not the prices received by the suppliers of the services. A set of price ratios designed to induce "efficient" use patterns by consumers may be precisely that set of price ratios which induces "inefficient" production by suppliers. To the extent that the price ratios designed to face the suppliers (the reimbursement formulae) are, over time, reflected in prices faced by consumers (the premia), the problem, under existing institutional arrangements, may well be insurmountable.

Consider a fragmented system of ambulatory and inpatient care. Suppose the objective is to reduce the utilization of resource-intensive patterns, namely, to reduce the rate of hospitalization. Those who would argue for using the price mechanism as the instrumentality for attaining objectives, would then have to suggest that the price of hospitalization facing the consumer should be increased relative to that of ambulatory care. But to induce providers to produce more ambulatory and less inpatient care, the prices facing suppliers would have to be adjusted in the opposite direction: the price of services, to the suppliers, on an ambulatory basis would have to be higher than the prices on an inpatient basis.

If the dual-pricing were effective over some period of time, changes in the pattern of care in the desired direction could be expected. That means that some excess capacity in the production of services on an inpatient basis would be created. If such excess capacities were to exist, utilization on an inpatient basis would be less expensive in real (resource) terms in the short run. If the excess capacities were not utilized, over time one would expect a reduction in the capacity to provide services on an inpatient basis. This reduction, in the long run, would drive up the supply price of inpatient services.

Behavior of the adjustment mechanisms, even in well-functioning markets, but where forward-trading is not feasible, is, at best, difficult to isolate and to analyze. Here, however, we must also consider that the "demand determinants" are also likely to be shifting around over time. Incomes, demographic patterns, conceptions of what medical science can and cannot accomplish, and should or should not do, notions of "demand vs. right," environmental factors, in other words, all the structural and behavioral parameters of the system change over time. Further, as we have shown, at least some elements of demand are endogenous. In a system of such complexity "efficient" pricing is not simple.

Pricing Proposals: Marginal Cost and Peak-Load Pricing

There have been many other suggestions but few more explicit and informed by worldly wisdom than that by Baird, who argues for marginal cost pricing and informed competition (32). He is firmly convinced that "the Thomistic notion of a 'just' or 'fair' or 'reasonable' price has no role to play in the allocation of scarce resources" (p. 127). Competition is the answer. Competition would eliminate "shortages" in the medical care sector, such as that of physicians. Here the answer is so obvious and simple that it might not have occurred to anyone. Baird advocates the establishment of a uniform licensing examination which anyone should be allowed to take without any prerequisites in terms of prior preparation. It would be both unfair and a barrier to entry to prevent anyone from practicing medicine, hence anyone who has taken the comprehensive licensing examination should be allowed to practice. Information on qualifications, of course, should be made publicly available, hence everyone ought to be graded rather precisely, "on a scale from A to F," and then be required to print his grade on his "stationery, medical forms, and prescription blanks, and all in the same place" (p. 129). This, of course, would enable consumers to maximize their independent and inviolable preferences. "If any buyer knowingly chose to purchase services from a grade F physician, that's his business" (p. 129). Competition would also solve the problems of the hospital sector, and it could best be encouraged by the entry of profit-making institutions. Using special logic and a libertarian value system, Baird then suggests as a good free enterpriser, that entry could be encouraged by granting government subsidies to "hospital entrepreneurs" (p. 127).

Other suggestions for marginal cost pricing have been developed by Weisbrod (431), Ro (348), and to some extent, P. Feldstein (139). In the proposals it is not always obvious whether the analysts are proposing a dual-price system or a single-price system, to be faced by consumers and suppliers alike. To what extent the proposals, in their present forms, should be seriously evaluated is also not obvious. Consider the meaning, in the light of our previous discussion, and of the citations on the difficulties of efficiency pricing, of the following statement by Ro:

> In order to avoid confusion the hospital should distinguish its function as a production unit of health services from that as a public agency. As a production unit of health care, a hospital should strive for economic efficiency using pricing as a means for this purpose as well as others. . .
>
> There appears to be a general agreement that the rate structure in the hospitals reflects a number of significant departures from the norm of competitive pricing. . . . However, the *obvious and simple means of correction–incremental pricing–* has seldom been advocated. . . (348, pp. 28-29, emphasis added).

We wonder why. The rest of the analysis is of the same simplistic nature. There is no apparent awareness of the interactions, and in addition, some of the economic concepts employed are put to debatable use. We have already shown that Ro thinks optimum utilization is full utilization, 100 percent occupancy rate. This is again advocated as one of the objectives of marginal cost pricing. This, of course, means that "optimum" means the use to the fullest extent of whatever capacity happens to exist at the time. The absurdity of this notion from every point of view is easily demonstrated: much work has been done by RAND and others on optimal nuclear delivery capability. Only fools would argue that the optimal use of whatever capability exists at a given time is to utilize it to deliver "the services" to maximum capacity.[g]

It is also suggested that "a price policy based solely on economic considerations not only enhances the efficiency of hospitals, but also consumer satisfactions. Individual patients can now have a wider choice. A consumer can now choose a hospital, through his doctor, on an economic basis" (p. 34). One small problem might be, however, that not all physicians have admitting privileges in

[g]This example also demonstrates the difficulties engendered by imprecise definition of terms. It is clear that nuclear delivery capability has multiple "uses." One, if not the major one, is said to be its "deterrent capability." The analogy to medical care happens to be quite accurate: medical care is most effective when its preventive and early diagnostic effects minimize the need for its more intensive utilization. In fact, an analysis in terms of "preemptive medicine" and "second strike capability" might be quite interesting.

all hospitals. Nor is it clear that the potential patient is cognizant of the possible price variations, nor that equal levels of quality would correspond to different prices and hence that the attending physician would be willing to "buy" (through his patient) an increased likelihood of treatment failure at the lower price. His suggestions for efficient training can only be appropriately appreciated when read in full. An excerpt gives the flavor:

> An autonomous body within hospitals should be made responsible for running various training programs in coordination with the activities involved in providing patient care. As would two independent business enterprises, such a body should pay competitive prices for the use of hospital facilities and charge to the hospital the value of the services the trainees provide at competitive prices. (Ro, 348, p. 35)

Does this imply that if Columbia-Presbyterian is not about to pay "competitive prices" to the interns, residents, and nurses, the "autonomous body" responsible for their training should pack up and move to Queen's Medical Center in Honolulu, which might? Should the "autonomous body" pay for the "use" of the emergency room while the first year residents are on duty, or should the hospital pay "competitive prices" for the resident's services to patients? Or should there be a paper transaction? And what are the prices "competitive" with? The opportunity cost of the residents, or the opportunity costs of the hospital in terms of full-time equivalents of fully salaried staff physicians? Some hospitals have leased emergency room operations to ad hoc medical "groups." In this case the opportunity cost, from the hospital's point of view, of employing residents is negative, and the residents, or the "autonomous body" on their behalf, should pay the hospital for the services they deliver on the hospital's behalf to the patients.[h]

Weisbrod (431) also advocates marginal cost pricing, in somewhat less strident terms. One of the major problems isolated by Weisbrod is instability in demand facing a given hospital. He suggests that prices should reflect occupancy rates: "If patients entered the hospital with the lowest occupancy, aggregate hospital costs would be reduced to some extent in the short run by cutting certain staff requirements, and in the long run by reducing capacity requirements (431, p. 23)."

There are problems here with the necessary assumptions as well as with the

[h]Some of Ro's statements are theoretically incorrect, e.g., "In welfare economics . . . it has been demonstrated that . . . an explicit system of subsidies or penalties is preferable to a covert one." That this is not generally correct is shown in detail by Musgrave (288), and also Newhouse (304). That no general statement is directly applicable to a particular situation without at least one particular premise is elementary logic.

logic of the argument. It must be assumed that hospitals are substitutable homogeneous units, or that the distribution within all hospitals of beds between services is the same. A low occupancy rate of a given hospital, to some extent specializing in maternity care, is not quite the substitute for the high occupancy in another hospital, to some extent specializing in diseases of the heart. Within the set of hospitals with the same or similar service-facility mix, we have already argued, surgical, medical, maternity, pediatric, obstetrical, and intensive care beds are not by any means perfect substitutes, if any substitutability exists. The logic of the argument is not precisely clear either. Why would increased occupancy reduce costs "by cutting staff requirements"? Those who argue that the constraint is beds, and that beds well-enough represent all other inputs, maintain that really what they have in mind are "staffed beds," or "available beds." Further, we have already shown that in fact an overwhelming proportion of labor is by its nature fixed, or quasi-fixed.

Empirically, or institutionally, the argument also disregards, like Ro, the fact that the referral patterns of physicians and their admitting privileges are neither independent of each other nor equally distributed over specialists and hospitals. Physicians admit patients to hospitals where they have attending privileges, and refer patients to those specialists who practice in the hospitals in which they have attending privileges. One of the major reasons for this pattern is that the physician does not want to take the chance of "losing" his patient to some other physician once admitted. (See e.g., Shortell and Anderson, 386.) The current organization of medical care *outside* the hospital is just as relevant for meaningful analysis as that within the hospital.

The suggestion of the advisability of some central admitting service to serve all hospitals in a given community (431, p. 26) is both interesting and probably would enhance the equalization of occupancy rates, *if* the patterns of referral and attending privileges were simultaneously changed. One problem with the "allocation board," however, might be that the existing facilities are *locationally* inefficient. Quite aside from the physicians, who, as another analyst suggests, should be "directed and programmed" (Johnson, 199, p. 66), "to accommodate the workflow of the hospital," neither the potential patients nor their families in Westchester might be enthusiastic about being placed in Bellvue in Manhattan because the occupancy rate is lower there. Of course, it may be argued that not only physicians but patients should be "directed and programmed . . . to accommodate the workflow of the hospital." Quite aside from the fundamental question of what is to be maximized, hospital "efficiency" or patient satisfaction, the analytics are simply technically deficient in not considering the marginal transportation costs as well as the possible, and quite likely, differentials between private and social benefits accruing from such proposed policies. This is a rather obvious example of the Lipsey-Lancaster "second-best" problem: if hospitals are already inefficient in the locational sense, interference to make them "economically" efficient in their inefficient locations is likely to produce a worse, rather than a better, overall result.[i]

The relationships between *allocative* and *distributive* efficiency receive short shrift from Weisbrod in his 1965 article (431). Consider the statement: "This assumes that both patients are willing and able to pay the hospital price. The case of a patient with great 'need' for care but insufficient ability to pay is an income distribution matter that will not be discussed here (431, p. 27, n. 21).

That this dichotomy is untenable has been shown many times. Economists have concerned themselves with incorporating *both* allocative and distributive effects into the development of efficient pricing principles (Freeman, 151). It can be easily shown that each specific pricing system will have a specific set of distributional effects, and the two must be analyzed together. We need not belabor the point. It has been better made by Ruth Mack: "Failure of economists to grapple with the distributional effects of public expenditures accounts for the fact that 'economists are often disappointed that their advice carries little weight' " (264, p. 213).

P. Feldstein makes somewhat similar arguments (139). "Efficient utilization," he says, "will exist only when the price is equal to marginal cost" (p. 65). Presumably, "efficient utilization" is that level of utilization which is observed "when price is equal to marginal cost."[j] His major contribution to the discussion is his clear and explicit recognition of some of the obstacles in the path of the marginalist principles (pp. 71-72).

It is notable that neither Ro nor Weisbrod, the two champions of marginal cost pricing, devote any analytic effort to the interaction between patient and physician preferences; the stochastic nature of demand; the ubiquity of uncertainty; the interdependence between ambulatory and inpatient utilization; the interdependence between physician income, hospital "prestige," and inpatient utilization; option demand; standby capacity; economic vs. technical efficiency; private vs. social efficiency; the oligopolist nature of the market in just about *any* given community; the incompatibility between price competition and an oligopolistic non-profit "industry"; that some hospitals are tax-financed and some for profit; the relevance of price competition between some tax-paying and some tax-exempt organizations; that private physicians in some sense "compete" with outpatient clinics, or should, and pay taxes, while voluntaries do not, to

---

[i]The appreciation of this argument, as well as of the proposals, is quite simple. Consider that the "occupancy rate," in this case capacity utilization, were to be equalized between two airports ostensibly serving the same community, without any consideration of other transport and inconvenience costs, as well as consumer satisfactions. Now make that argument for Washington's Metropolitan and Dulles International.

[j]"Then you should say what you mean," the March Hare went on.

"I do," Alice hastily replied: "at least—at least I mean what I say—that's the same thing, you know."

"Not the same thing a bit," said the Hatter. "Why you might just as well say that 'I see what I eat' is the same thing as 'I eat what I see'." (Lewis Carroll)

mention a few of those problems that are specific to the hospital sector and which must all be assumed away if "the obvious and simple means of correction–incremental pricing" is to have any validity at all.

It is generally recognized that one of the obstacles to utilization of existing capacity is the uneven distribution of demand over time: there are peaks associated with the time of the day, day of the week, special days, such as holidays, month of the year, not to mention changes in disease incidence. To "smooth off" the peaks and "fill in" the troughs is the objective of peak-load pricing.[k] The applicability of the theoretical discussion on peak-load pricing is at least questionable, since the generally made assumption is that while there may be problems in the sector under discussion, Pareto Optimality exists throughout the rest of the economy (e.g., Williamson, 435, p. 811).[l]

In terms of hospital utilization, Long and P. Feldstein have made the most comprehensive analysis and suggestion that to ration capacity, peak-load pricing should be practiced (257). While they advocate this pricing scheme for all services, the discussion and specific example they use is obstetrical care only. The argument is subject to precisely the same criticisms applicable to marginal cost pricing. This particular suffers from some additional inconsistencies. For example, the implicit assumption is made that the demand for obstetrical beds is perfectly inelastic (p. 120, n. 8). If the demand is price-inelastic, how can it be shifted by price changes? An additional, unrecognized problem arises if peak-load pricing is instituted–and then shifts the peak. Suppose the argument is made that since maternity ward capacity is only 65 percent utilized between Friday noon and Sunday noon, the marginal cost of treating a patient (of delivery?) is then lower than at other times, and hence this should be reflected in a lower price during such off-peak periods. Now, it is easy and relatively safe to induce birth in the final week of the third trimester. Suppose all *Homo economikai* then decide to have delivery induced during the off-peak period. If the system is effective, the peak might shift: Only on Sunday. Of course, this example is *ad extremum*. But managers in the Bell System may not think so.[m] Experimentation, of course, could establish somewhat of an evening out. How much would be "efficient" is not that simple. It is generally recognized that

[k]The theoretical discussion of peak-load pricing is very extensive. So is the discussion of its empirical applicability, but not to medical care. For a recent theoretical contribution as well as a source of references to the discussion, see Williamson (435).

[l]This assumption has some rather interesting medical equivalents. Suppose a 67-year-old female patient enters the hospital with a diagnosis of ovarian cysts. Suppose also that she is a diabetic with elevated urea nitrogen, anemic with low hemoglobin, and demonstrates severe fibrillation of undetermined etiology. The medical equivalent of "Pareto Optimality exists throughout the rest of the system" would then be to decide on a therapeutic procedure for the ovarian cysts on the assumption that that is the unique diagnosis, and that otherwise the patient is healthy.

[m]Consider what happened when peak-load pricing was first introduced. No trunk lines were available between 9:00 and 10:00 p.m. The peak shifted. Only after further experimentation was the shifting peak fairly evenly distributed, to everyone's benefit.

demand peaks are significantly influenced by *supply peaks.*[n] Admission variations with time of day and day of week are not only reflective of the admitting physician's convenience, but of his appreciation that during certain periods the likelihood of using ancillary facilities and personnel is very much reduced. To maintain at full steam the laboratories, X-ray departments, operating rooms and the full nursing staff—all of which tend to "slow down" after 5:00 p.m. and on the weekends—would involve either additional personnel, a second and/or a second and third shift, or the payment of overtime. In either case, it would not be costless. In fact, there is no available analysis to judge whether supply-induced demand peak elimination would be more or less costly than its accommodation. Most of the analyses of peak load pricing in other sectors have been concerned with production processes in which the major inputs are fixed: electricity generation, bridges, telephones, etc. In the hospital, where 60 percent or more of the input cost are the variable costs of labor, the shifting or smoothing of peaks is not obviously a move toward economic efficiency.

What, then, would be an appropriate pricing policy? It may seem like unnecessary repetition again to stress, as we have in the analysis of objective functions and of costs, that the first prerequisite is an operational concept of what is desired, of what the objectives are. The major concern in pricing strategy is to devise a set of prices that accurately reflect resource costs so that rational allocative decisions can be made. In a market network shot through with oligopolies, legal and institutional restrictions, public and third party funding, not-for-profit operations, and all of the other complexities we have previously discussed, existing market prices do not even approximately reflect resource scarcities. They do accurately reflect the effects of existing institutional arrangements and the apparent objectives of some of the actors to get on the public gravy train.

To know resource costs requires more than knowing resource equivalents. In partial analysis, where the rest of the system can be assumed to operate with reasonable efficiency, resource prices in the rest of the system can be taken to reflect their productivities there. "System" can be narrowly defined to mean, for example, the ambulatory activities of hospitals and the non-hospital medical sector. Since neither of them can be assumed to operate efficiently and hence in neither do prices reflect resource costs, market resource cost identification is not enough. What is required is a complete specification of objectives in terms of outputs; a method to weight the multiple objectives, to attach relative values to them in order to enable us to rank them; the identification of the technology matrix, the technological relationship of resource inputs to the specified

[n]"... It is also imprudent to fall sick or die between 6:00 p.m. on a Friday evening and 9:00 a.m. on a Monday morning. If you fall sick between those hours, you may get no medical attention; and if, in consequence, you die, you will certainly not be able to get yourself buried till Monday comes." (Arnold Toynbee, *Change and Habit*, (Oxford: Oxford University Press, 1966), p. 220).

outputs, and then a set of shadow prices, the prices of the outputs in terms of other outputs. Then we would be in a position to devise a pricing scheme for *suppliers* which would reflect the real costs of each of their individual outputs. Supplier prices should reflect opportunity costs. Allocative efficiency cannot be achieved by other means.

But allocative efficiency cannot be divorced from distributive efficiency and from questions of equity. Hence the prices *facing suppliers* need not, and probably should not, be the same as prices *facing consumers*, or patients. In devising consumer prices the objectives involve encouragement of utilization appropriate to patient preferences and to medical need, the elimination of price barriers to medically appropriate use of services, rationing the availabe services where this is not medically contradicted, and to encourage a utilization pattern that would correspond, within these limits, to the economically efficient utilization of alternative sources of supply, whether the alternatives be defined in terms of physical units or in terms of the time dimensionality of use.

Prices are used to allocate resources, to ration resources among both users and producers, and to provide incentives toward their economically efficient uses. In a complex system of inefficiencies and little understood interactions, no single pricing rule will do the three jobs simultaneously.

Proposals for changes to attain better, more desirable, "efficient," or less costly operating procedures must bear in mind Reder's injunction that "it is a truism, or should be, that . . . it is necessary to have an explicit model of the economy or economic sector under consideration" (337, p. 121). The champions of marginal cost and/or peak-load pricing have no model, or even a theorem. What they have is a postulate. And it is generally a single postulate: marginal cost and/or peak load pricing will lead to the efficient use of resources. Note that we say postulate, because it is not derived from within the analysis itself, but is taken from the conclusion of a general theory, that general theory which we have shown to require as necessary conditions precisely those characteristics which do not obtain in the hospital sector. Since in normative analysis, which this surely is, "the recommendation is as good as the postulates from which it is correctly derived," there appears to be only one valid conclusion: the case for marginal cost pricing has not been made.

The problem of devising incentives for efficient operations has been at the center of the discussion of reimbursement schemes, which is considered next.

Reimbursement and Incentives

The basis on which the supplier of the services covered by insurance, private or public, or financed contractually or otherwise by public bodies, should receive payment for the provision of such services has been, and is, the subject of much discussion. Although the problem is neither new, nor unique to the area of hospital and medical care services, once again, the literature does not take advantage of the findings in other applied fields, such as weapons systems acquisition.[o] There are some rather important similarities: the importance of the careful definition of all relevant output dimensions; product performance criteria (end results); process performance criteria (process oriented quality); the irrelevance of market prices as indicators of either product or process dimensions; the lack of price competition; contractee dependence on contract funding; the timing of delivery; provision for option demand; problems of developing incentive mechanisms in the absence of market signals and the presence of non-financial rewards; and the biases introduced by contractor-contractee interreliance. Since our purpose here is not to examine in detail the reimbursement mechanism and its ramifications, nor to develop an incentive scheme, but rather to review briefly its impact on efficiency, only a few of these problem areas will be mentioned.

Our discussion so far has demonstrated that the information required for the definition of the product "specs" is not available; product specifications, in whatever terms are applicable to the relevant product dimension to be specified, whether engineering performance standards, economic performance criteria, or time dimensionality, require that the contractor be able to define the product to be delivered in all its relevant dimensions. We have seen that "patient days" is the usual product definition, with specific ancillary services, surgical and medical procedures, nursing care levels, and other covered product dimensions specified. However, no qualitative and sometimes no quantitative dimensions are specified. Where alternative treatment processes, regardless of their medical or economic efficacy, are possible substitutes, for example on an inpatient only basis, and various lengths of stay are conceivable, neither a choice of the former nor of the latter is specified. It is as if in the Department of Defense contracting for a jet trainer, only "guidance systems" and "approximate weight" were specified: the choice of which guidance system, internal or external, mechanical or electronic, regardless of its cost and performance capability, as well as the determination of the exact weight of the plane, were left up to the contractor—for each and every plane. Each plane, that is, could vastly differ from the one before and all those thereafter, and still the terms of the contract would be fulfilled. Further, the contractor could subcontract just about at will, pay managerial salaries and provide stock options at his pleasure, change his production process at will, use whatever inputs of whatever quality he desires, load his product with a wide variety of "extras"—as long as some person, whose special technical qualifications are legally recognized, considers them to be desirable, in which category there are some 300,000 persons with different training and orientation, whose incomes partly depend on what they consider desirable extras—locate, relocate, or alter his facilities and equipment, thereby changing his cost structure at will, and so on. Neither any reasonably rational and honest contracting officer, and

[o]For an early example, see Miller (276), and for a fairly late one, Peck and Scherer (323).

certainly not the General Accounting Office would, for a moment, consider the management of such a system possible. But it is really just a little worse: prior to the entry of the federal government through Medicare and Medicaid, the group composed basically of the contractees themselves, along with some of the specially technically qualified people, and some token representatives of the "public," decided what the prices would be. Blue Cross was and is a creature of the hospitals, and when the federal programs were introduced on a large scale, Blue Cross became the dominant carrier. When exemplified in terms of military procurement, the irrationality of current reimbursement mechanisms is too apparent to need comment.

That waste, inefficiency, however defined, duplication, poor performance, the possibility of fraud and deception, as well as a "bottomless pit," are built in as if by design is clear to see, and has been recognized by many. "Reimbursement based on guaranteed full cost pricing," say Ro and Auster, "is an open invitation to waste" (351, p. 177). It is an invitation to waste in many pervasive respects: "In short, the method of payment is not just a neutral financial mechanism to 'pay the bills'. For good or for ill, it inescapably affects costs, quality, and patterns of service" (Somers and Somers, 401, p. 154).[p] It is notable that it is precisely the operational, and conceptually meaningful, definitions of "costs, quality, and patterns of care" that are altogether absent, not only in reimbursement mechanisms, but in the entire hospital literature. In the language of input-output analysis, the final bill of goods is unspecified and the matrix of technical coefficients unknown. There are additional problems relating to the nature of the "industry." Discussing different reimbursement mechanisms, and proposals for new ones, A. Somers has said:

> But none of these have gone far enough into the "gut" questions of what makes a hospital tick, how you build concern for efficiency and economy into a professionally oriented nonprofit institution, how you relate payment for services to institutional goals and management performance, and how you get responsible management in a dual-control situation. (397, p. 359)

Several reimbursement mechanisms incorporating incentives for the attainment of certain goals have been offered, some of which we next discuss.[q]

P. Feldstein proposed that a number of incentive mechanisms be considered. He correctly distinguishes between two kinds of goals and hence two kinds of incentives designed to elicit their attainment: (a) "process incentives," designed

[p]See also Schultz (374, p. 114), and Ref. 340, vol. I, pp. 45-48.

[q]For the most thorough conceptual discussion of reimbursement plans in the literature, see Leveson (247). See also *Report of the National Advisory Commission on Health Manpower*, vol. II, pp. 143-48. For the historical development see Wolkstein (442). On reimbursement in *Medicare*, a comprehensive discussion is available in Feingold (131), as well as Somers and Somers (401). See also *Intergovernmental Problems in Medicaid*, (196). Other extensive analyses will be found in Pauly (317), Klarman (212), and Wolkstein (441).

to encourage desired changes in the process of care, such as the establishment of a tissue committee; and (b) "output incentives," designed to reward the production of specified output dimensions (137a, p. 19). Four specific incentive plans are then proposed: (a) reimbursement on the basis of the mean of the average costs of all hospitals in a given community; (b) payments based on individual hospital performance; (c) payments based inversely on the length of stay; and (d) schemes based on targeted quality criteria (pp. 23-36). Still, certain difficulties remain with each, namely, that for example, unless (c) and (d) were combined, high patient turnover, very short length of stay, and very poor quality would be rewarded. Use of the mean of average costs is meaningful only if hospitals of similar facility service mix are compared, if then. A further difficulty lurks in the assumptions underlying the schemes: that both the short-run and long-run cost curves are U-shaped, that there is some optimal short-run capacity and operating level, that economies of scale exist (pp. 20-25). Our previous discussion has shown that there is neither strong evidence nor agreement in the literature that these assumptions are tenable.

Waldman has proposed the "average increase plan," in which each hospital would be reimbursed for cost increases, regardless of their actual magnitude in the given hospital, in the amount corresponding to the average of cost increases for all hospitals in the same classification in the relevant community (425). Neither output nor quality are specified; the impact of outpatient and training programs is not considered (unless included in the "same classification"). In general, it is hard to know what this means other than some incentive to incur cost increases below that of the average. One problem may be posed by the size of the given hospital relative to that of others, even in the same classification, in the relevant community. The larger the size relative to others of a hospital, measured, say in beds, the weaker the incentive effect of the plan, unless the standard is the "average of all excluding the specimen." And many communities with one or two acute hospitals would not fit the scheme at all.

A somewhat similar plan, but for physicians, has been proposed by McNerney (295). He suggests the reimbursement be based on area averages, where costs larger than 15 percent in excess of the area average would have to be medically justified, or be disallowed. Why this would differ, and how, from the "usual and customary" basis now in use is hard to see. Further, given the role of the county medical societies, the areawide average could increase by 100 percent in a given year, in which case costs only in excess of 115 percent would have to be justified. While Waldman's plan would, in certain situations, have some, if not much, of a breaking effect on cost increases, McNerney's plan has none. It is really "more of the same and more regularly so."

One incentive reimbursement scheme, if it can be called that, has been at the center of much recent discussion: prospective budgeting. In this scheme each hospital would be required to estimate its expected budget for some near future period. Using uniform accounting techniques, the hospital would be required to propose some months prior to the beginning of the fiscal year its budget for that coming fiscal year, and be expected to live with it. Given expected rates of outputs in its several departments and their associated unit costs, the rates of reimbursement for the relevant period would be established. In principle this is a fixed price contract with the hospital assuming the risks associated with larger than expected increases in the prices of its inputs and possible unexpected variations in utilization. But quite aside from the difficulty of accurately predicting the values of all the variables which influence the cost of operations, the estimates may be systematically biased either up or down depending on the hospital managers' estimate of the payoffs associated with each procedure. If it can be assumed that the contracting or monitoring agencies would exhibit the same zeal to control costs as they do now, there is no reason to expect an improvement in results. Particularly in the case of third parties, such as insurance carriers, which do not operate within strict financial resource constraints but can stretch them by increasing premiums, we have the phenomenon of "cost pass-through." Increased operating costs are translated into increased financing costs where the pool of insured pays the bill. The cost pass-through is aggravated by the mode of payment to carriers which is usually on the basis of a percentage of payout or volume. Hence there are no incentives on private insurers, including the Blues, to attempt to hold down prices and costs. The Blue plans, which must receive state approval for proposed premium increases are somewhat constrained, but less so than publicly funded programs such as Medicare. Hence it is difficult to envisage a behavioral transformation brought about by the imposition of prospective budgeting.[r]

Prospective budgeting is one form of fixed price contracting, prospective reimbursement on a capitation basis is another. In the latter form, the contracting organization agrees to deliver whatever services are needed to the person or group which is covered by the contract, within a prespecified scope of services, for a fixed, per capita fee per month, or year. In a comprehensive group practice, for example, the contracting group will usually agree to deliver all home, ambulatory, and inpatient diagnostic and therapeutic services, but generally excluding dental, psychiatric, and ambulatory drug services, for a capitation fee. The population, or membership of the plan or group is not de jure constrained to seek care only from the group, but since no payment for services received elsewhere will be made on their behalf (except when traveling and under other prespecified circumstances), they are provided with a strong financial incentive to limit their "outside" utilization. Application of the capitation scheme to hospitals has been proposed by two analysts.

Expansion of the capitation form of prospective fixed price contracting to hospitals has been suggested by Feldstein (137) and Sigmond (390). The *hospital* would be reimbursed on a capitation basis, as proposed by Sigmond. One

[r]An excellent formal analysis of this as well as of other incentive schemes is found in McCall (292).

difficulty would be the establishment of "patient lists," since potential patients would be expected to, and would have to, associate with a given hospital on a more or less permanent basis. This proposal appears untenable on its face. P. Feldstein, on the other hand, would reimburse on a capitation basis not hospitals, but *medical groups*. Hospitals would be expected to be associated with medical groups, or perhaps not, but in any case the estimated yearly costs for complete services to be provided by the group, including hospitalization, would be paid to the group on a capitation basis. The group, then, would become responsible for the medical management of the patient. The underlying assumption is that the organization of prepaid group practice leads to the more efficient practice of medicine. In addition, this would clearly reduce the incentive to hospitalize.

The suggestion merits attention even though some difficulties remain. This is the *only* one which is based on the realization that incentives to attain hospital "efficiency," usually defined simply in terms of reduced costs, or at least costs not greater than the average, or cost increases no greater than average increases, can not be seriously proposed without considering that hospital utilization, on both ambulatory and inpatient basis, is not independent of the organization of medical care service outside the hospital. The major premise is that unless the *system* for delivering care *as a whole* is made rational, the hospital can not be. It further assumes that the attainment of acceptable or better quality would be enhanced or guaranteed by the internal medical controls characteristics of large group practice. The proposal, however, does not consider how hospitals could or should set prices to the groups. Nevertheless, it must be stressed, again, that this is the only proposal which considers the entire medical care system and does not attempt an artificial isolation of the hospital.

Ro and Auster develop a method by which reimbursement would be made a function of the difference between the standard cost of treating a well-defined diagnosis in a relevant area and the realized cost of the hospital (351). It is actually a weighted average reimbursement formula with variable weights by which both the "incentive" and "penalty" factors could be changed, depending on the degree of deviation from standard cost and its definition. The standard cost is defined in terms of the mean of observed costs and deviations around it (pp. 178-84). In addition to the fact that this plan also considers that the hospital is an isolable unit within the medical care system, the other problems arise in terms of what is the "relevant area," and which factors of interhospital variation are to be included in standard cost and which not. Nevertheless, it is an imaginative step in the direction of devising efficiency-enhancing alternatives to the full cost formuli now in use.

Some of the changes on a similar plan are rung by the National Advisory Commission on Health Manpower. They propose a "Variable Incentive Payment," "V.I.P.," which would be "a percentage figure and its size would depend on the categorization of the hospital on the basis of its standard of care." In the category for the lowest standard of care V.I.P. would be set equal to zero, and in the highest category might be as high as 15 percent (340, vol. II, p. 147). Why this would attain anything other than the maximization of the quality element in the decision makers' objective function is hard to see. An additional proposal is to reimburse the hospital on last year's cost, plus a V.I.P. component, plus the average increase in per diem during the current year in an "appropriate" group of hospitals. This appears to mean: the average of usual and customary plus something extra for better quality. It can be properly viewed as a quality incentive, but otherwise its incentive effects are minimal, particularly since its basis is the per diem. It might even encourage longer stays, if, as the conventional wisdom holds, the last few days of care are less expensive than the first few. Even if they were not, under the present system, the impact of the plan might well be to induce a few extra days of stay during which few or no ancillary services are provided, reduce the turnover, and thereby reduce the average per diem for a given hospital. Since per diem below that of the average for all hospitals, is "rewarded," whatever the relevant area and "appropriate" groups for comparative bases may be, the longer stays would be rewarded. Attending physicians might not be averse to this plan either, since the longer their patients were hospitalized, and the more patients, the more the physician's earnings would be increased.

An additional problem with this plan, as well as all others with the possible exception of the group plan of P. Feldstein, is that the hospitals would still be completely free to allocate costs, and charge fees, at will.

These and similar incentive reimbursement schemes are devised on the postulate that patient choice with respect to which hospital to enter is either weakly expressed or not translatable. Hence the incentives are meant to operate on the suppliers and not on the consumers. A set of proposals which assume that patient choice is translatable into differential utilization among hospitals, address themselves to devising incentives to act upon the potential patients. One such incentive proposal is developed by Newhouse and Taylor (305 and 306). The basic assumption is that while the demand for inpatient care may be price inelastic, the demand for the quality dimensions of care is not. Assuming, as we have seen before, that the current scheme of insurance reimbursement encourages the production of excessively high levels of quality and absence of quality variation, they propose what is essentially an indemnity type of reimbursement wherein the payment in lump sum would be a function of total treatment costs independently of which individual hospital the insured entered. To permit individual choice with respect to quality contingent upon payment for quality variation, they propose the "Variable Cost Insurance" scheme, where "(1) hospitals in a community are given 'expense ratings' reflecting their relative level of charges; (2) the individual designates an expense-class rating for which he would like to insure himself; higher expense-class ratings are associated with higher premiums; (3) the proportion of a subscriber's hospital bill paid by insurance is inversely proportional to the expense rating of the hospital and directly proportional to the expense-class rating of his insurance" (305, p. 454). If what they have in mind by quality strictly refers to the non-medical aspects of care, such as room accommodations and choice of menu, the suggestion is plausible. It would be even more robust if the suggestion for variable cost insurance were coupled with standards of minimally acceptable levels of quality, promulgated, monitored, and enforced by a public body, an agency of "certified medical auditors." For as we have argued in the discussion of quality, the problem is not too high a level or lack of variability, but rather the ubiquity of poor quality reflected in unnecessary or improperly performed procedures, and nonperformance of required procedures, neglect. When quality is defined in medical terms, where variations in quality are associated with different probabilities of successful outcome, it is difficult to envisage anyone who according to the "place-taking test" would willingly choose lower quality.

It has also been suggested that it is not cost reimbursement itself which has a distortive effect, but rather the question is what percentage of hospital costs are so reimbursed. Hospital costs will not be increased unless patients covered by third party schemes that reimburse hospital costs exceed 95 percent of all patients. The hypothesis is tested by the use of a one equation model which, Davis claims, "Unlike previous statistical hospital costs analyses, [it] includes factor costs, complexity of case-mix, and extent of cost reimbursement as explanatory variables" (99, p. 10). When we inspect the "model," however, we find that "complexity of case-mix" is measured by "mean length of stay" and "factor costs" are represented by the average hospital wage rate (p. 10). The regressions are difficult to interpret unambiguously for "cost reimbursement" (measured as a proportion of hospital costs reimbursed on costs basis to total expenses) is insignificant when single year and pooled data with a time dummy are used, but very significant when pooled data without a time variable is employed (table 1). A further difficulty is posed by the procedure which considers reimbursement on the bases of charges as totally different from reimbursement on the bases of costs. The argument is made that "in 1965, the percent of hospital expenses covered by cost reimbursement varied from zero in states in which Blue Cross reimbursed on the bases of charges to 52.4 percent in Rhode Island" (p. 15). But one must assume, for the argument to hold, that there is no relationship between charges and costs. In fact, unless there exists the kind of strong charge control by third parties, which is conspicuously lacking at present, there is no reason to assume that cost changes are not rapidly reflected in charges. Thus one would expect that it is not whether reimbursement is made on the basis of costs or of charges that would be significant, but rather the proportion of patients under essentially uncontrolled third party reimbursement schemes of any sort.

There are very few empirical studies of the differential impacts of various reimbursement schemes, partly because there isn't very much variation in them.

Pauly and Drake conclude a study of four plans which are all on a cost basis, but vary from 97 percent of billed charges to 105 percent of costs or charges, with the statement that "... whether hospitals are paid on the basis of costs or of charges does not seem to affect costs per patient day" (320, p. 17). That costs "per patient day" is a very inaccurate measure at best is one thing. The fact that under "full cost" pricing one would not expect any difference between costs and charges is another. That is, if indeed hospitals charge fees on the bases of setting them equal to their allocated full costs, why would one expect any difference at all? What hypothesis is being tested? What is being measured?

One source of difficulty in existing as well as proposed reimbursement mechanism is the treatment of depreciation, capital funds.[s] Both in private insurance plans and the federal programs, one of the areas of basic disagreement between hospitals and the carriers is the treatment of depreciation. That this is a sensitive issue is indicated by the fact that philanthropy, for voluntaries, is a decreasing source of funds. "Interest and depreciation allowances are the present day counterpart of community campaigns. They create a living endowment fund for prepayment of capital costs in advance of their need by the community" (Rorem, 358, p. 26). The director of Mount Sinai in New York City has said that "If we were forced to rely on patient charges for [capital] funds, then we'd no longer be worrying about rates of $100 to $150 a day, but about rates of $250 to $300 a day" (405, p. 229). For public non-federal hospitals, the major and growing source has been bonded indebtedness by taxing authorities (403). Somers and Somers have argued that the accumulation of depreciation allowances via reimbursement by the individual hospital is likely to result in long-run inefficiency (401, pp. 217-25). Individual hospital accumulation does not assure that future capital and facility distribution are going to coincide with community requirements. They suggest, therefore, that depreciation allowances be paid into a "pooled" capital fund from which allocation would be made by regional planning agencies. Leveson also discusses this plan and shows how certain incentives for short-term efficiency could be incorporated into the "pooled capital" plan (247). One advantage of the "pooled capital" plan is that it goes part of the way toward P. Feldstein's group capitation scheme: it realizes that the individual hospital is part of a set of hospitals, and hence its behavior can not be analyzed and influenced without considering the effects on the other members. It doesn't go all the way because it still considers that the hospital subset can be excised from the whole set of medical care providers, outside the hospital as well as in it.

It appears that under current reimbursement the hospitals have fared rather well. Medicare has helped hospitals substantially to increase their net revenues, although not by as much as during its first year (142; 143). The impact was somewhat differentiated by the approximate proportion of the aged in the total patient load, hence smaller hospitals benefited relatively more than larger ones.

[s]For a discussion of capital funding issues, see Rorem (358), as well as Stambaugh (403).

This also shows in the differential occupancy rate changes, which were substantial for hospitals with less than 100 beds, and negligible for large ones (143, p. 22, table 5). P. Feldstein and Waldman offer three hypotheses about the causes of both charge and net revenue increases: (a) previously uncharged services to some patients were eliminated and collection rates increased; (b) increased rates of occupancy; and (c) both because the period was viewed appropriate for a restructuring of charge schedules and because of incorrect expectations of less than full reimbursement under Medicare, charge schedules were not only increased but increased to overcompensate for the latter expectation.[t]

One generally held implicit assumption appears to be that the price system is the uniquely available mechanism by which to attain whatever changes in behavior are specified. This assumption also appears to be present in some current suggestions that to reduce cost increases in the future, a ceiling must be imposed. While it might well be that a "cost ceiling" in the context of the current void of knowledge may be the least harmful, it has been demonstrated that changes in managerial behavior as well as in productive processes can be induced by non-price mechanisms. ". . . There is clear evidence that management practices and technologies have been voluntarily adopted as a result of experience with government contracts. In short, government contracting appears to be a vehicle for technological changes" (Black, 49, p. 217).

Summary

The discussion of pricing, reimbursement, and incentives, as we have seen, is generally in terms of the applicability and desirability of marginal cost and peak load pricing with some recent forays into some aspects of fixed price contracts such as prospective budgeting or capitation prepayment.

In this chapter we emphasized the conditions under which either marginal cost or peak load pricing may lead to better rather than worse results. A willing suspension of disbelief, and a complete renunciation of the reality principle does allow one to conclude that incremental pricing is "the obvious and simple means of correction" of inefficiency, fragmentation, objective conflicts, shortages, cost pass-throughs, demand unpredictability, and the other problems of the hospital sector.

Incentives are means to encourage behavior conformance with predetermined standards. The standards are predetermined to lead to the achievement of

---

[t]For a review of some problems and the impact of Medicaid on a prepaid plan, see Shapiro and Brindle (383). Colombo, et al., discuss the incorporation of an O.E.O. program into a prepaid plan, Kaiser Permanente, Portland (88). See also, Kisch, et al. (208). A fascinating evaluation of both Medicare and Medicaid is the Staff Report, Committee on Finance, U.S. Senate (272).

desirable objectives. Objectives are never one dimensional. The efficient allocation of resources is one objective, but seldom the ultimate and never the unique one. Hence no pricing strategy and no system of incentives can be designed unless the objectives are known. What we have seen in the literature is an attempt to design a pricing rule first, assuming that whatever objectives it would maximize are the appropriate objectives to strive for. Marginal cost pricing, tonsillectomy, and the weekend bender may be the appropriate procedures for certain ills, but none are all purpose cure-alls.

The concern with high and rapidly rising hospital costs, with public program cost overruns, with increasing premiums, with vaguely conceived inefficiencies, and with the poorly understood and ill defined "crisis" in the medical care sector, have lead to hasty attempts at correction, such as the phases of price control. Prices allocate resources among suppliers and outputs among consumers. If prices are not allowed to perform these functions, something else will. It may be administrative fiat, queues, of black markets.

In this chapter we have attempted to show that if the current state of pricing, reimbursement, and incentive practice and analysis is deficient, it is too early to throw in the towel. The operationally meaningful definition of objectives and outputs, the identification of the technical and economic production processes, and the mapping of the intrasector interdependencies are required to devise pricing and incentive mechanisms to move us close to the achievement of our objectives with the most efficient economic use of resources.

Hospitals are plagued with many problems, of which economic inefficiency is but one. Conflicts in objectives, contradictions in output decisions, poor quality, expanding competing demands are but a few of the problems hospitals face. There is a special set of hospitals which have all these difficulties and more. We consider next the plight of the urban public hospitals, the municipals.

8 The Municipal Hospital

> What separated this world most distinctly from the other one across the landing was the smell, the all-pervading, overpowering stench of poverty, sickness, neglect, unwashed feet, unwashed clothes, foul breath, the stench of vomit and diarrhea . . . My mind commanded "hospital," my senses "stockyard."
>
> —Jan De Hartog, 180, pp. 22-24

In the preceding six chapters we have considered in some detail the nature of the outputs and of the objectives of hospitals, measures of their productivity, efficiency, and costs, the nature of the complex demands they seek to satisfy, as well as the pricing and reimbursement mechanisms that have been suggested to encourage the economically efficient utilization of resources. We have attempted to encompass these areas within a framework, set out in the first chapter, which seeks to interrelate the variables and parameters that constitute the system of complex interactions that constitute the hospital, while placing it squarely within the larger medical care sector. We now turn our attention to a special segment of the hospital system.

Analytic detachment becomes increasingly more difficult to maintain as one approaches the story of degradation presented by the urban governmental hospital set. We shall find poor quality of care, medical and financial neglect, overburdened facilities striving to meet the medical needs of populations without alternatives, half-hearted attempts at reform doomed to failure by inability or unwillingness to see the system for what it is, a catchall for what "mainstream medicine" leaves out, neglects or rejects.

We approach the plight of the urban public hospitals, the municipals, by first describing some of their characteristics and special functions. Both their functions and their difficulties are shown to be related to the nature of the demands placed upon them, particularly their role of meeting the medical care needs, at whatever low level, of what one might call people without alternatives: the poor, the ghetto dwellers, the social misfits and outcasts. The municipals attempt to do this while constrained by the political purse strings attached to public funds. After discussing in general the funding issues, with their concomitant multiplicity of bureaucratic controls, we turn to the consideration of the outcome of these two pressures in terms of their outputs and their dispiriting quality.

There seems little disagreement that indeed we are faced with the most sordid segment of the short-term hospital sector. A variety of solutions have been tried, from affiliation with leading teaching hospitals to the creation of quasi-autonomous public agencies for their operation, as in the case of New York City's Health and Hospitals Corporation. It is with a bitter taste that we demonstrate that even as general a model as ours in chapter 1 would have been sufficient to predict that the attempted solutions will not and cannot work. The weekly reports in the *New York Times* on the sit-ins at Lincoln Hospital, the strike of physicians at Sea View, the law suits at St. Vincent's, the crash program in Upper Manhattan, continually reaffirm that just as affiliation failed, the quasi-public corporation approach is also but a waystation to an eventual solution not in terms of municipals, but in terms of the entire interlaced system of medical care in the urban community. We try to demonstrate this by considering the goal conflicts, the competing output conflicts, the role of internally generated demands, as well as the inefficacy of present planning goals and procedures.

In this chapter, also, we introduce some of the flesh and bone reality of a system which, after all, deals with torn flesh and broken bones. We urge the fortunate reader whose experience with hospitals is limited or second hand to clothe the impersonal data of his analysis with the avoidable dehumanization, suffering, and death we here report. For it need not be thus.

The special subset of hospitals which exhibit all the problems of hospitals, and which, in addition, bear the triple burden of urban plight, neglect, and poverty; the special subset which has been designed to assuage the "social conscience" of the *past*, to catch, if not to redeem, the human waste of the social system; that special subset which has borne the brunt in medical care, as the ghetto school in education, of the effects of racial discrimination, sometimes separate and unequal, sometimes not separate but always unequal; that special set of hospitals whose wards provided the fodder for the training of medical students who were not members of the community nor became so after their training; that special subset which serves communities bereft of other medical services, where the physician's office is a rarity; that set of hospitals to whose door the patients come on foot and the ambulance is the police van; that special subset which today is the focus of criticism for not having erased in a few years, and without much help, the imprint of its sordid past, but without which the past may have been more so, is the set known as the municipal hospitals.

The cathedral, the "object of civic pride" (see p. xv of this volume), is in a state of disrepair. The Piel Report summarized some of the major problems of the New York City municipals this way:

"Crowded wards
"nursing staffs desperately short-handed
"buildings dirty, crumbling and dreary
"sullen, dispirited people, waiting by the hundreds in ill-lit, noisy corridors of the OPD's

"administrators disgruntled and dejected–fighting piles of paperwork and warring with their opposite numbers (equally dejected) in the central offices and the affiliate voluntaries." (326, p. 103)

The human reality lurks behind the words of official reports. "Nursing staffs desperately short-handed." Well, there are shortages of auto mechanics too; and when the staff gets short-handed, some of the "amenity" levels can be squeezed, but the "quality" of care will be maintained. That is to be accepted, even, perhaps, expected: "one accepts deficiencies in the comforts, amenities, and courtesies afforded to patients who do not pay for their care" (Klarman, 219, p. 117).

"Deficiencies in the comforts, amenities," the flavor of reality is lost, lost perhaps even to those who write the words. To get a whiff of the human reality one needs the eye-witness:

> Bedpans with stools, uncovered, stood on bedside tables next to water pitchers and trays with food. Orderlies and aids, forever at a run, walked across dirty bandages on the floor, around piles of soiled linen. Urine drainage bottles, kicked over, were left where they rolled. Dirty dressings were found in the beds; underneath the beds were dark stains where bloody drainage had run from the ends of chest tubes, dropped on the floor. Amidst all this, sick people had to be cared for.
>
> They were not, not even to minimal standards. Bedside care was supposed to be given by the orderlies and the aids; RNs and LVNs were so snowed under with administrative duties that they rarely left the nurses station. But the recurrent mechanical chores took up all of the aids' and orderlies' time; the taking of vital signs was an impersonal ratrace in which they whisked from one bed to the other, breathlessly; I often saw them just estimate pulse and respiration in passing and fill in a "likely" blood pressure on the treatment sheet for those patients who were not critical. Nursing procedures prescribed by doctors were frequently ignored, medications not given, elaborate and delicate machinery . . . stood idle during entire shifts or were left on long beyond the prescribed limit of time, thus turning from instruments of mercy into tools of torture.
>
> As a rule, the only people available to give the patients bedside nursing care were their fellows in misfortune. Old men, who could barely stand on their feet, tried to shave their helpless neighbors. Patients in wheelchairs would labor back and forth between the drinking fountains and the bedside tables trying to keep the pitchers filled. If someone was in critical need of attention, a call for help would be cried from bed to bed until it reached the nurses' station. One night, when the shift had just come on and the nurses were checking the charts at the desk, there came from the silent ward a feeble cry, "Nurse . . . Help . . ." at which someone replied from the desk, "Shut up!" When the voice went on calling, she repeated, "Be quiet!" and was obeyed. (180, pp. 329-31)

Is this a description of the Middle Ages or perhaps of the nineteenth century when "the hospital was generally a shelter for the socially unfit?" (385, p. 27).

No. It is a description of the only municipal hospital in one of America's major cities, in the 1960s. And it is a description of some municipal hospitals in New York, Chicago, and Detroit today.

From time to time, in the analytic discussion of "occupancy rates," "reimbursement incentives," "quality can't be measured," "price elasticity of demand," "efficiency," "rising costs," from time to time, one needs be reminded that lost in the cacophony of analytic abstractions is a human reality. The student needs to remember that the subject of the studies is an institution attempting to deal with *human* disease, misery, pain, and fear; an institution which often and for many, the poor, the black, the helpless, and for many reasons, has turned "from instruments of mercy into tools of torture."

Hartog's description is of one municipal hospital. Short-term, non-federal, governmental hospitals (the category comprised of city, county, city-county, and some few state operated units, most of which are city) have just around 25 percent of short-term beds, 20 percent of admissions, and account for just over 22 percent of all short-term hospital expenditures in the United States in the late 1960s.[a]

The national figures do not fully reveal the significance of municipals in terms of urban medical care. In New York City, for example, in a recent year, about 40 percent of beds and of patient days were in municipals, as well as 49 percent of ambulatory care provided through the OPDs and 53 percent of ambulatory care provided through the emergency room. Of emergency ambulance calls, the municipals had 59 percent (Klarman, 219, p. 34).

In fiscal year 1967-68, of the total city executive budget of $5.18 billion, $794 million or 15.5 percent was for "health care." This is something like $227 *per capita*, about 60 percent above the national average. Of the almost $800 million in tax supported funds, 55 percent ($440 million) was for inpatient and 31 percent ($248 million) for ambulatory care. Not only did this support the care provided in municipals, but fully 11 percent of the almost $800 million total ($89 million) was spent for public support beneficiaries in "charitable" institutions, the voluntaries. The city's share of the total tax supported expenditures was 42 percent ($331 million) while New York State accounted for 23 percent ($182 million), and the federal contribution was 31 percent ($245 million). The remaining $15 million was from other sources.[b]

The fiscal 1968-69 health budget was similar. In tables 8-1 and 8-2, we present the allocation of expenditures by function as a percentage of the total (table 8-1) and in dollar amounts. Note that the 1968-69 budget represents a 37 percent increase over the previous year.

The health budget is distributed by six federal, five state, and fourteen municipal agencies: twenty-five agencies are directly involved. While New York City has the highest level of *per capita* expenditures administered, until the

[a]Annual current figures are available in *Hospitals, Guide Issue* (189).

[b]The figures are from Ref. 326, pp. 76-79, 116-17.

Table 8-1
New York City Personal Health Services Expense Budgets by Program Distribution 1967-68 and 1968-69 Request

Program Budget Category	Per Centum of Total Personal Health Services	
	1967-68	1968-69
Personal Health	100	100
Inpatient Care	63	57
Ambulatory Care	24	32
Home Care	1	1
Ambulance Services	1	1
Mental Health	10	8.5
Addiction Treatment	1	0.5

Source: Clarence Teng, "The New York City Health Budget in Program Terms," RM-5774-NYC, May 1969, tables 24 and 25.

Table 8-2
New York City Health Services 1968-69 Request Expense Budget in Program Terms ($ in thousands)

Program Budget Category	Total Request
I. Personal Health	$ 952,780
A. In-Patient Care	544,678
B. Ambulatory Care	300,145
C. Home Care	8,392
D. Ambulance Services	7,277
E. Mental Health	81,181
F. Addiction Treatment	10,837
II. Investigation into Causes of Death	1,719
III. Environmental Health	7,753
IV. Health Education	17,145
V. Research	7,801
VI. Support	100,844
Total	$1,088,042

reorganizations of 1969-70, by the most complex set of partially coordinated agencies, the situation in other urban centers is different only in degree.[c]

We next consider utilization patterns, some of their special problems, the concept of what is "public," and some suggested organizational alternatives.

[c]For a study of Chicago, see Gibson (164), and other papers and references; Bugbee (63), and Caldwell et al. (71).

Urban Utilization Patterns and Some Special Problems

The municipal hospitals, "large metropolitan institutions that historically were established and operated to provide care for indigent patients" (163, p. 680), at the same time "served as training centers for large numbers of physicians and surgeons attracted by the rich assortment of medical and surgical disease in patients they treated" (334, p. 328). At least one meaning is clear: the poor are rich in diseases.[d]

Maybe we no longer need be reminded that "it is in the cities . . . that new problems of public health and chronic illness, of medical indigence, and of crucial issues related to the financing of medical care and the structure of the medical care establishment are most visible and pressing" (Piore, 329, p. 61). But while in the early 1960s about a third of personal health care received in New York City was paid for by public funds, by the late 1960s, fully 50 percent of the city's population met the standards of "medical indigency" as established by state and federal regulations. That these standards, while having a higher cut off point than in all other states, are rather low is demonstrable, for example, by the city's own "How to Measure the Ability to Pay for Social and Health Services" (191). A family of four, with three children under six years of age and no wage earner in the family is considered to need, to meet a "basic budget" inclusive of rent and taxes, a gross weekly income of $108 (p. 20). The implicit "cost of work," is indicated by the fact that the same family, *with* a wage earner is considered to need an additional $16 per week in gross income.

For the United States as a whole there is credible evidence that the color of a patient is well correlated with the institutional setting where he seeks, and receives, primary care (112). For all income groups, and both sexes, only 7.7 percent of whites received their primary care from a hospital OPD or ER during the 1965-67 period for which the latest data are available (112, p. 32). In the same period, however, 25.8 percent of non-whites received their primary care from either a hospital OPD or ER. This difference is somewhat reduced when income is taken into account, but not by much. Among the poor, those living in families (unspecified size) with a family income of less than $3,000, the percentages are 10.4 for whites, and, more than double that, 26 percent for non-whites (Ibid.).

So-called "white" and "non-white" comparisons are dangerous at best, particularly if the reasons for the assumed validity of the comparison are not made clear. Hypotheses about different incidence rates may be made, but then the two samples must be standardized for income, age, sex, education, as well as any other characteristics which are known or assumed to have an effect on the

[d]For a general discussion of trends in the development of public hospitals from 1956 to the present, see Gerdes (163). The New York City case is perhaps best represented by Klarman (219), the Piel Report (326), and Burlage (65). See Burlage also for extensive references to the study, analysis, report-ridden New York period from the late 1950s to the present.

phenomenon whose differences are being measured. How income is defined is also relevant. We have shown above the implied "cost of working." For "white" and "non-white" families in the $7,000-$8,000 group, the careful comparisons would take into account explicitly that while for the "white" families the usual number of wage earners is one, for the "non-white" family in that same income group the number of wage earners is more like three. For medical care utilization purposes the difference in the number of wage earners is meaningful, not only because the net income is reduced as the number of people working to earn it is increased, but also because, and partly depending on the occupation, the incidence of certain diseases, as well as of accidents, is related to working. An unusually careful and disaggregated study of health status differentials by race is presented by Breslow (55) who considers a variety of indicators in California for four "racial" categories, Japanese, Chinese, white, and black. On every index from infant mortality through adult disability to life expectancy, the Japanese rank the best and blacks the worst. Infant death rates per 1,000 births, for example, are 13.2 for Japanese, 15.8 for Chinese, 18.8 for whites, and 30.1 for blacks (55, p. 767). Among other fascinating things, what this implies is that when blacks, Japanese, and Chinese, along with Spanish-speaking people are aggregated into the all-inclusive "non-white" category (as is usually done in national statistics), the reported health indices for blacks are biased upward. They are worse off than the data show.

The differences by color are not diminished as family income increases: for individuals in families with income between $3,000 and $6,999, 9.3 percent of whites and 28.4% of non-whites receive primary care from hospital OPD and ER facilities. Above $7,000, the percentage for both groups is decreased, but the differential, if anything, is increased: 6.3 percent whites, 18.8 percent non-whites. The evidence is also overwhelming that while whites have a higher rate of hospitalization, the non-whites have longer average stays (see tables 8-3 and 8-4).

Further, the whites and the non-whites do not go to the same hospitals for either primary or for inpatient care.

For New York City, Klarman has shown that the distribution for whites hospitalized is: 65 percent in voluntaries, 21 percent in proprietaries, and 14 percent in municipals. The distribution for Puerto Ricans is quite different: 30 percent to voluntaries, 12 percent to proprietaries, and 58 percent to municipals.

Table 8-3
Percentage of Persons with Short Stay Hospital Days, 7/65-6/67 Both Sexes

	White	Non-White
All ages	10.2	8.2
Age 65 and over	14.0	8.5

Source: (Table S, p. 20) *Differentials in Health Characteristics by Color*. National Center for Health Statistics, Series 10, No. 56, Washington,D.C.: U.S. H.E.W., October 1969.

Table 8-4
Percentage Distribution of Persons with Short-Term Hospital Day by Number of Hospital Days, 7/65-6/67

Length of Stay	Both Sexes		Males Only	
	White	Non-White	White	Non-White
1-7 days	65.5	63.1	60.8	50.1
8-14 days	18.9	18.2	19.4	22.2
15 or more	15.6	18.6	19.9	22.7

Source: Table T, p. 21. *Differentials in Health Characteristics by Color.* National Center for Health Statistics, Series 10, No. 56, Washington, D.C.: U.S.H.E.W., October 1969.

The remaining non-white category is now largely black, and the distribution changes shape again: to voluntaries, 23 percent; to proprietaries, 0.9 percent; to municipals, 76 percent. The data are for 1951 (Klarman, 219, p. 97). The municipals, as early as 1951, were serving the black and Puerto Rican communities, the "non-whites." When total admissions for each type of hospital by control are considered, this again shows. In 1951, in all of the proprietaries, of 100 percent admissions, 96.7 percent were white, and 0.6 percent were black. In voluntaries, 93 percent were white, and 5 percent were black, the rest Puerto Ricans. In municipals, however, 50 percent were white, 41 percent black, and 9 percent Puerto Ricans (p. 98). Later data, for 1957, shows a similar pattern (see tables 8-5 and 8-6).

When the distribution of patients by type of accommodation is considered in all hospitals regardless of control, it is found that 88 percent of the blacks, 90

Table 8-5
Distribution of Admissions to Type of Hospital and Type of Accommodation, Whites, Blacks, and Puerto Ricans, New York City, 1957

Hospital Control	Total	White	Black	Puerto Rican
		(in percentages)*		
All Hospitals	100	100	100	100
Voluntary	61	67	37	44
Proprietary	18	22	3	2
Municipal	22	12	60	54
Voluntary				
Private & Semi	41	50	9	8
Ward	20	17	28	38

Source: H.E. Klarman, *Hospital Care in New York City* (New York: Columbia University Press, 1963), p. 99, table 3.6.
*The percentages are rounded.

Table 8-6
Distribution by "Ethnic" Categories to Hospitals by Type of Control, New York City, 1957

Hospital Control	Total	White	Black (in percentages)	Puerto Rican
All Hospitals	100	78	14	8
Voluntary	100	86	8	6
Proprietary	100	97	3	1
Municipal	100	42	38	20
Voluntary				
Private & Semi	100	96	3	1
Ward	100	66	19	15

Source: H.E. Klarman, *Hospital Care in New York City* (New York: Columbia University Press, 1963), p. 100, table 3-7.

percent of the Puerto Ricans, and 28 percent of the whites were in wards (p. 100). But of the white ward patients, 40 percent were in municipal wards, of the blacks, 70 percent, and of the Puerto Ricans, 60 percent. The non-white patient, therefore, will tend to be found in a municipal hospital, and within the municipal, on a ward.

In an attempt to account for the possible influence of income differentials, Klarman considers the admission patterns of patients from a group of housing projects. This of course is a rather rough measure of income, but probably quite meaningful nevertheless. If we expect a relationship between type of accommodation and income, then this measure of income appears to be quite good, for Klarman found that now 80 percent of the whites are admitted to wards, along with 90 percent each for the other categories. Of all admissions to wards, those to municipals were 42 percent for whites, 40 percent for Puerto Ricans, and 72 percent for blacks. This certainly implies that even when there is an attempt to account for income differentials, black admissions will be more frequently made to municipals. Not only is there a racial pattern on a cross-section basis, there is a longitudinal pattern as well. Of all patient days, in 1940, 72 percent were in wards; by 1958, 51 percent. The reduction in ward patient days, however, came about as a result of decreasing ward capacity in the voluntaries, and increasing ward capacities in the municipals. In voluntaries, from 1940 to 1958, the percentage of ward beds declined from 52 percent to 45 percent, while in municipals it increased from 48 percent to over 54 percent (Klarman, pp. 45-56). One implication of these shifts is that as some of the financial barriers–via inpatient coverage–to those patients who prior to the introduction of insurance were using ward facilities in the municipals were removed, they shifted from municipal ward beds to semi-private beds in the voluntaries. In addition, while the municipals during this period increased hardly at all, private and semi-private facilities in the voluntaries increased significantly (p. 87).[e]

That systematic racial and economic patterns exist is also demonstrated by the Chicago Study of Cardwell, Reid, and Shain. There, for example, no less than 66 percent of the variations in length of stay are "explained" in terms of socioeconomic variables (71, pp. 129-30).[f]

There is also some evidence that at least some aspects of analyzed care differ between private and municipal hospitals. Muller found that patients in New York City voluntaries received more drugs per day, and more intravenous drugs, than patients in municipals (287). But since there are no analyses by diagnostic category, the results cannot be evaluated in terms of quality. In another study, Muller had found that outpatients in municipals receive fewer drugs, and usually less expensive ones, which then accounts for lower general drug costs (283).

We have suggested in the development of our analytic framework, as well as in our discussion of demand and utilization, that to disregard the ambulatory services of hospitals, or to relegate them to the "unmeasurable" category and hence to exclude them, is to disregard one of their most important functions. This is certainly the case for the municipals which tend to be major sources of outpatient care. In both the analysis of demand and utilization of inpatient as well as outpatient care, "accessibility" is a relevant factor which the economic analyses do not directly consider. In large urban centers such as New York, Chicago, Detroit, alternative outpatient facilities in terms of private physician's offices or private clinics are at best scarce, and generally non-existent.

The Bruckner-Soundview area of New York City is a community of 35,000 people. There are no medical facilities, clinics, physicians, or whatever (326, p. 134). "The clinics, emergency rooms and wards of the municipal and voluntary hospitals are the 'family doctor' for most of the Negro and Puerto Rican population" (66, p. 174). The outpatient departments and the emergency rooms not only in New York, but in urban areas in general, have become the major source of primary care for the poor and the black (Weinerman, 429). Again, for New York City, in the year 1966 there were just under nine million visits, at roughly three visits per person, to the OPD and ER facilities of all hospitals. Of these, however, six million were to OPD and three million to the emergency room. More than a third of the total ambulatory visits, 3.4 million, were to municipals. What is striking is that almost a half of these ambulatory visits, a little over 44 percent, were to the emergency rooms of the municipal

[e]Klarman calls attention to the fact that when utilization analysis is based on hospital data reported by accommodation, ward occupancy rates tend to be understated, and semi-private overstated: when a semi-private patient is admitted without a semi-private bed being available, he is admitted to ward, classified as semi-private, and attended, usually by a private physician. (219, p. 48)

[f]For evidence of racial discrimination in medical care in general, and in hospitals in particular, see Nash and Gregg (297).

hospitals (245).[g] Of these, it can be estimated that perhaps two-thirds were for a non-emergent medical condition. For the State of New York as a whole, a recent survey shows that 70 percent of the visits to the emergency room were *non*-emergent (326, p. 326). Could it be that the emergency room is a nice place to visit?

Crowding in the ER has added to its problems. For example, the three-sided examination rooms provide little enough privacy for patients, but the situation is made worse when the waiting patients must sit in an area where they have a full view of patient examinations. Unless curtains are carefully drawn, patients being treated are not hidden from this "audience." (It was observed that lighting is better if the curtains are *not* pulled.) (326, p. 277, emphasis in the original)

Briefly, the emergency room is very crowded. No privacy is allowed patients. Apparently there is not sufficient police coverage or hospital security, and thievery is common. The staff is obviously too small and the space problem is undeniable. In the corridor at the time of the interviews were sick people, a man on a stretcher (an "overdose" case), friends and relatives looking lost and desperate, and general chaos and confusion. There was even a prisoner in the holding ward with a guard (when acutely ill, prisoners cannot go to the regular prison ward but must stay in the ER under guard). To quote one of the staff, "This really is where the buck stops" (326, p. 265-66).

It is noteworthy that in the municipal hospital referred to in the first quotation, the 1966 ER census was 127,262, and in the second municipal, 150,000. That emergency room conditions remain still today consistently below "Cadillac only" care, demonstrating that variation in quality whose absence some analysts decry, is shown in a recent investigative report from the *Wall Street Journal.*

Hence, it's not surprising that recent studies suggest a significant portion of the 700,000 medical and surgical emergencies that occur in the United States every year are mishandled in some way that often results in preventable death or permanent injury. In the emergency room of one Chicago private hospital, a 12-year-old boy with an open fracture of the right arm had to wait so long for treatment that gas gangrene developed in the wound and his arm had to be amputated.

In New York, a 35-year-old unemployed man went to a hospital emergency room and complained of stomach pains. He was given a painkiller and sent

[g]In terms of ambulatory care provided through the OPD and ER, the share of the municipals has increased significantly over time, with a corresponding decrease in the share of the voluntaries. This occurred during the period when the inpatient load of the municipals was also increasing, thus creating additional demands on municipal facilities. In general, see Klarman, 219, chapter 2. For evidence that both OPD and ER visits about trebled between 1948 and 1965, and that the overwhelming proportion, over 90 percent of these, were by the poor whites, blacks, and Puerto Ricans, see Lerner, Kirchner, and Dieckman (243; 244; 245).

home. He died 24 hours later, in another hospital, from massive hemorrhaging of stomach ulcers. A Dallas nurse is still haunted by memories of an episode in a local hospital one night. An accident victim, brought to the hospital was admitted as dead on arrival on the word of the ambulance attendants. The emergency room was so crowded that night, according to the nurse on duty, that no one bothered to examine the man. Several hours later, the supposed corpse coughed. The victim survived, but with serious brain damage apparently caused by the delay in treatment.

In a shocking number of cases, blatant incompetence by medical people is indicated. In Tennessee a few years ago, for instance, a teenage boy died of a ruptured liver after interns in a crowded emergency room diagnosed him as drunk and sent him away. Nurses in Mississippi ignored a man who was bleeding to death. Near Chicago, a college football player broke his leg during a game. The general practitioner on duty at the hospital emergency room put the cast on so tightly that the boy's leg later had to be amputated above the knee. (R.A. Shaffer, "Grim Diagnosis," *Wall Street Journal*, 51, 1 [October 5, 1971].)

This is not to imply that emergency room practice is without attraction to all physicians:

In a properly organized group, however, E.R. practice offers many advantages to the physician, including regular hours, a variety of patients, *freedom from continuing responsibility for patient care*, and reduction of administrative burdens, along with professional satisfaction and financial rewards. (Carlova, 72, p. 134, emphasis added)

Several reasons have been adduced for the increased utilization of the emergency room. Weinerman has suggested that the inadequacy of alternative facilities as well as the changing practice patterns of private physicians are both contributory factors (428). Another factor to consider is that, on the whole, municipal hospitals do not have separate admitting facilities, no admissions desk, and hence admissions take place through the OPD and ER. This leads the Piel Report to conclude that "the emergency room *is* the hospital" (326, p. 326, emphasis in original). Outpatient departments are similarly overcrowded, and hence while they offer no attractive substitute sources of care during the hours when they are open, they tend to be run on an 8:00 to 5:00 basis. Furthermore, the OPDs impose eligibility standards, with the implied requisite paper work, while the emergency room in the municipals is generally required by law to treat whoever enters, regardless of financial eligibility. It is also continuously open.

That the quality of care delivered in the municipals is a problem has long been recognized. Ravitch has argued that ". . . Maintenance of city hospitals as charity institutions for one segment of the population is not likely to result in anything but inferior care under inferior circumstances" (334, p. 331). Since traditionally and still today they have been serving the poor, the result is a set of "caste distinctions that now so invidiously segregate the city hospitals from the rest of the hospital system" (327, p. 383).[h] There is no agreement on the factors which account for the agreed upon fact that quality is inferior and that "the patient in the municipal hospital system experiences difficulties from the time he attempts to enter a hospital for treatment up to and including the time he leaves the hospital" (326, p. 324). Three general categories of factors are most generally discussed: (a) resource constraints in the past and in the present which have resulted in obsolete, inefficient, and antiquated physical facilities as well as material and personnel shortages; (b) intrahospital and municipal government organizational inadequacies, with overlapping and conflicting lines of authority, bureaucratic enterpreneurship as well as delays; and (c) general social factors both in terms of patient characteristics, the special role of municipal hospitals, and social attitudes toward medical care in general, and publicly provided care in particular.

Both of the first two factors, resource constraints and organizational conflicts and inefficiencies, may be discussed and documented in detail.[i] The various studies, proposals, and commission reports are generally in terms of antiquated facilities, "nurse and physician shortages," "inefficient management," "lack of clear decision-making powers," "administrator-municipal government conflicts," "delays," or in terms of organizational analysis, group interaction, small group dynamics. It is not our purpose to review that literature here. Within a framework of analysis that conceives of the public hospitals, the municipals, as a subset of a larger set, namely all hospitals within a relevant community, the difficulties mostly randomly discussed in the literature can be subsumed under two basic categories: objective function definitions, and supply-demand interrelations between the private and public sectors.

We have already shown that *what* the hospital attempts to maximize, and by whom, through what processes the objective function is derived, has not yet been established in the literature. Confounding that already complex issue is the introduction of yet another set of objectives: those of the political decision makers, at both the elective and appointive level, who bear legal and political responsibility for the functioning of the municipal hospitals. That their objectives cannot simply be defined in terms of the "quantity and quality of patient care" is intuitively obvious. That conflicts between their objectives and those of the administrators and medical staffs should exist, while not obvious, is both expectable, and documented.

Operating subject to financial constraints imposed by tax generated revenues

[h]On this point, see Willis as well (436). Hartog, whom we have quoted at some length, is instructive. A good discussion of the quality implications of hierarchical care, that is, different classes of treatment for different socioeconomic groups, is found in 270. The Piel Report (326, passim), is perhaps the best source of general discussion.

[i]See, for example, Burlage (65 and 66); Manning (266); the Piel Report (326); Freidson (152); and Haldeman (175).

as well as alternative demands for public funds, and subject, further, to political pressures by groups with yet another set of often differing objectives, the political decision maker must, necessarily, consider the municipal hospitals as merely one, if a significant one, potential recipient of public funds, and source of political embarrassment. Directors of Departments of Hospitals, hospital administrators, and medical staffs, on the other hand, within their narrower scope of concerns and responsibilities, focus on the hospital not as one of alternative sources of public service, but as *the* provider of that service to which they see no alternatives.[j] The degree to which the medical care oriented latter set is correct, to a significant extent, is determined by the public-private hospital, and hospital-private practice interdependencies. When one-half of the population is considered to be medically indigent in communities where alternative private facilities for medical care are largely absent, when the municipal hospital in fact becomes the "family doctor," the traditional conception of the municipal hospital as the source of care for the acutely ill indigent in need of hospitalization is no longer in accord with reality. Under current conditions the municipal hospitals no longer "fill the gaps" in the private system for a small percentage of the population. They are the sole source of care for the majority of population subsets. Thus it is that the conjunction of decisions made under that assumption, with changing population patterns and medical practice, resulted in the multiplication of binding resource constraints. That is to say, a system designed marginally to complement a larger private system, considered to be operating well for the majority of the population, has become itself the major system for a large minority in the cities as a whole, and in some cases, a majority. Facilities and operating levels designed with the prior purpose in mind have become inadequate. And while the municipal systems experienced increases in demands for their services, the private system itself, for a variety of social and economic reasons, became the object of rapidly increasing demands. While "inefficiencies" in both systems may well be present, excess capacity in service capability is not. Given the mobility of medical resources, relative nurse "shortages" in private and in municipal hospitals are interrelated: the municipals could not, even if administrative procedures were streamlined, enter a surplus labor market. In fact, it may well be that the nurse shortage in municipals can be analyzed in terms of feedback effects: given the inadequacy of facilities and the nature of diseases and of patients in municipals, as well as their organizational rigidities, any increase in the shortage of nurses further deteriorates working conditions relative to the voluntaries, and hence the maintenance of current personnel and

---

[j]It can be argued, and persuasively, that for the poor and especially for the ghetto dweller, medical problems are so intertwined with social, political, environmental, and economic factors that they cannot be easily separated (see Norman, 311). If we then use as the next step in the argument the relative availability of resources and organizational machinery in the personal medical care sector, it appears natural to emphasize its function as both fulcrum and lever.

the hiring of additional nurses becomes even more difficult, resulting in a further increase in the shortage, and a further deterioration of working conditions.

Not only the special role of the municipals and the characteristics of their patients, but social attitudes toward medical care, and social values regarding the role and determinants of income distribution in society, are also relevant to an understanding of current phenomena.

Implicit in the statement, which we have earlier quoted, that "One accepts deficiencies in the comforts, amenities, and courtesies afforded patients who do not pay for their care" (219, p. 117), is the assumption that medical care is one member in the complex set of rewards the economic system offers its productive members. This is made explicit by Fuchs:

> . . . I would also urge that we declare a moratorium on misleading talk about complete equality of medical care. This is technically not a realistic possibility, and in my view it is not a desirable objective as long as there is substantial inequality in the distribution of other goods or services. (160, p. 29)

The emphasis on equality, as well as on quality, is likely to reduce actual quality, as well as quantity, in this line of not clearly specified argument. The observed result, "Cadillac only care," is then held to be less desirable than more care, even if quality would vary: "Let's Make Volkswagen Medicine Compulsory" (Fuchs, 157). What levels of reduced quality, in any of its dimensions, would be acceptable to its advocates is not specified.

Since neither the economic considerations nor other analytic aspects are discussed by the advocates of quality variation, it is taken to be a basically ideological argument. However, there are certain aspects in which the arguments are nevertheless deficient. Namely, aside from the fact that we have already shown in some detail just what "lowered amenity standards" in reality imply, even before drastic reductions are obtained, there exist the complex interrelations between physiological, psychological, and social factors in the treatment and healing process, which are the subject of much debate (see, e.g., Donabedian, 119). Thus, if "reduced amenity" standards in fact contribute, for some conditions, to extensions in the medically required length of stay, the result opposite from that desired will be achieved.

The ideological attitude is also reflected in the legal patterns of care. While, with some local exceptions, the private hospitals are not legally obligated to admit any patient, the municipal hospitals are. Thus it is that the "dumping" of severe or complex cases, who can neither pay nor are medically "interesting," is an often deplored by nonetheless standard practice.

> Stories abound of patients who've been insulted because of their race, or turned away because of inability to pay. One notorious case occurred in a Midwest hospital, where a woman who had given birth in a car during rush-hour traffic was refused emergency care. In another case, a baby boy who'd fallen off a

porch and suffered brain concussion was denied admission to an E.R. because his family was on welfare; his mother had to carry him all the way across a large city to the county hospital. (Carlova, 72, p. 103)

Poor practice in the emergency room is dangerous, warns a cardiologist, because it can't be hidden:

The emergency room is a window to a hospital. When something disastrous happens to a patient there, its often a case for the coroner—*and* the local press. So the medical profession suffers another black eye. [And the patient dies.] (Quoted from a cardiologist whom we shall not name, in Carlova 72, at p. 116, emphasis in original. See also 245, p. XII).

The dumping of severe cases in municipal hospitals, in addition to the municipals' inability to control admissions through OPD and ER, leads to overcrowding. Given the patterns of demand, when facilities are expanded, the demand grows with it. In one municipal hospital, for example, when as a result of overcrowding in general OPD a separate pediatric OPD was established, within five days it, too, was overcrowded (326). Perhaps it can be argued that "overcrowding" is another of the discomforts that a municipal system can afford. But what degree of decrease in "amenity levels" or "overcrowding" is acceptable?

As in all the OPD's and ER's, space is a dominant problem. . . Apparently patients had to wait six to eight hours, during which time some children became dehydrated and other serious consequences developed. (326, p. 264)

Indubitably, the advocates of "deficiencies in the comforts, amenities, and courtesies," and of "Volkswagen medicine," would find this level both medically and socially unacceptable. The point we wish to make here is this: generalized value statements in terms of acceptable inequalities not only disregard the reality of the underlying phenomena, but permit the proliferation of facile solutions of equal imprecision and unreality.

What is "Public" and What Should Be: Definitions and Some Suggestions

Consider a professor holding an endowed chair in a private university, legally owned by a private corporation, who carries out a research project under contract to a government body, with government equipment. Or consider that the same man performs private industry sponsored research in a state university, with state ancillary equipment for whose use he reimburses the state university.

Consider further that the private university is chartered by the relevant state authority to grant degrees and is also exempt from both local and federal taxation. Students with privately granted scholarships attend state universities, while publicly granted scholarship programs are available in private institutions. Or consider that the professor doing research on a government contract holds a chair in a private medical school which is affiliated with a voluntary hospital. Suppose a necessary part of his research involves patient care, which at the same time he uses to facilitate his teaching of medical students. The professor on the federal contract may then provide care in the private hospital with the aid of his private medical students to patients who are beneficiaries of public programs. The private hospital, however, is subject to a wide variety of statutory regulations as well as to a large and expanding application of the laws of tort and contract. Further, to qualify for participation in both privately and publicly financed reimbursement schemes, the private hospital is also subject to a variety of public accreditation regulations, as well as quite specific and detailed rules in terms of acceptable bookkeeping and recordkeeping procedures, and cost allocation formuli. And to carry out his government contract research, the professor had to get clearance from a committee on human subjects research whose members are all private members of the private medical school, but which clearance was required by a government agency. Or the hospital with which the medical school is affiliated is a municipal hospital, legally owned by a city corporation, and the patient service may be provided to a private patient who pays for it himself. Any variation is possible; any number can play.

The continuum along which "publicness" or "privateness" is measured may be defined for different purposes in different terms. It can be defined in terms of *function*, in terms of *funding*, in terms of *accountability*, in terms of *operating control*. For our purposes here, and to consider the case of municipal hospitals, it is sufficient to say that function and funding may be considered *economic* criteria while accountability and operating control, *legal* criteria. Within the category of economic criteria, however, we must further distinguish between the "publicness," in the Samuelsonian sense, of the services performed, technical externalities, externalities through interactions in preference functions, as well as between public provision and public consumption. In legal terms, the question quickly becomes *not* is there public accountability, but rather how direct and for which functions under what circumstances.

It might be argued that the distinctions drawn are scholastic, the result of quibbling. It can be argued that the real question is: are there tax funds involved, is it on the public payroll? Indeed, because most of the suggested solutions to the problems of the municipal hospitals have been offered in those terms, either "get it all on the public payroll, but not the local level, make it state or federal," or "get it off the public payroll, let the private, or quasi-private, sector handle it," that we wish to indicate the intricate complexities of deciding what is, and what is not, public, or private.

Of the services provided to patients in hospitals, voluntary, proprietary, or municipal, a very small subset can be said to be purely Samuelsonian public. A purely Samuelsonian public good is that whose consumption in any amount by any given individual does not reduce the amount available for consumption to all other individuals who wish to do so. There are indeed very few such commodities anywhere, and certainly not in medical care. Public knowledge, such as freely published and available research results, may qualify. Thus research done within hospitals may yield a truly public good. But since in the treatment process of patients that knowledge comes embodied in identifiable personnel, equipment, and materials, it is no longer a truly public good: more care to some set of patients can be gained only at the cost of less care to some others. Under some special conditions, some of which we have discussed in the section on capacity, when the relevant constraints are not binding, that is, there is excess capacity, there need be no trade-off. That, however, is a function of excess capacity and not of the publicness of the good.

Externalities in the provision of patient services abound. There obtain externalities (a) between teaching and patient service, (b) between research and patient service, (c) between teaching and research, (d) between disease and disease, (e) between treatment and treatment, (f) between disease and economic productivity, and (g) between health status and crime levels, to mention a few.[k] While some interesting attempts have been made to identify the externalities and to estimate their economic consequences, not enough is known about them, theoretically or empirically.[l]

It can be shown that even if externalities exist, not all of them need be taken into account: only externalities not "captured" by some economic unit, that is, not counted simultaneously as someone's benefit and some other's cost, will create a divergence between private and social costs. However, the validity of the argument depends on the nature of the market: if market signals in terms of prices and costs are used and the allocation of resources takes place through the market mechanism, then it can be shown that only "significant" unaccounted for externalities may justify interferences with the market. Since in the hospital sector such market signals are either wholly absent, or if present, can not be taken as accurate indicators of relative social preferences, it would appear that any identifiable externalities would be relevant for purposes of decision making.

An additional type of interaction, or externality, may also be relevant: that which obtains via the interdependence of preference functions. The existence of "charity" institutions in the past may be "explained" by a variety of disciplinary approaches. For the purposes of economic analysis it is useful to postulate that

[k]An obvious example of the last is drug addiction, if that is taken to be a "disease," or at least diminished health.

[l]For a discussion in terms of economic theory, see Mishan (274 and 275); Coase (80); Turvey (421). With respect to medical care in general, externalities are discussed by Mushkin (289 and 290); as well as by Rice (343 and 344). Attempts at application to specific diseases are many, one of the earliest is Rice (345); arthritis (113), cancer (114), and kidney disease (207), costs have been analyzed in these terms.

the preference functions of most members of society incorporate the welfare levels of others. The medical condition of others, and the likelihood of their receiving adequate care, the argument goes, is not viewed neutrally, or with utter indifference. Quite the opposite: it is postulated that when some members of society are in need of care, but are unable to receive it for a variety of reasons, society conceives itself as a whole and most individual members of it who are not directly affected as well, to be worse off. No man is an island.

Needless to say, not everyone agrees. If not an island, at least a peninsula, say some economists. Pauly has argued that medical care is a normal good, just like all other goods. He, therefore, argues that the attainment of overall efficiency conditions requires the selective public provision of medical care *only* in those cases where identifiable externalities in consumption are present, *and so recognized by the relevant community* (319, p. 242). Such recognition is a function of both the medical condition and the income of the subject individual. This leads him to conclude that "there are many individuals with respect to whose consumption of many types of medical care, externalities are zero or insignificant . . . For other types of expense, such as physician's office visits and dental care, marginal externalities may be generated only by the consumption of the very poorest in the community, so that public provision for all would be clearly inefficient" (p. 242). Other than merely disregarding the technical medical relationships between different types of care, prevention, early diagnosis, etc., Pauly also doesn't consider the fact that *what* level of poverty is defined as that level at which externalities are generated is also a question of social values. Even if in the rarified abstractions of some economists that question is not permissible, that is precisely what the changing definitions of "medical indigence" indicate. Social policy at both the federal and state and local levels has indeed concerned itself to translate into policy *social* evaluation of that level of indigence at which externality is generated by both the consumption and non-consumption of medical care.

We have discussed before in some detail the conditions under which markets are said to operate well. Both because in many instances the markets do not work, or do not even exist, or if they exist they are effectively barred to price competition, entry by new "firms," or by potential patients, it seems to us that the question is not whether social action is required, but in what form, through what kinds of institutional arrangements, for what ends.

Social recognition of the desirability of social control in some form for certain purposes and under specific conditions is indicated by the discussion of "what is a public hospital."

To start from the "private" terminus of the continuum, some analysts maintain that in fact the "purely private" institution does not exist (Somers, 397). Why should that be so?

> In fact, of course, for many years, the so-called "voluntary hospital" has not been purely, or even predominantly "voluntary," if by this is meant supported by philanthropic contributions and fees from private patients. The voluntary

hospital of today would be incapable of operating without support from the public sector. This support is not merely financial, although this is highly important, taking the form of tax privileges allowed taxpayers' contributions to the support of the hospital, financial aid for construction costs and capital needs, as well as the ever-growing grants for research, mainly from the Federal government. Equally important is the symbiotic relationship of the voluntary hospitals to the public system . . . The city, by financing the supply of charity patients and by operating public hospitals for the poor, has provided the medical schools and voluntary teaching hospitals with badly needed teaching material . . . The existence of the public system has served as a screen to protect the voluntary system as a whole . . . from the public criticism that would otherwise have been directed at (1) its operation of a highly selective admission system . . . directed primarily by the institutions' needs as research and teaching agencies, (2) its lack of concern with what happens to the patient once he leaves the hospital premises . . . and (3) the failure of the voluntary system to give leadership in the realm of prevention. (326, p. 94-95)

They are "uniquely endowed with the public interest" (Somers, 397, p. 353). That they are "uniquely" so endowed is of course questionable, but that the private hospitals are in fact highly regulated is not.

Current public regulation of voluntary hospitals is broad in scope, but chaotic both in its origins and function. Labor law, common law, tax law, licensure of personnel and of facilities, certification directly by public bodies and through power delegated to quasi-public bodies, the case law of negligence as well as of antitrust, are applied to many of its organizational and functional attributes, without clearly specified objectives. A.R. Somers, in the most complete review and analysis of this heterogeneous body of regulatory devices, has said:

Many kinds of law are involved–public and private, statutory and common. All levels of government–federal, state, and local–and all branches–the legislature, the judiciary and the administrative agencies–are passing laws, handing down rulings, and making rules; in short bringing their separate and often conflicting pressures to bear on the hospital. The AHA study lists sixteen different federal agencies involved and twelve government bodies. (397, p. 16)

Some maintain that the voluntary hospital "is a special kind of public utility which remains for the most part in private hands, yet provides service to all the people" (Hamilton, 177, p. 395). Some would have it that they are "quasi-public bodies" (Burns, 67, p. 28). Somers and Somers maintain that even if the hospitals are not quite there, "they are recognizing their inescapable role as 'public utilities' and the desirability of some coordinated and knowledgeable regulation. . ." (401, p. 287). Shain and Roemer thought as far back as 1961 that "hospitals are essentially public utilities" because of "the obligation of the community to protect the health of its members" (380, p. 403, 401). Note how the conceptualization of the function of hospitals differs here from our discussion in chapter 1 and 2. The objectives that hospitals attempt to maximize, as we have seen, were defined in terms of "quantity and quality" or "profit" or "expansion." Social needs, community health levels, which we suggested as appropriate objectives depending on how and by whom the objective function is to be defined, now are entered. Note also how far this differs from conceptions of the hospital as the "physician's workshop."[m]

We have discussed some of the major distinguishing characteristics of basically publicly owned, in a legal sense, hospitals in terms of their specialized functions. A second line of distinction is based on the argument that it is the public hospital alone which is directly tax dependent (see, e.g., Gerdes, 163, esp. p. 685). Implicit in this, as well as in the previous arguments, is what we have attempted to make explicit above: the mixture of private and public funding, control, indirect and direct subsidies, and externalities is such that the private-public distinction is blurred. Why it should be even raised is the question. We have attempted an answer to this by indirection: because the private-public distinction was based on the socioeconomic characteristics of their potential patients, resulting in a double standard of care, which is no longer acceptable. The next question then becomes: What is to be done?

Suggestions for changing the system range the gamut from a complete restructuring of the medical care system to elimination of public institutions and increased reliance on profit motivated private ones. We have distinguished above between *economic* and *legal* criteria for differentiating private and public functions and institutions. The few proposed alternative reorganizational schemes we next consider do not always specify separately the questions of economic efficiency and public accountability, nor are the goals to be attained clearly defined. There seems to be general agreement on one issue: more money is not the answer. There are numerous suggestions, though not by hospital administrators, that "money" is not the solution required. The frequently cited quotation, in part, is that by Dunlap, who incisively argues that what is needed is not more resources but a restructuring of the existing system into a more efficient one:[n]

> . . . But my point is, given the country and its resources, the major problems lie outside of merely more money . . . The paramount problem . . . is the need for more productivity . . . Nothing could be worse than to say we need another three or five billion dollars for medical care, and then simply to duplicate or multiply the arrangements we now have. (quoted in 97, p. 1236)

---

[m]For an interesting discussion of some other factors blurring the "public-private" distinctions, see Friedman (153). A suggestion for a form of public utility regulation is made by Kissick (209). But see Stigler's warning that "as a rule, regulation is acquired by the industry and is designed and operated primarily for its own benefit" (410, p. 3). This is a good source for an incisive and elegant discussion of the economics of regulation.

[n]Barr (34) also agrees with this position.

Consider, however, three examples of the endemic situation in municipal hospitals:

Of four elevators in the plant, two are running. Generators installed in 1927 cannot handle the electrical loads. Furnaces are coal fired. Air-conditioners in the surgical recovery rooms do not work . . . The lights above the pediatric examining tables were bought several years ago by Dr.---- out of his own pocket. Otherwise only the ceiling lights in the room would have been available for examinations . . . Dr.---- also won a crash repainting of the pediatric service, after fruitless requests and follow-ups, by producing a chemical analysis showing the existing paint to be 28% lead. (326, p. 266)

. . . The obstetrics department has a medical consultation one day a week during which X-rays are examined. For years they have been requesting a viewing box; at present examinations have had to be made by holding the films up to the lights. (326, p. 285)

The correspondence division of the medical records department is not adequately staffed; correspondence is slipping further behind each day . . . Resolution of these problems requires at least two more typists, two more clerks, and new typewriters. (326, p. 277-78)

That these examples are far from isolated exaggerations, but rather mild representatives of a generic condition in municipal hospitals, has been documented; that they are intractable to solutions by more money has not.

The following report of today's conditions in municipals in New York City in terms of waiting time addresses the issue of money and costs directly.

On the basis of a one-week survey involving more than 20,000 visits, the staff report states that 76 percent of outpatients wait more than 30 minutes and that 49 percent of emergency room patients wait more than 15 minutes to see a doctor. In outpatient departments, waiting time ranged from nearly zero to 6 hours 45 minutes, with an average of 1 hour 14 minutes. In emergency rooms, the range was from nearly zero to 8 hours 10 minutes, with an average of 31 minutes.

According to . . . [the] staff report, it might cost as much as $45.5 million to implement the waiting time resolution alone. In that resolution, the board voted to "take whatever steps are necessary" to insure that patients are seen by a physician within 15 minutes of their arrival in any of the 14 emergency rooms, and within 30 minutes in any of the 800 outpatient clinics. (John Sibley, "Hospitals Lagging on New Programs," *New York Times*, 121:72, November 7, 1971.)

In the absence of any meaningful definition of "productivity" in hospitals and in view of the shortages of those crippling items, such as typewriters, examining lights, and viewing-boxes, which are so simple and so basic that the guardians of the public purse might well assume them to be in surplus, the argument that for the municipal hospitals money is not the answer is probably correct—in the long run. But that long run in which "we are all dead" will come much sooner for many unless money *is* the answer in the short run.[o] For the proposals are all basically long-run proposals.

The suggestions could be categorized as follows:

1. Basically the system functions, but it can be improved by
   a. affiliation with medical schools
   b. the introduction of competition through bargaining.
2. The dual system of municipal-voluntary does not work. It should be *all* private. It should be
   a. for profit
   b. all voluntary
   c. all voluntary with a public "model" hospital.
3. The fragmented system does not work, there should be a complete reorganization
   a. on a city level, by the creation of a Public Service Corporation
   b. on a state level, by the creation of a "Revitalized Federal-State" system.

Affiliation contracting. This was perhaps first offered as the general solution for the problems of the municipal hospitals by the Hospital Council of Greater New York (310). In affiliation contracting the municipal hospital affiliates with a medical school, or with an established voluntary hospital which is already affiliated with a medical school. The municipal authority contracts to provide, in addition to the physical plant, a specified level of general financial support as well as support for specified functions, such as OPD. The contract may also incorporate a provision requiring the municipal authority to maintain specific services, such as surgery, at standards acceptable to the affiliating non-municipal party. The non-municipal party in turn agrees to provide the staffing requirements and at times other specified services (326, pp. 301-24). The major explicit objective of the plan was, and is, to improve the quality of care in the municipal hospitals through the provision of medical care by physicians associated with the teaching institution. It was also expected that the municipal hospitals' attractiveness to potential residents would be increased, and hence some of the manpower shortages could be eased. The elimination of the dual system de facto if not de

[o]It might be suggested that the shortage of typewriters is an unhappy if not trivial example. There is overwhelming evidence, in the same source, that in many large municipal hospitals in New York City record keeping suffers from a *five year* lag. There is also overwhelming evidence in the Teamster Reports, from which our examples of "poor quality" were drawn, that poor records and inadequate diagnosis and treatment are frequently encountered together. While on the surface, recordkeeping and correspondence may not appear to be significant medical problems, when the records get five years behind, and hence are unavailable when the patient subsequently returns, the solution by new history taking is not likely to be achieved in the rushed conditions of the municipals.

jure was claimed as one of its major benefits. The non-municipal affiliating organizations, medical schools and affiliated hospitals, were to benefit by the increased "teaching material" as well as the "opportunity" to perform a community service.

Within the analytic framework developed in chapter 1, the a priori shortcomings of the affiliation system may be seen in terms of (a) the objective function, (b) internally generated demand interaction with externally generated demands, (c) production criteria, and (d) the pricing mechanism.

With the addition of teaching and research as the primary objectives of the affiliating organization, the hospital's goals are enlarged and become the subject for definition by an expanded set of interests and motivations embodied in groups and in individuals with differentiated and unequal status within the organizational hierarchy. While the administrator and the pre-affiliation staff may view as their primary objective the maximization of the *quantity* of patient service with some minimum quality constraint, the medical school connected medical director and the members of the post-affiliation staff drawn from the teaching institution view both the *quality* of care and professional, or institutional prestige as their dominant objectives. In addition to internal organizational stress and dysfunctional conflicts over goal definition, this will also reflect itself in the greater weight placed on the new element of internally generated demand for a patient mix appropriate for teaching and research purposes. The consequent deemphasis of patient care *qua* patient care, and emphasis on case selectivity with higher quality, will, in turn, tend to isolate the affiliated hospital from whatever pattern of medical care existed in the community pre-affiliation. The implications for the optimal production process given the changed objectives will be reflected in the deemphasis of processes yielding high quantity if low quality, in favor of processes designed to treat complex diagnoses with the newest technological configurations. But since the municipals were not originally designed to perform this set of functions, and no new pricing mechanisms were implemented to correspond with the altered objectives, the shift in the production processes toward the more resource-intensive production rays will imply an increased shortage of operating revenues.

In fact, this is what happened. Even those who consider the affiliation contract a desirable mechanism to attain certain goals have identified as serious shortcomings such factors as "staff discrimination" in favor of the post-affiliation medical school connected staff, emphasis on the teaching and research "needs" of the affiliated staff, "inattention" to community needs, and the generation of continual deficits (Piel, 326, pp. 301-24). The critics, the most comprehensive and analytical of whom is Burlage (65; 66), see the shortcomings in somewhat personalistic terms: the "exploitation" of the colonized communities for the private purposes (teaching and research) of the private affiliators, not to mention the "scandalous" expropriation of public resources, in facilities and operating funds, for private ends. The existing patterns of care were disrupted. A large percentage of private physicians, who pre-affiliation had attending privileges, or other, more comprehensive relationships, with the municipals, lost their privileges after affiliation, presumably because of quality considerations (401, p. 105).[p] Three municipals were closed, and those that affiliated shifted their focus from the community within which they were located to the larger "community of physicians." The planning and operational functions were shifted to the private institutions, without any attempt to delineate the contours of objectives to be attained, and without any mechanism to provide for the accountability of the private institution.

The difficulties generated by the affiliation-contract plan were inherent in the plan itself. The specification of objectives, their evaluation, their relation to the relevant community, implications for practice patterns within and outside the hospital, none of those factors that can be identified as crucial elements in any meaningful analysis of hospital operations, were considered in the "planning" of affiliation. While it may well be that certain private interests did in fact significantly benefit from the plan at the expense of communities previously served by the municipals, neither individual "devils" nor a "devil's theory" is required to analyze and to understand the complex difficulties of affiliation-contracting. The major reason was the attempt to "get the municipals off the city's back" in the absence of *any* analysis of the likely impacts on the systems of care. Patterns of care within and outside of the hospitals were changed in what turned out to be undesirable, and sometimes intolerable directions, while the deficits mounted and patients were turned away from crowded hospitals. This is a prime example of the validity of the argument we have previously suggested: ad hoc interference in a complex system characterized by multiple imperfections to obtain change in one identified imperfection (quality in this case), but without the ability to predict system wide repercussions, is as likely to lead to a worse, as to a better overall result.

Competition through bargaining. The introduction into the system of some elements of "countervailing power," is suggested by Ehrenreich (121). The major groups of purchasers are seen as the vehicles by which such "bargaining power" representing patient and community objectives in terms of costs and quality can be attained. The argument, though not completely detailed, is appealing, partly for that reason. To assume that "consumer interests" can in fact be represented, and via "bargaining" attained, must assume the existence of some viable market mechanism which is capable of responding. It must also be assumed that the inpatient-ambulatory, private-public, insured-noninsured, personal-community, quantity-quality, private-social interdependencies and some-

[p]While only 14.3 percent of physicians in private practice in southern New York do not have hospital affiliations, not less than 39.6 percent of general practitioners whose offices are located in areas with the lowest economic status have no association with hospitals (Johnson et al., 202).

times conflicts are capable of self-resolution via bargaining. Not only must there be a mechanism that responds to bargaining pressures, but all the various interests must be represented, and if no one else, at least the "arbitrator" must be able to see the system clearly as a whole in all its dimensions. We have demonstrated that the present state of knowledge does not permit that.

Profit Motive. The introduction of the *profit motive* is seen by some as the panacea. Constraints on for profit operations are sometimes envisaged, as by Johnson who suggests that while they should be permitted to "skim," that is, to admit selectively the more "profitable" cases, they should at the same time be required to provide some services, such as emergency and obstetric care "even if they must operate at a loss" (201, p. 107).

In a most draconian if simplistic reach for the competitive Nirvana, Feldstein and Long recommend restructuring the system to one of unconstrained profit oriented hospitals.

> One alternative to the present organization of hospitals would be a system of profit maximizing, proprietary units. In such a system hospitals would charge higher prices to ration places when crowded; market signals would then indicate the desirability of expanding or contracting facilities. (Long and Feldstein, 257, p. 119)

That this suggestion cannot be taken seriously on its face has been shown in several places (e.g., Somers, 396; 397; 401). The probable results of actually implementing it are shown in the recent Staff Report to the Senate Committee on Finance (272, esp. pp. 135-42).[q] We have shown in great detail that those conditions required to assure the acceptable operation of a free market do not obtain in medical care. Any solution, therefore, which takes as its assumption that the optimality conditions exist or can be attained, which the proposal for a "system of profit maximizing, proprietary units" must, is irrelevant on theoretical grounds alone.

All Volunteer. A system of *all voluntary hospitals* is recommended by several analysts on the plausible ground that since the financing of care is now largely a federal and state responsibility, the rationale for local ownership and control no longer exists (163, esp. p. 685 ff; 60). Since local governments face an increasing tax burden (while, it may be added, their tax base is continually eroded), they should be quite ardent "to transfer their public institutions to voluntary control and ownership" (163, p. 686). The argument is also made that "there is nothing inherent in public or voluntary ownership which necessarily means that a better quality of care will be rendered by a public or voluntary organization" (Ibid.).

[q]Current for-profit hospitals have not been much analyzed. A good source of data on their operations is available in Ferber (145).

The assumption is that in such a system, interhospital competition in terms of quality, accommodations, amenities, etc., will not only develop, but assure the attainment of a single high quality system. The otherwise undeveloped argument gains a degree of credibility if we consider that the basic distinction between "private" and "public" has been and is made in terms of the incomes of the potential patients of each. If through the introduction of private or social insurance the income constraint for purposes of medical care consumption is replaced by a single consumption-enabling mechanism, *and if* admitting and referral patterns shift accordingly, a redistribution from the municipal to the voluntary is predictable. The perceptible shift in demand from some of the worst municipals in New York City attendant upon the introduction of Medicare and Medicaid to some of the voluntaries perceived to be accessible was not only predictable in these terms, but lends a degree of validity to the proposition. The problems of racial discrimination, as well as self-segregation, the forces operating for community control and involvement in community decision making, as well as all those in terms of conflicting objectives, however, are unlikely to be capable of solution by this method.

All Voluntary with a public "model" hospital. A system of *all voluntary* hospitals *with a "model"* is advocated by Ravitch (334). The objective, once again, is the elimination of the dual system of care, the establishment of a single hospital system within which the only difference between hospitals would be the source of financing, which, as we have seen, is some difference. Ravitch advocates that municipalities relieve themselves of the burden of maintaining their own hospitals, turning their facilities over to organizations which then would operate them as private, voluntary hospitals. To accommodate the "needy" there would be a return to the concept of "charity." The voluntaries would be required to maintain "free beds" for the indigent. The problem of attaining and maintaining high quality of care would be handled by the novel and possibly quite tenable proposal to establish, in each community of sufficient size, a large experimental municipal hospital to serve as the "model" for the system of voluntaries. The mechanisms by which "model" levels of care developed in the experimental hospital would be diffused voluntarily, or enforced, are not discussed, and perhaps for a good reason. There do exist currently large experimental hospitals which could indeed perform the "model" function for the rest of the voluntary as well as the municipal system, at least in terms of personal care (see, for example, Wilson, 437). They have not been "imitated." This suggestion for a "demonstration project writ large" should not be dismissed, for it would have interesting implications and a significant degree of validity—within a very different general system.

On a City Level. The fragmented system of medical care in the large cities is an anachronism in the context of complex technology and inadequate market mechanisms. "We don't, in our country, leave it to the consumer to assemble his own automobile with this manufacturer's motor and that manufacturer's fenders" (Piel, 327, p. 382). The objective is to establish continuous, coordinated, personal, or family care. An entirely *new, integrated, system* on the *city level* is needed to assure "the delivery of health services to the population as a whole. It would eliminate the classical dichotomy that separates the individual patient and the face-to-face physician contact on the one hand—and the public health concerns on the other—fusing them into a single moral and effective political concern . . . (T)o deploy the city's considerable assets to promote the restructuring of the entire health service system in the community; to give the system a structure appropriate to the modern medical technology, and to make it responsive to human need" (327, pp. 384 and 383).

The most comprehensive study of urban health problems related to the role of municipal hospitals, the Piel Report, takes specific cognizance of some of the interrelations we specified in chapter 1. The interdependencies between the role of the private physician and the hospitals are recognized, as well as the difficulties in arriving at socially acceptable private objectives for hospitals. The recommendation is made to establish a functional hierarchy: goal setting and the operationalization of the established goals are to be divorced. A *Health Services Administration* (since implemented in New York City) is to establish community needs, set specific program objectives, and within established constraints, is to approve budgets designed to achieve program objectives as specified. A separate quasi-public *Health Services Corporation* is to design the specific programs and their specific budgets to attain the objectives established by the Health Services Administration, which programs and budgets would then have to be approved by the H.S.A. Upon approval, the Health Services Corporation would perform the objective-specific tasks.[r]

The municipal authorities would "turn over" to the Corporation the municipal hospitals, thereby discharging them "from the constraints of the checks and balances system of city government . . . [which] most effectively promotes waste, delay, frustraction, procrastination, incompetence, and impotence" (Piel, 327, p. 383). What is to bring about the invigorated potency of the reborn system? "Voluntary initiative in the delivery of public health services" (Piel, 327, p. 348).

This system is now in operation in New York City. It can be shown, a priori, that its viability will depend on six factors, within our framework of analysis:

[r]The details are specified and explained in the Piel Report (pp. 3-83), with additional detailed analyses and specific organizational structures discussed and evaluated in the Staff Studies (esp. pp. 489-514, 520-30, 560-79). A somewhat similar proposal has been made, in less detail, by Somers, 397. The general idea, and objectives to be achieved are summarized by Piel (327). The argument for the quasi-public organization in favor of a public utility scheme is perhaps best made by Somers (396). Good summary discussions of the New York City model with its Health Services Administration and the quasi-independent Health and Hospitals Corporation are Terenzio (418), and Ellwood (124). The results, or some of them, of objective conflicts are discussed in Bernstein (45).

(a) the successful definition of system goals acceptable to private practitioners, hospital staffs, teaching institutions, hospital administrators, and above all, the public who uses the facilities; (b) the development of mechanisms, in terms of incentives as well as direct and indirect controls, to assure that the established objectives will be attained; (c) institutional restructuring such that newly specified tasks can be accommodated; (d) sufficient funding to permit the attainment of goal-specific tasks; (e) the development of both analytic and operational systems to permit the identification and correction of inefficiencies, consistent with community and medical care goal attainment; and (f) the development of social value systems which differentiate medical care from the other socioeconomic rewards now considered to be functions of private economic productivity.

The extent to which the faults of the affiliation-contracting scheme will be repeated or avoided remains a question. The mechanism by which private ambulatory care is to be tied into the system is not discussed. The attendant problems of differential payoffs, and hence differential demands, for ambulatory versus inpatient care are not discussed, nor is it clear how the "Public Service Corporation" is to remedy them. The method by which responsiveness to "human needs" and community controls is to be achieved is, at best, vague. In fact, after all the rhetoric, the plan is, in its essentials, "affiliation with coordination."

On a State Level. A somewhat similar scheme, but on *a broader regional scale* is suggested by A. Somers under the name of "revitalized state-federal system" (396, pp. 192-233). Recognizing that "the hospital can no longer operate in splendid isolation from other health programs" (p. 217), general proposals are made to tie hospital regulation "into the total health machinery including environmental and public health services." The most direct interconnections are perceived to exist between the hospital and public sector and the private sector providing personal care, and hence that is where the "ties" are to be sought. The specification of the elements to be "tied" together and of the nature of the "ties" cannot at this point be provided for they are not presently understood. In fact, the studies we have reviewed fit rather well the categorization of the problems by A. Somers: no one "has come to grips with the heart of the matter, the physician-hospital relationship . . ." (p. 223). Some suggestions, however, are offered, with an attempt to develop a system well within the "mainstream" of American economic thinking, "a creative mix." This "creative mix" is to be in terms of "controls plus incentives."

The rationalization of "regional planning," regulation along the "New York model," state-federal relations, are all discussed by Somers and Somers in several places and with great comprehensiveness.[s] But neither they, who cite this approvingly, nor anyone else, has offered anything other than broad generaliza-

[s]For example, 396; 397; 398; 401, esp. pp. 200-202, 213-25; as well as 402, esp. pp. 502-34. For a U.S.-U.K. comparison, see Brown and Chester (57).

tions to what we consider the pivotal question, as phrased by the president of the Blue Cross Association:

> If the assumption is true that our health system is not sufficiently animated by competition and informed demand to be left without planned incentives and controls, it follows that concerted attention must be given to goals and objectives. Greater effectiveness and efficiency without reference to targets is not very meaningful. (McNerney, 295, p. 19)

In the absence of specified "goals and objectives," without "targets" to be attained, plans for reorganization, either on a piecemeal or system-wide basis, are bound to fail. They are bound to fail *even if* the underlying technical relationships were understood. They are not. That is why the suggestion that "money is not the answer," at least for the short run, is not acceptable. The present crushing conditions in municipal hospitals, in all likelihood, could be eased by minor organizational changes and more than minor infusion of resources. Long-run changes, if they are to be effective in terms of agreed upon goals, must await the articulation of the goals and the specification of the technical, medical, social, and economic relationships of the system.

Existing planning mechanisms embodied in local, regional, and state planning agencies, federally mandated and subsidized, engage in a special kind of planning known as "Walter Mitty Planning," but not as well as he did. For while Walter Mitty merely daydreamed, he at least projected not only his own roles, but a situational context as well. Current planning in the hospital, and the euphemistically called "health care" area, is focused on the hospital as if it were an isolated entity in an otherwise amorphous vacuum. And perhaps that is all to the good, for given the control and incentive mechanisms the planning agencies have at their disposal to operationalize their plans, a more comprehensive perspective would only entail a higher degree of frustration. The agencies are paper tigers when it comes to having any effect on future physical hospital developments, since their roar is limited to granting or denying certification for physical expansion, particularly in terms of new beds. When it comes to the present operation of hospitals, their inter-organization, the development of networks of coordination, the limitation or the expansion of the scope of services, the hospitals' relation to the other elements of the medical care sector, they are not even smiling kittens. They do not exist.

Their principal mode of operation is "round table planning." The notion appears to be that if only "everyone" concerned with "efficient" hospital planning, the administrators, the representatives of the medical staff, community "representatives," and the fiscal agents, as well as local governmental agencies, can get into the same room and, presumably leaning on the fundamental findings of small group dynamics, sit around a round table, the public interest will be achieved by the force of persuasion operating on men of good will. That there is more than $30 billion at stake at the national level (expenditures for hospitals), that the hospitals' internal and external constituencies in fact represent conflicting interest groupings, that to achieve a modicum of success would require a thorough restructuring of the system and its constituent elements, seem not to be reflected in the control mechanisms available to the planners. The obstacles are assumed to yield to the power of jaw-boning. But unlike Samson and his jawbone, they have not smitten even one philistine (see Judges, 15; 15-20).

Presenting a case study of organizational ineffectiveness resulting from mandated reliance on the power of whispered rhetoric, the planning agencies are an interesting study for sociologists and political scientists with a curiosity focused on bootstrap attempts at community planning without controls. For the economist interested in hospital organization, they are irrelevant; for the hospital administrator, merely a tangential nuisance. Hence we do not consider them.

A less generous view of the origins, functions, and effectiveness of planning agencies would maintain that they are an example, weak as they may be, of the demand for regulation (see Stigler, 410, and Carr, 73). In this perspective, existing voluntary hospitals and governmental institutions, as well as the insurance carriers and public funding agencies, realized the threat posed to them by unfettered expansion of the hospital sector stimulated by the infusion of additional private and public funds starting in the 1960s. The threats were seen in terms of developing overcapacity and the attendant financial difficulties to be faced by existing institutions. Hence the dominant interest groups, both to prevent possible future regulation of the public utility type and to insure the future utilization of their own institutions, turned to the alternative of "planning" as a mechanism to "regularize" their own bailiwick. In this view, the agencies are seen as comprising a kind of publicly approved cartel, successful in erecting barriers to entry while safeguarding the existing institutions and legitimizing the dominant role of the hospital-carrier coalition.

A third and even less generous, if more popular, view would maintain that the current state of planning in the health care area is an example of the American penchant for muddling through by legislating goals at the federal level while leaving implementation without resources to the local level.

Whatever one's view of the origins and purposes of regional and community health planning, old and "new," their effectiveness remains to be demonstrated. It also remains to be demonstrated that any meaningful reorganization of the hospital subset is possible without first considering that we are faced with an institutional and organizational system incapable of meeting the demands and expectations placed upon it.

Summary

In this chapter we have attempted to demonstrate that of all hospitals the urban public institutions are faced with the most serious of problems, perhaps practicing good "medicine," but providing less than acceptable levels of medical care. Good medicine, for the research and teaching functions place a high premium on technical skills applied to organs, particularly if the condition challenges the pride of workmanship in the clinician. But if medical care is care of the patient as a human being, the urban public hospitals are institutions of dehumanization, only a few steps ahead of the so-called "long-term mental institutions," which are but holding bins for their inmates who, often smeared with their own feces, moaningly await the merciless end.

The urban public hospital, as we have seen, has become the major and often only source of whatever medical care the poor, the disadvantaged, the ghetto dweller can secure. Its emergency rooms and outpatient clinics are the equivalent of the friendly physician's office for people without alternatives. In their deteriorating and underequipped facilities they dispense care of poor quality, dehumanizing both the patient and the provider. Encrusted with bureaucratic controls and embroiled in goal conflicts, they are the finger in the dam. They provide for those whom "mainstream medicine" leaves out.

Numerous proposals have been made to try to remedy some of the worst elements of this system of noncare. But few, as we have seen, consider that while one of the sources of difficulties is the constraining public purse, the public urban hospitals can not with any degree of realism be seen as separated or separable from the rest of the hospital and medical care system. Hence, if any solutions are to come, they will have to address not only issues specific to urban public hospitals. The attempts at solutions will have to address the issue of how to reorganize, and under what auspices, that interconnecting institutional system which now fails at the cost of some $70 billion to ensure that anyone in need of medical attention can in fact receive it with an assurance of good quality in decent circumstances.

We shall return to this point in our next chapter where we summarize our conclusions.

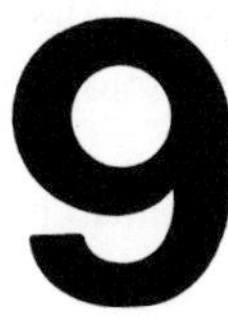

Conclusions: The Road Ahead

"Would you tell me, please, which way I ought to go from here?"
"That depends a good deal on where you want to get to," said the Cat.
"I don't much care where—" said Alice.
"Then it doesn't matter which way you go," said the Cat.

—Lewis Carroll

The way we go does matter. And where we ought to get to seems clear enough. Our long-run objective should be the establishment of an environment that fosters and maintains physical, mental, and social health where disease is a geriatric, genetic, and stochastic residue. How many of us live to see progress toward that goal will partly depend on how well in the short run our institutions of sickness care do their jobs. Our immediate proximate objective, therefore, should be to restructure the medical care system and within it the hospital sector so that:

1. Barriers to access to medically useful treatment are eliminated whether those barriers are posed by personal financial limitations, resource constraints, systematic disorganization leading to multiple and conflicting entry points, racial and ethnic discrimination, or by the existing culture gap between providers and much of the client population.

2. Those who can benefit from medical intervention do in fact receive it. As in the field of elementary education, both private and public interest would be served by vesting legal accountability for health levels, preventive and early diagnostic programs, and management of chronic conditions in a public body. That experience with analogous programs, such as those administered by the Food and Drug Administration and the Bureau of Biological Standards, give cause for some pessimism about the attainability of these ends simply places a greater burden on imaginative new approaches.

3. Minimum acceptable standards of quality, established by the use of professional medical knowledge and a humane approach to the anxiety attendant on disease, are everywhere assured. This requires the development of administrative mechanisms that would operationalize the public accountability of providers by a system of monitoring, auditing, and reporting the quality of care. Internal audits, peer review, process controls, and other present mechanisms, while major improvements, rely on intraprofessional controls and hence are prone to the pitfalls brought about by professional colleaguality, while failing to provide a mechanism of public accountability with sanctions.

4. The human factor is placed at the center of the process of care, recognizing that the patient is not a set of organs and biologic process networks, but a person in a social system.

5. The organizational units of the system, hospitals, be they private or public, physicians regardless of their form of practice, and the ancillary providers such as laboratories, are restructured and formally interrelated to eliminate the presently inhibiting factors of fragmentation, discontinuities and duplication flowing from the absence of the integration of technically and medically interdependent functions and from conflicting incentives.

6. The production process for each alternative medical intervention procedure is the most economically efficient one to achieve the outcome specified in all its relevant dimensions, including quality. This requires the ability to identify the relevant production functions in terms of completely specified outputs and knowledge of their shapes sufficient to introduce them at the economically best scale of operations. The interrelations among the various production processes, again in terms of completely specified outputs, must be understood to exploit the advantages of technical integration.

7. A system of incentives, regulations, and sanctions acting upon decision makers assure the choice of the most economically efficient process from among the medically appropriate alternatives. Faced with the complex and interacting objectives of providers, sole reliance on the price system without changing existing institutional arrangements is not sufficient to bring about the adoption of resource saving alternatives.

8. A system of price and nonprice rationing to allocate among potential users medical resource capabilities with a commitment to expand such resources to the point where anyone who may benefit from medical intervention in fact will.

9. An adequate financial base is established. The cry ought not to be "off the tax rolls," but rather "onto a financial base, public and private, adequate to the needs." The problem of local governmental units is not merely the increasing financial burden they represent but the eroding tax base combined with many communities' unwillingness to bear the tax costs of achieving the social objectives of equal access and equal care, in medical care as in education, affirmed in party platforms. This requires both a rationalization of the health care sector and the appropriation to it of an increasing proportion of the national product. The argument that the United States spends more per capita than any other country in the world for medical care is irrelevant since it disregards the fact that we also spend more, on the same basis or absolutely, on cosmetics, chewing gum, and dog food. If the pronounced priorities are to be met,[a] the appropriate financial base must be provided and it cannot be without significantly greater reliance on federal general tax revenues.

---

[a]"Just as our National Government has moved to provide equal opportunity in areas such as education, employment, and voting, so we must now work to expand the opportunity for all our citizens to obtain a decent standard of medical care. We must do all we can to remove any racial, economic, social, or geographic barriers which now prevent any of our

10. Medical care is recognized for what it is, an ameliorative, restorative, palliative function, and not a panacea. The solution of all environmental and social ills, from poverty through racism to alienation, cannot be achieved by using the medical care sector as the lever. Nor can the attainment of significantly better performance of the usual health status indicators, such as infant neonatal mortality and life expectancy, be predicated upon the improvement or expansion of the medical care sector alone. Where the contributing factors are poor nutrition, poverty, debilitating working conditions, the stresses of achievement in an industrialized society, and dysfunctional life styles, medical care can perform only a residual function. But that it should perform well.

These are the objectives we should strive for and implicit in them is a large role for the economist, hospital administrator, and health analyst. But even those who, for whatever reasons, would disagree with our rather explicit value orientation in which equal access to high quality care is the primary goal, would subscribe to the subsidiary goal of striving for economic efficiency as set out in points 5 through 8 above. And the literature shows this.

We have reviewed the literature on what could be called the hospital and hospital related operations. This was done within an analytic framework, set out in chapter 1, in which the hospital is seen as a complex economic organization with some complex objective function expressed in quantity, quality, and prestige terms, responding to a set of internally and externally generated demands along some set of production functions. Our review shows that there is little agreement, and little empirical or conceptual work, on what it is that hospitals attempt to maximize, and how that objective is established by whom. We have seen that the conceptualization and measurement of "output" is inadequate for meaningful analysis and that this makes the study of cost behavior at best difficult, if not impossible. Thus it is that different students of the field can come to such glaringly different notions on whether economies of scale exist, and if so, at what undefined size. The analysis of demand and utilization is equally tentative.

In our analytic framework, as well as in our subsequent discussion, we have argued that as each hospital is a member of some set of hospitals, so the set of hospitals form a subset, if a substantial one, of the large set composed of all medical care suppliers. The interactions, in terms of alternative treatment processes, interrelated demands, intersecting interests, are not always clear in the literature, but enough empirical evidence exists to lend a degree of "real world" validity to our theoretical formulation of them. The brief discussions of alternative pricing and reimbursement schemes have shown them to be

citizens from obtaining adequate health care protection. For without good health, no man can fully utilize his other opportunities." President Nixon's "Health–A Message from the President of the United States Relative to Building a National Health Strategy," 92d Congress, 1st Session, House Document No. 92-49, February 18, 1971, p. 2.

largely deficient, vain attempts at partial solutions to dimly perceived problems.

Some promising approaches have recently begun. The detailed analyses of case mix and its relationship to hospital characteristics, pioneered by Martin Feldstein and refined by Lave and Lave, and Rafferty, and Dowling, sometimes to the point of precise diagnostic specification, indicate the fruitfulness of so specifying hospital outputs, in the inpatient categories, for purposes of cost analysis. This approach should be expanded by incorporating into the specifically recognized output set the output dimensions we specify in chapter 2, especially ambulatory care. This might well be attempted by using a formulation similar to Kovner's to identify and weight its individual medical procedures. None of the analysts, however, have given sufficient attention to a complete specification of all relevant output dimensions, including medical quality and patient satisfaction. If services flowing to patients in diagnostic categories are conceived to be the relevant outputs, as they should be, the application of quality scalars as developed by Payne, the Yale studies, and elsewhere, should be incorporated into the economic analyses.

Using the well-defined output measures which now appear to be methodologically feasible and conceptually satisfying, there needs to be much greater effort devoted to the identification of the engineering production functions, their interrelations within the various hospital departments, and the implied cost patterns. The seemingly endless search for economies of scale appears to be a quixotic attempt to identify certain aspects of cost behavior without being able to identify what is produced, what should be produced and for whom. Since for reorganization and planning functions one would wish to know what scale of hospital operations yield the greatest economies, we should be first concerned with identifying just what the "hospital" is, what functions it performs where, for whom, and how those multiples of functions can best be integrated in an economically efficient organization. Once again, expansion into the many areas of hospital functions of the refined case mix approach to output identification is a prerequisite.

The pathbreaking conceptual reformulation of demand theory by Lancaster is a good place to begin thinking anew about what "demand" for medical care really constitutes. There is minimally a five element demand set, which we show in chapter 6 to be related to multiple and possibly conflicting demand determinants. Both conceptual work and empirical analyses incorporating the findings of learning behavior will have to be done before we can with any degree of certainty predict expected demand reactions to price and income changes. Current attempts, with the exception of Andersen and Benham, to identify price and income elasticities fail both because the demand determinants are inadequately identified and because the quantity measures are replaced by expenditure proxies. The role of the physician in demand determination is sometimes recognized, as we have seen, but seldom placed in that central locus we suggest is its proper place.

Though some recent work by Lee, M. Feldstein, and Newhouse provide some beginnings, one of our major conclusions must be that nothing is known about what hospitals conceive as their objective function and how this relates to what the community, or larger society would wish. Given the complete absence of a meaningful specification of objectives at the institutional and societal levels, it is not surprising that efficiency appears as a chimera, or as salvation, which we all define differently, none of us know how to measure, all seek, but none can achieve. A new approach is required; an approach which takes well-defined outputs and weighs them by a revealed social preference function, though more revealed than that used by at least one student in the past, and relates them to identified production functions. This would enable us to identify organizational efficiency. Social efficiency must be measured in terms of social costs, and benefits, and since market prices do not reflect these, recourse must be had both to the process analysis we suggest and to the development of imputed costs.

There are two other fundamental shortcomings exhibited by all of the studies in the field, one conceptual and the other attitudinal. The basic conceptual fault stems from the view of the hospital as an isolated unit. While production and cost functions can be adequately analyzed in a microscopic slice from the complex system of simultaneous interdependencies that the medical care sector represents, the questions revolving around demand formation, organizational and social efficiency, alternative institutional arrangements, desirable pricing strategies, incentive schemes, the role of insurance, and other economically interesting issues do not yield to an approach which abstracts from the overwhelming realities.

We have seen that with a few exceptions even the interdependencies within the hospital as the unit of analysis are not recognized, much less its relation to the rest of the medical care sector in terms of alternative sources of care, physician referral patterns, the role of admitting privileges and staff appointments, the use of emergency rooms as weekend extensions of the private office, the differential impacts of selective, partial insurance coverage, multiple objectives expressed within the hospital and by its several external constituencies, all of them factors which, like umbilicals of steel, bind the hospital to the rest of the system. The fact that reliable data do not readily exist to estimate the parameters and variables of such a complex interdependent model should not prevent the initiation of the analytic effort required to construct it.

The attitudinal fault, in our view, is the disregard of the human realities underlying the abstractions of a system which, as we have stressed, does deal in torn flesh and broken bones and misery, suffering, and death. Thus the cavalier treatment of quality and "quality variations."

This brings us to the issue of why the current state of the literature can be reasonably characterized as one of chaotic ignorance with a few rays of light. There is a prevalence of ad hoc theorizing upon conclusions derived by often sloppy methodology from bad data; alternatively, there are numerous cases of empty theoretical gymnastics used to rationalize the application of sophisticated methodology to admittedly inappropriate data, only to yield conclusions which even their authors smother in the protecting shield of caveats.

Why such a state of affairs? Consider the insights of Mack:

But just as real as any bias in data gathering are those biases which are theoretical and substantive: pressures which influence the selection of a research problem, the formulation of a research design, and the interpretation of data. I want to address several of these biases:

1. Ethnocentricism, including the aggrandizement effect;
2. Tool bias, or problem selection on the basis of tool availability;
3. Fiduciary drift, or monetary magnetism in problem selection;
4. The debunking bias, or gee-whiz approach to social science;
5. Theory-shyness, or the false modesty cop-out; and
6. Theoretical inefficiency: labels and nonvariable frames of reference. (Mack, 263, p. 53-54)

To this list of biases, or variables, must be added one more: the facility factor as the basis of academic rewards. Theoretical and/or methodological facility, particularly when applied to data manipulation, yields publishable articles which both demonstrate the sought after abilities and reward their perpetrators. That the studies, analyses, investigations, research reports, while ad hoc, limited in scope and range, spasmodic, unrelated to previous and/or parallel efforts and hence noncumulative, of limited or no generalizability, touch empirical reality at best tangentially, matters not. In the reality of phenomenologically empty but elegant theory the name of the game is acrobatics and as with all acrobats, the further away the feet from the ground, the higher up in the air the abstractions, the better the performance. But as acrobats are nurtured and rewarded, so the current academic setting encourages the most nimble of its denizens to demonstrate the skills that bring the rewards.

It is now clear that there are a number of students of the field who, while capable of performing on the rings, are doing the legwork of conceptual and empirical analysis required to address the major issues. What is needed is good theory building and large-scale cooperative empirical research, on agreed upon issues, in an environment that encourages careful, detailed, long-term studies on specified problems. Academic institutions with their multiple demands do not appear to be well suited for this purpose. The medical care field does not have its own RAND, or Brookings. It should.

It is not our function here to outline in detail the organizational characteristics of such a research organization. But four major characteristics that such an organization should have to facilitate the successful implementation of meaningful research must be considered: (1) It must be large enough to provide a minimum critical mass. One principal investigator and two research associates along with a cadre of research assistants, the present mode of operation, is not enough. (2) Theoretic work and the related empirical research as well as other methodological approaches such as simulation (for example of physician decision making) should be focused on prespecified (policy relevant) problems. The theoretic and research problems should be identified with a view to understanding empirical, social, operating problems and issues, and not with the principal objective of expanding the core theory of any social science discipline. The major goal, that is, should be applied theory and applied research. (3) The program should be long term, with the key personnel making a long-term and full-time commitment to the objectives. (4) Protection against insularity, dogmatism, and careerism can be provided by various methods, among them periodic changes of leadership, one to two year visiting appointments to promising scholars *and* to field experienced administrators and policy makers.

The cost of such a major undertaking would not exceed that of the "multidisciplinary" Health Services Research Centers established some five years ago by the National Center for Health Services Research and Development. The results could not be fewer.

It is de rigueur to conclude with "more research is indicated." And that is certainly accurate in the whole field of medical care and especially in the case of hospital economics. But none of what we have said should be taken to denote or to suggest that solutions to all the problems we have pointed to must await prior research findings. Many of the most fundamental problems, those which plague the urban governmental hospitals in particular, are known, are there to be seen, are understood, documented in tons of reports. They should not be exploited for purposes of "research." They should be solved. But the solution constraints are not strictly economic factors: they are the professional jealousies, the national and local politics, the racism, and the poverty that countenance and fester the urban mess. Economists and economic analyses are not likely to shed much light on the solutions. But then, consider the alternatives.

References

References

Abbreviations frequently used

A.E.R. *American Economic Review*
A.J.P.H. *American Journal of Public Health*
H.S.R. *Health Services Research*
MMFQ *Milbank Memorial Fund Quarterly*

1. *A Decade of Change in U.S. Hospitals, 1953-63.* A Study Comparing Utilization, Staffing and Cost Trends in Civilian and CONUS Army Hospitals. Washington, D.C.: Office of the Surgeon General, D.O.A. May 1965.

2. *A National Program to Conquer Heart Disease, Cancer and Stroke*, vol. II, Report to the President, The President's Commission on Heart Disease, Cancer and Stroke. Washington, D.C., 1965.

3. *A Program For Research in Health Economics.* Health Economics Series No. 7. (By H.M. Somers and A.R. Somers) Washington, D.C.: U.S. Dept. of H.E.W., P.H.S., 1967.

4. *A Study of Operating Costs in 199 Hospitals, 1965-66.* Springfield, Illinois: State of Illinois, Dept. of Public Health, n.d.

5. Abbott, M., and Alkane, J.F. "Transport of Intrathecal I 125 RISA To Circulating Plasma." *Neurology*, Sept. 1968, pp. 870-74.

6. Abel-Smith, B. *Paying for Health Services.* Geneva: Public Health Papers 17, World Health Organization, 1963.

7. ——— *An International Study of Health Expenditure.* Geneva: Public Health Papers 32, World Health Organization, 1967.

8. *Cost Finding For Hospitals.* Chicago: American Hospital Association, 1957.

9. American Medical Association. *Report of the Commission on the Cost of Medical Care*, vol. 4. *Changing Patterns of Hospital Care.* Chicago, Ill.: A.M.A., 1964.

10. Andersen, R. *A Behavioral Model of Families' Use of Health Services.* Research Series 25. Chicago: Center For Health Administration Studies, 1968.

11. Andersen, Ronald, and Benham, Lee. "Factors Affecting the Relationship Between Family Income and Medical Care Consumption." In Herbert E. Klarman (ed.) with assistance of Helen H. Jaszi, *Empirical Studies in Health Economics*, Proceedings of the Second Conference on the Economics of Health. Baltimore, Md.: The Johns Hopkins Press, 1970, pp. 73-95.

12. Andersen, R., and Hull, J.T. "Hospital Utilization and Cost Trends in Canada and the United States." *H.S.R.*, Fall 1969, pp. 198-222.

13. Andersen, R., and Anderson, O.W. *A Decade of Health Services.* Chicago: University of Chicago Press, 1967.

14. Anderson, O.W. "Two Surveys Show Trends in U.S. Hospital Charges." *Hospitals*, May 16, 1962, p. 35.

15. _____ "Research in Hospital Use and Expenditures." *J. Chronic. Dis.*, Sept. 1964, pp. 727-33.

16. _____ *Health Services in a Land of Plenty*. Health Administration Perspectives Number A7. Chicago: Center for Health Administration Studies, 1968.

17. Anderson, O.W., and Neuhauser, D. "Rising Costs Are Inherent in Modern Health Care Systems." *Hospitals, J.A.H.A.*, Feb. 16, 1969, p. 50.

18. Anderson, O.W., and Sheatsley, P.B. *Hospital Use–A Survey of Patient and Physician Decisions*. Center for Health Administration Studies, Research Series 24, 1967.

19. Apple, D. (ed.) *Sociological Studies of Health and Sickness*. New York: McGraw-Hill Book Co., Inc., 1960.

20. Archibald, G.C. "Profit-Maximizing and Non-Price Competition." *Economica,* N.S., February 1964, pp. 13-22.

21. *Areawide Planning For Hospitals and Health Related Facilities*. P.H.S. Publication No. 855. Washington, D.C.: U.S. Dept. of H.E.W., 1961.

22. Arrow, K.J. "Uncertainty and the Welfare Economics of Medical Care." *A.E.R.*, Dec. 1963, pp. 941-73.

23. _____ "Public and Private Values." In S. Hook (ed.) *Human Values and Economic Policy*. New York: New York University Press, 1967, pp. 3-21.

24. _____ "The Economics of Moral Hazard: Further Comment." *A.E.R.*, June 1968, pp. 537-38.

25. Auster, Richard; Leveson, Irving; and Sarachek, Deborah. "The Production of Health, an Exploratory Study." *The Journal of Human Resources* 4, 4 (Fall 1969): 411-36.

26. Babnew, D., Jr. "Can the Profit-Motivated Center Stop the Medical Cost Spiral." *Hospital Management* 108 (August 1969): 40-44.

27. Bailey, R.M. "An Economist's View of the Health Services Industry." *Inquiry*, March 1969, p. 3.

28. _____ "Economies of Scale in Medical Practice." In Herbert E. Klarman (ed.) with assistance of Helen H. Jaszi. *Empirical Studies in Health Economics*, Proceedings of the Second Conference on the Economics of Health. Baltimore, Md.: The Johns Hopkins Press, 1970, pp. 255-73.

29. _____ "Philosophy, Faith, Fact and Fiction in the Production of Medical Services." *Inquiry* 8, 1 (March 1970): 37-53.

30. _____ "Potential Economies in Medical Practice." Resource Paper for Discussion Group A-4, AMA National Congress on Health Manpower, October 22-24, 1970, Chicago, Illinois.

31. Bain, J.S. *Industrial Organization*. New York: Wiley, 1959.

32. Baird, Charles W. "A Market Solution to Medical Inflation: A Reply." *Journal of Human Resources* 6, 1 (Winter 1971): 125-29.

33. Baligh, H.H., and Laughhunn, D.J. "An Economic and Linear Model of the Hospital." *Health Services Research* 4 (Winter 1971): 293-303.

34. Barr, A. "Value For Money In Hospitals." *Lancet*, Feb. 17, 1968, pp. 353-55.

35. Barzel, Yoram. "Productivity and the Price of Medical Services." *Journal of Political Economy* 77, 6 (November/December 1969): 1014-27.

36. Bator, F.M. "The Simple Analytics of Welfare Maximization." *A.E.R.*, March 1957, pp. 22-59.

37. Baum, Allyn Z. "ER Patients: How Many Are Yours?" *Medical Economics*, August 5, 1968, pp. 100-105.

38. Baumol, W.J. *Welfare Economics and the Theory of the State*. 2nd ed. Cambridge, Mass.: Harvard University Press, 1965.

39. ______"Macroeconomics of Unbalanced Growth: The Anatomy of Urban Crisis." *A.E.R.*, June 1967, pp. 415-26.

40. ______"Reasonable Rules for Rate Regulation: Plausible Policies for an Imperfect World." In A. Phillips, and O.E. Williamson (eds.) *Prices: Issues in Theory, Practice, and Public Policy*. Philadelphia: University of Pennsylvania Press, 1967, pp. 108-23.

41. Baumol, W.J., and Bowen, W.G. "On the Performing Arts: The Anatomy of Their Economic Problems." *A.E.R.*, May 1965, pp. 495-502.

42. Baumol, W.J., and Bradford, David F. "Optimal Departures from Marginal Cost Pricing." *A.E.R.* 60, 3 (June 1970): 265-83.

43. Beesley, M.E. "The Value of Time Spent in Traveling: Some New Evidence." *Economica,* N.S., May 1965, pp. 174-85.

44. Bellin, S.S.; Geiger, H.J.; and Gibson, Count D. "Impact of Ambulatory-Health-Care Services on the Demand for Hospital Beds." *The New England Journal of Medicine* 280, 15 (April 10, 1969): 808-12.

45. Bernstein, Betty J. "What Happened to 'Ghetto Medicine' in New York State?" *American Journal of Public Health* 61, 7 (July 1971): 1287-93.

46. Berry, R.E. "Returns to Scale in the Production of Hospital Services." *H.S.R.*, Summer 1967, pp. 123-39.

47.____"Product Heterogeneity and Hospital Cost Analysis." *Inquiry* 7, 1 (March 1970): 67-75.

48. Bice, Thomas W.; and White, Kerr L. "Cross-National Comparative Research on the Utilization of Medical Services." *Medical Care* 9, 3 (May-June 1971): 253-71.

49. Black, G. "The Effect of Government Funding on Commercial R and D." In W.H. Gruber and D.G. Marquis (eds.) *Factors in the Transfer of Technology*. Cambridge, Mass.: The M.I.T. Press, 1969.

50. Block, Louis. "Proprietary Hospitals–Threat or Challenge." *Hospital Progress* 51 (June 1970): 61-63.

51. Blumberg, M.S. " 'DPF' Concept Helps Predict Bed Needs." *The Modern Hospital*, December 1961, p. 75.

52. Boan, J.A. *Group Practice*. Ottawa, Canada: Royal Commission on Health Services, 1966.

53. Boulding, K.E. "The Concept of Need for Health Services." *M.M.F.Q.*, October 1966, Part 2, pp. 202-21.

54. Breslow, Lester. "Role of the Public Hospital." *Hospitals* 44, 13 (July 1, 1970): 44-46.

55. Breslow, Lester, and Klein, Bonnie. "Health and Race in California." *A.J.P.H.* 61, 4 (April 1971): 763-75.

56. Brissenden, Robert W., and Lennard, Henry L. "Hospitals as 'Family Physician'." *Hospitals* 44 (May 16, 1970): 55-57.

57. Brown, Douglas R., and Chester, Theodore E. "Hospital Planning in Practice: A Cross National Study." *Hospital Administration*, Fall 1969, pp. 99-113.

58. Brown, R.E. "Let the Public Control Utilization Through Planning." *Hospitals*, December 1, 1959, p. 34 ff.

59. ______ "The Health Care Facilities System: Influences on Facility Construction Costs." In *Costs of Health Care Facilities*. Report of a Conference Convened by the National Academy of Engineering, National Academy of Sciences, Washington, 1968, pp. 57-65.

60. _____ "The Public Hospital." *Hospitals* 44, 13 (July 1, 1970): 40-43.

61. _____ "The New Pressures Will Be Social, Not Technical." *Modern Hospital* 117, 2 (August 1971): 111-14.

62. Bugbee, G. et al. "Panel Discussion: Organizing the Hospital for Care of the Poor." *Inquiry*, March 1968, Special Issue, pp. 49-64.

63. Bugbee, George (ed.). *Urban Community Hospital in Transition*. Proceedings of the Twelfth Annual Symposium on Hospital Affairs, April 1970, Conducted by the Graduate Program in Hospital Administration and Center for Health Administration Studies, Graduate School of Business, University of Chicago.

64. Bunker, J.P. "Surgical Manpower: A Comparison of Operations and Surgeons in the United States and in England and Wales." *New Eng. Jour. Med.*, Jan. 15, 1970, pp. 135-44.

65. Burlage, R.K. *New York City's Municipal Hospitals: A Policy Review*. Washington, D.C.: Institute for Policy Studies, 1967.

66. ______ "The Municipal Hospital Affiliation Plan in New York City. A Case Study and Critique." *M.M.F.Q.*, v. 46, Supplement, January 1968, pp. 171-201.

67. Burns, E. *Social Policy and the Health Services: The Choices Ahead*. 6th Bronfman Lecture, A.P.H.A., 1967.

68. Butter, I. "Health Manpower Research: A Survey." *Inquiry*, Dec. 1967, pp. 5-41.

69. Callahan, P.H., and Kabat, H.F. "Experiences with a Bid System of Purchasing in a Private Hospital." *Am. Jour. Hosp. Pharm.*, August 1965, p. 471.

70. Campbell, T.J. *Program Cost Allocation in Seven Medical Centers: A Pilot Study*. Association of American Medical Colleges, 1969.

71. Cardwell, R.L.; Reid, M.G.; and Shain, M. "Hospital Utilization in a Major Metropolitan Area." Chicago: Hospital Planning Council for Metropolitan Chicago, 1964.

72. Carlova, John. "The Widening E.R. Crisis." *Medical Economics*, January 4, 1971, pp. 97-155.

73. Carr, W. John. "Central Planning vs. Evolutionary Development." In Herbert E. Klarman (ed.) with assistance of Helen H. Jaszi. *Empirical Studies in Health Economics*. Proceedings of the Second Conference on the Economics of Health. Baltimore and London: The Johns Hopkins Press, 1970, pp. 195-221.

74. Carr, W.J., and Feldstein, P.J. "The Relationship of Cost to Hospital Size." *Inquiry*, June 1967, pp. 45-65.

75. Carroll, A.J. *Program Cost Estimating in a Teaching Hospital: A Pilot Study*. Association of American Medical Colleges, 1969.

76. Cherkasky, Martin. "The Hospital as a Social Instrument: Recent Experiences at Montefiore Hospital." In John H. Knowles (ed.) *Hospitals, Doctors, and the Public Interest*. Cambridge, Mass.: Harvard University Press, 1965, pp. 93-110.

77. Chiang, C.L. *An Index of Health: Mathematical Models*. N.C.H.S. Series 2, No. 5. Washington, D.C.: U.S. Dept. of H.E.W., P.H.S., 1965.

78. Christ, C.F. *Econometric Models and Methods*. New York: Wiley, 1966.

79. Ciriacy-Wanthrup, S.V. "Water Policy and Economic Optimizing: Some Conceptual Problems in Water Research." *A.E.R.*, May 1967, pp. 179-89.

80. Coase, R.H. "The Problem of Social Cost." *Jour. Law. and Econ.*, October 1960, pp. 1-44.

81. ——"The Theory of Public Utility Pricing and Its Application." *The Bell Journal of Economics and Management Science* 1, 1 (Spring 1970): 113-28.

82. Codman, E.A. "The Product of a Hospital." *Surgery, Gynecology and Obstetrics*. Jan.-June 1914, pp. 491-96.

83. Coe, R.M.; Friedman, E.A.; et al. "The Impact of Medicare on the Utilization and Provision of Health Care Facilities." *Inquiry*, December 1967, p. 42.

84. Cohen, H.A. "Variations in Cost Among Hospitals of Different Sizes." Paper presented at the Southern Economic Association Meeting, Nov. 12, 1965. Published in *Southern Econ. Jour.*, Jan. 1967, p. 355.

85. ——"Costs and Efficiency: A Study of Short-Term General Hospitals." Ph.D. dissertation, Cornell University, 1967.

86. ——"Hospital Cost Curves with Emphasis on Measuring Patient Care Output." Paper delivered at the Second Conference on the Economics of Health. Subsequently published in Herbert E. Klarman (ed.) with assistance of Helen H. Jaszi. *Empirical Studies in Health Economics*. Proceedings of the Second Conference on the Economics of Health. Baltimore, Md.: The Johns Hopkins Press, 1970, pp. 279-93.

87. Colman, J.D. "An Analysis of the Components of Rising Costs." In *Report of the National Conference on Medical Costs*. Washington, D.C.: U.S. Dept. of H.E.W., pp. 91-133.

88. Colombo, T.J.; Saward, E.W.; and Greenlick, M.R. "The Integration of an OEO Health Program Into a Prepaid Comprehensive Group Practice Plan." *A.J.P.H.*, April 1969, pp. 642-50.

89. *Comprehensive Health Planning, A Selected Annotated Bibliography*. P.H.S. Publication No. 1753. Washington, D.C.: U.S. Dept. of H.E.W., 1968.

90. *Conference on Research in Hospital Use*. Report and Proceedings of a Conference Sponsored by the American Hospital Association and the Public Health Service. Hospital and Medical Facilities Series. Washington, D.C.: U.S. Dept. of H.E.W., P.H.S., 1963.

91. *Costs of Health Care Facilities*. Washington, D.C.: National Academy of Sciences, 1968.

92. Coughlin, R.E. "Hospital Complex Analysis: An Approach To Analysis and Planning a Metropolitan System of Service Facilities." Ph.D. dissertation, University of Pennsylvania, 1965.

93. Cowling, Keith, and Rayner, A.J. "Price, Quality, and Market Share." *Journal of Political Economy* 78, 6 (November/December 1970): 1292-1309.

94. Cruikshank, Nelson H. "Delivery of Health Care: Do We Know Where We Are Going? Comment." In George F. Rohrlich (ed.) *Social Economics for the 1970's*. Cambridge: University Press of Cambridge, Mass. and New York: The Dunellen Company, Inc., 1970, pp. 131-41.

95. Dahlgren, T.E. "Six Hospitals Share a Central Laboratory–And Save Money." *Modern Hospital* 112 (April 1969): 92-93.

96. Daniels, Robert S. "Physician Productivity and the Hospital: A Physician's View." *Inquiry* 6 (September 1969): 70-78.

97. Darley, W., and Somers, A.R. "Medicine, Money and Manpower–The Challenge to Professional Education. I. The Affluent New Health-Care Economy." *New Eng. J. Med.*, June 1, 1967, pp. 1234-38.

98. Davis, Karen. "Net Income of Hospitals 1961-1969." U.S. Dept. of H.E.W., Social Security Administration, Office of Research and Statistics, Staff Paper No. 6, 1970.

99. ______ "Impact of Cost Reimbursement Schemes on Hospital Costs." Social Security Administration, January 1971.

100. ______ "Economic Theories of Behavior in Nonprofit, Private Hospitals." Washington, D.C.: The Brookings Institute, February 1971.

101. ______ "Relationship of Hospital Prices to Costs." Brookings Economic Policy Fellow, 1970. *Applied Economics*, June 1971.

102. Davis, Karen, and Russell, Louise B. "The Demand for Hospital Outpatient Services." U.S. Dept. of H.E.W., Social Security Administration, Office of Research and Statistics, n.d.

103. ______ "The Substitution of Hospital Outpatient Care for Inpatient Care." Social Security Administration, December 1970.

104. De Geyndt, Willy. "Five Approaches for Assessing the Quality of Care." *Hospital Administration* 15 (Winter 1970): 21-42.

105. Deland, E.C.; Raub, W.F.; Stacy, R.W.; and Waxman, B.D. "Computers and the Delivery of Medical Care." Santa Monica: The RAND Corporation, P-4019, February 1969.

106. Deland, E.C., and Waxman, Bruce. "Technological Opportunities for the Delivery of Health Care." Santa Monica: The RAND Corporation, P-3947, October 1968.

107. *Delivery of Health Services for the Poor*. Program Analysis 1967-12, Human Investment Programs. Washington, D.C.: U.S. Dept. of H.E.W., Office of the Asst. Sec. Planning and Evaluation, December 1967.

108. Denison, E.F. *The Sources of Economic Growth in the United States*. New York: the Committee for Economic Development, 1962.

109. Densen, P.; Greene, D.; and Moskowitz, R. "Primary Medical Care for an Urban Population–A Survey of Present and Potential Utilization." *J. Med. Educ.*, December 1968, pp. 1244-49.

110. Densen, P.M.; Jones, E.W.; et al. "Prepaid Medical Care and Hospital Utilization in a Dual Choice Situation." *A.J.P.H.*, Nov. 1960, pp. 1710-26.

111. Densen, P.M.; Jones, E.W.; and Baldinger, I. "Prepaid Medical Care and Hospital Utilization." *Hospitals*, Nov. 16, 1962.

112. *Differentials in Health Characteristics by Color*. Vital and Health Statistics, Data from the National Health Survey, National Center for Health Statistics, Series 10, No. 56, Washington, D.C., October 1969.

113. *Disease Control Programs: Arthritis*. Program Analysis 1966-4. Washington, D.C.: H.E.W., Office of Asst. Sec. for Program Control, 1966.

114. *Disease Control Programs: Cancer*. Program Analysis 1966-3. Washington, D.C.: H.E.W., Office of Assistant Sec. for Program Coordination, 1966.

115. Donabedian, A. *A Review of Some Experience with Prepaid Group Practice*. Bureau of Public Health Economics Research Series No. 12. School of Public Health. Ann Arbor: University of Michigan, 1965.

116. ______ "Evaluating the Quality of Medical Care." *M.M.F.Q.*, July 1966, Part 2, pp. 166-203.

117. ______ "The Nature and Magnitude of Need and Unmet Need in Medical Care." In *Institute on Planning and Administration of Nursing Service in Medical Care Programs–Selected Papers*. Continuing Education Service, School of Public Health. Ann Arbor: University of Michigan, 1968, pp. 1-21.

118. ______ "An Evaluation of Prepaid Group Practice." *Inquiry*, Sept. 1969, pp. 17-27.

119. ______ *A Guide to Medical Care Administration, Vol. II: Medical Care Appraisal*. New York: American Public Health Association, 1969.

120. Dowling, William Laine. *A Linear Programming Approach to the*

Analysis of Hospital Production. Ph.D. dissertation, University of Michigan, 1970.

121. Ehrenreich, J.W. "Creating Competition in the Health Care Industry: Possible Impacts of Major Group Purchasers on Costs and Quality of Health Care." In *Private Health Insurance and Health Care*. Washington, D.C.: U.S. Dept. of H.E.W., S.S.A., O.R.S., 1968, p. 1.

122. Elliott, F.N. "Goals for Quality Must be Based on Values of Society." *Modern Hospital* 117, 2 (August 1971): 107-10.

123. Ellwood, Paul M., Jr. "Concept and Strategy." *Hospitals* 45, 6 (March 16, 1971): 53-56.

124. Ellwood, Paul M., and Hoagberg, Earl J. "Problems of the Public Hospital." *Hospitals* 44, 13 (July 1, 1970): pp. 47-52.

125. Ennes, Howard. "Delivery of Health Care: Do We Know Where We are Going? Comment." In George F. Rohrlich (ed.) *Social Economics for the 1970's*. Cambridge: University Press of Cambridge, Mass. and New York: The Dunellen Publishing Co., Inc., 1970, p. 114.

126. Erba, G., and Lombroso, C.T. "Detection of Ventricular Landmarks by Two Dimensional Ultrasonography." *J. Neurol. Neurosurg. Psychiat.* 31 (1968): 232-44.

127. Fahs, Ivan J.; Choi, Thomas; Barchas, Kathryn; and Zakariasen, Paula. "Indicators of Need for Health Care Personnel: The Concept of Need, Alternative Measures Employed to Determine Need, and a Suggested Model." *Medical Care* 9, 2 (March-April 1971): 144-51.

128. Falk, I.S.; Schoenfeld, H.K.; et al. "The Development of Standards for the Audit and Planning of Medical Care 1. Concepts, Research Design, and the Content of Primary Physician's Care." *A.J.P.H.*, July 1967, pp. 1118-36.

129. Fanshel, S., and Bush, J.W. "A Health-Status Index and its Application to Health-Services Outcomes." *Operations Research* 18, 6 (November-December 1970): 1021-66.

130. Fein, Rashi. "An Economic Analysis of Variations in Medical Expenses and Work-Loss Rates: Comment." In Herbert E. Klarman (ed.) with assistance of Helen H. Jaszi. *Empirical Studies in Health Economics*. Proceedings of the Second Conference on the Economics of Health. Baltimore, Md.: The Johns Hopkins Press, 1970, pp. 141-44.

131. Feingold, E. *Medicare: Policy and Politics*. San Francisco: Chandler Publishing Co., 1966.

132. Feldstein, M.S. "Effects of Differences in Hospital Bed Scarcity on Type of Use." *Brit. Med. Jour.*, August 29, 1964, pp. 561-64.

133.______ *Economic Analysis for Health Service Efficiency*. Chicago: Markham Publishing Co., 1968.

134.______"Discussion." In V.R. Fuchs (ed.) *Production and Productivity in the Service Industries.* New York: National Bureau of Economic Research, 1969, pp. 139-46.

135.______"Hospital Cost Inflation: A Study of Nonprofit Price Dynamics."

Cambridge, Mass.: Harvard Institute of Economic Research, Harvard University, Discussion Paper Number 139, October 1970.

136. Feldstein, Paul J. *Prepaid Group Practice: An Analysis and Review*. Bureau of Hospital Administration, School of Public Health. Ann Arbor, Michigan: The University of Michigan, June 1971.

137. Feldstein, P.J. "A Proposal for Capitation Reimbursement to Medical Groups for Total Medical Care." *Reimbursement Incentives for Hospital and Medical Care*, U.S. Dept. of H.E.W., S.S.A., Research Report No. 26. Washington, D.C., 1968, pp. 61-72.

137a. ______"An Analysis of Reimbursement Plans." *Reimbursement Incentives for Hospital and Medical Care*, U.S. Dept. of H.E.W., S.S.A., Research Report No. 26. Washington, D.C., 1968, pp. 17-38.

138. ______"Research on the Demand for Health Services." *M.M.F.Q.* July 1966, part 2, pp. 128-65.

139. ______*An Empirical Investigation of the Marginal Cost of Hospital Services*. Studies in Hospital Administration, Graduate Program in Hospital Administration. Chicago: University of Chicago, 1961.

140. Feldstein, P.J., and Carr, W.J. "The Effect of Income on Medical Care Spending." Paper delivered at the meeting of the American Statistical Association, December, 1964. Published in abbreviated form, *Jour. Am. Stat. Assoc., Proceedings*, Dec. 1964.

141. Feldstein, P.J., and German, J.J. "Predicting Hospital Utilization: An Evaluation of Three Approaches." *Inquiry*, June, 1965, pp. 13-36.

142. Feldstein, P.J., and Waldman, S. "Financial Position of Hospitals in the Early Medicare Period." *Social Security Bulletin*, Oct., 1968, pp. 18-23.

143. ______"The Financial Position of Hospitals in the First Two Years of Medicare." *Inquiry*, Mar. 1969, pp. 19-27.

144. Ferber, B. "The Relationship of Multiple Health Insurance Coverage and Hospital Utilization." *Inquiry*, Dec. 1966, pp. 14-27.

145. ______"An Analysis of Chain-Operated For-Profit Hospitals." *H.S.R.* 6,1 (Spring 1971): 49-60.

146. Fitzpatrick, T.B.; Riedel, D.C.; and Payne, B.C. "Character and Effectiveness of Hospital Use." In W.J. McNerney, *Hospital and Medical Economics*, Vol. 1. Chicago: Hospital Research and Educational Trust, 1962, pp. 361-588.

147. ______"Changing Patterns of Care." In W.J. McNerney, *Hospital and Medical Economics*, Vol. 1. Chicago: Hospital Research and Educational Trust, 1962.

148. Fitzpatrick, T.B.; Riedel, D.C.; Payne, B.C.; Hill, L.A.; and Grenholm, G.G. *Changing Patterns of Hospital Care*. Report of the Commission on the Cost of Medical Care, Vol. 4. Chicago: American Medical Association, 1964.

149. Foyle, W.F. "Accounting and Finance." In W.J. McNerney, *Hospital and Medical Economics*, Vol. II. Chicago: Hospital Research and Educational Trust, 1962.

150. Francisco, Edgar W. "Analysis of Cost Variations Among Short-Term General Hospitals." In Herbert E. Klarman (ed.) with assistance of Helen H.

Jaszi. *Empirical Studies in Health Economics*. Proceedings of the Second Conference on the Economics of Health. Baltimore and London: The Johns Hopkins Press, 1970, pp. 321-32.

151. Freeman, A.J., III. "Income Distribution and Planning for Social Investment." *A.E.R.*, June, 1967, pp. 495-508.

152. Freidson, E. (ed.) *The Hospital in Modern Society*. New York: The Free Press, 1963.

153. Friedman, J.W. "Multiple Determinants of Hospital Programs." *Soc. Sci. & Med.* 3 (1969): 49-62.

154. Friedman, M. "Comment." *Business Concentration and Price Policy*. Princeton: Princeton University Press, 1955, pp. 230-38.

155. Fry, J. "Operations Research in General Clinical Practice." *J. Chronic Dis*, Sept. 1964, pp. 803-13.

156. Fuchs, Victor R. "Hospital Services: Comment." In Herbert E. Klarman (ed.) with assistance of Helen H. Jaszi. *Empirical Studies in Health Economics*. Proceedings of the Second Conference on the Economics of Health. Baltimore and London: The Johns Hopkins Press, 1970, pp. 118-20.

157. ______ "Let's Make Volkswagen Medicine Compulsory." Interview in *Medical Economics*, Nov. 10, 1969, p. 110 ff.

158. ______ ed. *Production and Productivity in the Service Industries*. Studies in Income and Wealth, Vol. 34. New York: N.B.E.R., 1969.

159. ______ *The Service Economy*. New York: N.B.E.R., 1968.

160. ______ "The Basic Forces Influencing Costs of Medical Care." In *Report of the National Conference on Medical Costs*. Washington, D.C.: U.S. Dept. of H.E.W., 1967, pp. 16-31.

161. ______ "The Role of Economics." In *Conference on Research in Hospital Use*, Report and Proceedings of a Conference Sponsored by the American Hospital Association and the Public Health Service. Hospital and Medical Facilities Series. Washington, D.C.: U.S. Dept. of H.E.W., P.H.S., 1963, pp. 74-75.

162. Gee, D.A. "Cost Factors in a Hospital-Based Home Care Program." *Inquiry*, Oct. 1967, pp. 55-60.

163. Gerdes, J.W. "Anticipated Directions for the Future of Public General Hospitals." *A.J.P.H.*, Apr. 1969, pp. 680-88.

164. Gibson, Geoffrey. "Variations in the Delivery of Ambulatory Services by Urban Hospitals." In George Bugbee (ed.) *Urban Community Hospital in Transition*. Proceedings of the Twelfth Annual Symposium on Hospital Affairs, April 1970. Conducted by the Graduate Program in Hospital Administration and Center for Health Administration Studies, Graduate School of Business, University of Chicago.

165. Ginsburg, H. "Wage Differentials in Hospitals, 1956-1963: A Study Emphasizing the Wages of Nurses and Unskilled Workers in Nongovernmental Hospitals." Ph.D. dissertation, New School for Social Research, 1967.

166. Ginsburg, P. *Capital in Nonprofit Hospitals*. Ph.D. dissertation, Harvard University, 1970.

167. Glasser, Jay H. "The Selection of Statistical Techniques." In Merwyn R. Greenlick (ed.) *Conceptual Issues in the Analysis of Medical Care Utilization Behavior*. Dept. of H.E.W., Public Health Service, Hlth. Svcs. & Ment. Hlth. Admin., October, 1969, pp. 59-91.

168. Gold, E.M., and Stone, M.L. "Total Maternal and Infant Care: A Realistic Appraisal." *A.J.P.H.*, July, 1968, pp. 1219-29.

The Gorham Report–look under: *Medical Care Prices*. A Report to the President.

169. Gottlieb, M. "Discussion." *A.E.R.*, May, 1965, pp. 503-505.

170. Graff, J. deV. *Theoretical Welfare Economics*. Cambridge, Eng.: At the University Press 1957.

171. Greenberg, Ira G., and Rodburg, Michael L. "The Role of Prepaid Group Practice in Relieving the Medical Care Crisis." *Harvard Law Review* 84, 4 (Feb. 1971): 887-1001.

172. Greenlick, M.R.; Hurtado, A.V.; et al. "Determinants of Medical Care Utilization." *H.S.R.*, Winter, 1968, pp. 296-315.

173. Griffith, J.R.; Weeks, L.E.; Sullivan, J.H. *The McPherson Experiment*. Ann Arbor: Bureau of Hospital Administration, University of Michigan 1967.

174. Grossman, M. *The Demand for Health: A Theoretical and Empirical Investigation*. Ph.D. dissertation, Columbia University, 1970.

175. Haldeman, Jack C. "The Impact on the Hospital." In George Bugbee (ed.) *Urban Community Hospital in Transition*. Proceedings of the Twelfth Annual Symposium on Hospital Affairs, April 1970, Conducted by the Graduate Program in Hospital Administration and Center for Health Administration Studies, Graduate School of Business, University of Chicago.

176. ______ "Elements of Progressive Patient Care." In L.E. Weeks and J.R. Griffith (eds.) *Progressive Patient Care*. Ann Arbor: University of Michigan 1964.

177. Hamilton, E.L. "The Voluntary Hospital in America: Its Role, Economics, and Internal Structure." pp. 393-405. In R.W. Scott, and E.H. Volkart (eds.) *Medical Care*. New York: Wiley 1966.

178. Hansen, W. Lee, "An Appraisal of Physician Manpower Projections." *Inquiry* 7, 1 (March 1970): 102-13.

179. Harris, Allyn R. "Mergers are Made to Add Service and Save Money–And They Do." *Modern Hospital* 114 (May 1970): 92-96.

180. Hartog, J.De. *The Hospital*. New York: Atheneum 1964.

181. Haughton, J.G. "Can the Poor Use the Present Health Care System?" *Inquiry*, March 1968, pp. 31-36.

182. Hayes, J.E. (ed.) *Factors Effecting the Cost of Hospital Care*. Vol. 1. New York: Commission on the Costs of Hospital Care, 1954.

183. *Health Care Delivery in the 1970's*. Report, Findings, and Recom-

mendations of the Subcommittee on Health Care Delivery of the Committee on Medical Economics, Health Insurance Association of America, Oct., 28, 1969.

184. *Health Planning: A Programmed Instruction Course*. B.H.S. Programmed Instruction Series No. 2, P.H.S. Bulletin No. 1846. Washington, D.C.: Dept of H.E.W., P.H.S., 1968.

185. *Health Planning, Problems of Concept and Method*. Scientific Publication No. 111. Washington, D.C.: Pan American Health Organization, 1965.

186. Hefty, T.R. "Returns to Scale in Hospitals–A Critical Review of Recent Research." *H.S.R.* 4 (Winter 1969): 267-80.

187. Hill, L.A. "Hospital Costs and Controls in Canada and the United States." *H.S.R.*, Fall, 1969, pp. 170-76.

188. Hirshleifer, J. "An Exposition of the Equilibrium of the Firm: Symmetry Between Product and Factor Analyses." *Economica*, N.S., Aug., 1962, pp. 163-68.

189. *Hospitals. J.A.H.A.* Guide Issue. August, continuing.

190. *Hospital Profiles, A Decade of Change, 1953-1962, Non-Federal, Short-Term, General Hospitals*. Hospital and Medical Facilities Series. Washington, D.C.: U.S. Dept. of H.E.W., P.H.S., 1964.

191. *How to Measure Ability to Pay for Social and Health Services*, rev. ed. New York: The Community Council of Greater New York, 1967.

192. Hurtado, Arnold V.; Greenlick, Merwyn R.; McCabe, Marilyn; and Saward, Ernest W. "The Utilization and Cost of Home Care and Extended Care Facility Services in a Comprehensive, Prepaid Group Practice Program." Paper presented at the 98th Annual Meeting of the American Public Health Association, Houston, Texas, October 28, 1970.

193. Hyman, Martin D. "Some Links Between Economic Status and Untreated Illness." *Social Science and Medicine* 4 (1970): 387-99.

194. *Increasing Productivity in the Delivery of Ambulatory Health Services*, Report UR-033. Bethesda, Md.: Resource Management Corporation, May, 1968.

195. Ingbar, M.L., and Taylor, L.D. *Hospital Costs in Massachusetts*. Cambridge, Mass.: Harvard University Press 1968.

196. *Intergovernmental Problems in MEDICAID*. Washington, D.C.: Advisory Commission on Intergovernmental Relations, 1968.

197. Jeffers, James R.; Bognanno, Mario F.; and Bartlett, John C. "On the Demand Versus Need for Medical Services and the Concept of 'Shortage'." *A.J.P.H.* 61, 1 (January 1971): 46-63.

198. Jelinek, R.C. "An Operational Analysis of the Patient Care Function." *Inquiry*, June, 1969, pp. 53-61.

199. Johnson, Everett A. "Physician Productivity and the Hospital: A Hospital Administrator's View." *Inquiry* 6 (September 1969): 59-69.

200. Johnson, E.T. "The Delivery of Health Care in the Ghetto." *J. Nat. Med. Ass.* 69 (May 1969): 263-70.

201. Johnson, R.L. "How to Make Competition Fair–Have the Same Rules for all Hospitals." *Modern Hospital*, 113 (December 1969): 104 ff.

202. Johnson, Walter L.; Rosenfeld, Leonard S.; and Fernow, L. Carol. "Professional and Socio-Demographic Factors which Influence the Hospital Appointment Status of Private Practitioners in New York City and Surrounding Counties." Presentation made at American Public Health Association Annual Meeting, Houston, Texas, October 26, 1970, Medical Care Section, Contributed Papers I.

203. Johnston, J. *Econometric Methods*. New York: McGraw-Hill 1963.

204. Kaitz, E.M. *Pricing Policy and Cost Behavior in the Hospital Industry*. New York: Praeger Publishers 1968.

205. Kelman, Sander. *Utilization of and Investment in U.S. Short-Term Hospitals*. Ph.D. dissertation, University of Michigan, 1970.

206. Kennedy, R.B. "The Price of People–Crucial Quantity in Hospital Costs." *J. Mississippi Med. Ass.*, Aug. 1967, pp. 495-500.

207. *Kidney Disease. Program Analysis*. P.H.S. Publication, No. 1745, Washington, D.C.: 1968.

208. Kisch, A.I., and Gartside, F.E. "Use of a County Hospital Outpatient Department by Medi-Cal Patients." *Medical Care*, Nov.-Dec. 1968, pp. 516-23.

209. Kissick, William L. "Delivery of Health Care: Do We Know Where We Are Going? Comment." In George F. Rohrlich (ed.) *Social Economics for the 1970's*. Cambridge: University Press of Cambridge, Mass. and New York: The Dunellen Publishing Co., Inc., 1970, p. 122.

210. Klarman, Herbert E. (ed.) with the assistance of Helen H. Jaszi. *Empirical Studies in Health Economics*. Baltimore, Maryland: The Johns Hopkins Press, 1970.

211. ________ "Increases in the Cost of Physician and Hospital Services." *Inquiry* 7, 1 (March 1970): 22-36.

212. ________ "Effect of Third-Party Methods of Reimbursement on Hospital Performance: Comment." In Herbert Klarman (ed.) with assistance of Helen H. Jaszi. *Empirical Studies in Health Economics*. Proceedings of the Second Conference on the Economics of Health. Baltimore and London: The Johns Hopkins Press, 1970, pp. 315-19.

213. Klarman, H.E.; Rice, D.P.; Cooper, B.S.; and Stettler, H. Louis III. "Source of Increase in Selected Medical Care Expenditures, 1929-1969," U.S. Dept. of H.E.W., Office of Research and Statistics, Staff Paper No. 4, April, 1970.

214. Klarman, H.E. "Approaches to Moderating the Increases in Medical Care Costs." *Medical Care*, May-June 1969, pp. 179-84.

215. ________ "Economic Aspects of Projecting Requirements for Health Manpower." *The Journal of Human Resources* 4, 3 (Summer 1969): 360-76.

216. ________ *The Economics of Health*. New York: Columbia University Press, 1965.

217. ________ "The Increased Cost of Hospital Care." *The Economics of Health and Medical Care*. Ann Arbor: The University of Michigan 1964, pp. 227-54.

218. Klarman, H.E. "Some Technical Problems in Areawide Planning for Hospital Care." *J. Chronic Dis.*, Sept., 1964, pp. 735-47.

219. ______ *Hospital Care in New York City*. New York: Columbia University Press 1963.

220. Knowles, John H. (ed.) *Hospitals, Doctors, and the Public Interest.* Cambridge, Massachusetts: Harvard University Press, 1965.

221. ______ "Radiology–A Case Study in Technology and Manpower." *New England Jour. of Medicine* 280 (June 5, 1969): 1271-78.

222. Koopmans, T.C. *Three Essays on the State of Economic Science*. New York: McGraw-Hill 1957.

223. Kovner, J.W. "Measurement of Outpatient Office Visit Services." *H.S.R.*, Summer, 1969, pp. 112-27.

224. Kovner, J.W.; Browne, L.B.; and Kisch, A.I. "Income and the Use of Outpatient Medical Care by the Insured." *Inquiry*, June, 1969, pp. 27-34.

225. Kravis, I.B. "Discussion." In V.R. Fuchs (ed.) *Production and Productivity in the Service Industries*. New York: N.B.E.R. 1969, pp. 84-93.

226. Kroeger, Hilda H.; Altman, Isidore; Clark, Dean A.; Johnson, Allen C.; and Sheps, Cecil G. "The Office Practice of Internists I. The Feasibility of Evaluating Quality of Care." Reprinted from the Journal of the American Medical Association, August 2, 1965, Vol. 193, No. 5, pp. 371-376, Graduate School of Public Health, University of Pittsburgh, Summer, 1965.

227. Kushner, J. "Returns to Scale in Hospitals: Comment." *H.S.R.* 5, 4 (Winter, 1970): 370-77.

228. Lamson, Robert D. "Measured Productivity and Price Change: Some Empirical Evidence on Service Industry Bias, Motion Picture Theaters." *Jour. of Political Economy* 78, 2 (March/April 1970): 291-305.

229. Lancaster, K.J. "A New Approach to Consumer Theory." *Jour. Political Economy*, Apr. 1966, pp. 132-57.

230. Larmore, M.L. *An Inquiry into an Econometric Production Function for Health in the United States.* Ph.D. dissertation, Northwestern University, 1967.

231. Lave, Judith R., and Lave, Lester B. "The Extent of Role Differentiation Among Hospitals." *H.S.R.* 6, 1 (Spring 1971): 15-38.

232. ______ "Hospital Cost Functions." *A.E.R.* 60, 3 (June 1970): 379-95.

233. Lave, J. "A Review of Methods Used to Study Hospital Costs." *Inquiry*, May, 1966, pp. 57-81.

234. Lave, J.R., and Lave, L.B. "Hospital Cost Functions: Estimating Cost Functions for Multiproduct Firms." Graduate School of Industrial Administration, Carnegie-Mellon University, Dec., 1968, (Xeroxed).

235. Layton, L.E. *Medical Care and Economic Security: A Study of Selected Foreign Programs.* Ph.D. dissertation, University of Minnesota, 1967.

236. Lee, Maw Lin. "A Conspicuous Production Theory of Hospital Behavior." Paper presented at the Conference of the Western Economic Association, August, 1970.

237. Lembcke, P.A. "Medical Auditing by Scientific Methods." *J.A.M.A.*, Oct. 13, 1956, pp. 646-55.

238. Leontief, Wassily. "Theoretical Assumptions and Nonobserved Facts." *A.E.R.* 61, 1 (March 1971): 1-7.

239. Lerner, M. "Mortality and Morbidity in the United States as Basic Indices of Health Needs." *Annals of the American Academy of Political and Social Sciences*, Sept. 1961, pp. 1-10.

240. ______ *Hospital Use by Diagnosis*. Health Information Foundation, Research Series 19, 1961.

241. Lerner, M., and Fitzgerald, S.W. "A Comparative Study of Three Major Forms of Health Care Coverage: A review." *Inquiry*, June 1965, pp. 37-60.

242. Lerner, R.C., and Kirchner, C. "Social and Economic Characteristics of Municipal Hospital Outpatients." *A.J.P.H.* 59 (January, 1969): 29-39.

243. ______ *Municipal General Hospital Outpatient Population Study: Social and Economic Characteristics of Patients in New York City Outpatient Departments, 1965*, Report No. 1, School of Public Health and Administrative Medicine. New York: Columbia University, June 1967.

244. Lerner, R.C.; Kirchner, C.; and Dieckman, E. *Municipal General Hospital Outpatient Population Study: Social and Economic Characteristics of Patients in New York City Outpatient Departments, 1965*, Report No. 2, School of Public Health and Administrative Medicine. New York: Columbia University, December 1967.

245. ______ *Municipal General Hospital Outpatient Population Study: Social and Economic Characteristics of Patients in New York City Outpatient Departments, 1965*, Report No. 3, School of Public Health and Administrative Medicine. New York: Columbia University, December 1967.

246. Leveson, Irving. "The Demand for Neighborhood Medical Care." *Inquiry,* 7, 4 (December 1970): 17-24.

247. ______ "Medical Care Cost Incentives: Some Questions and Approaches for Research." *Inquiry*, Dec. 1968, pp. 3-13.

248. Lew, I. "Day of Week and Other Variables Affecting Hospital Admissions, Discharges, and Length of Stay for Patients in the Pittsburgh Area." *Inquiry*, Feb. 1966, p. 3-39.

249. Lin J.P-T; Goodkin, R.; et al. "Radioionated Serum Albumin (RISA) Cisternography in the Diagnosis of Incisural Block and Occult Hydrocephalus." *Radiology*, Jan. 1968, pp. 36-41.

250. Lindsay, C.M. "Option Demand and Consumer's Surplus." *Quarterly Jour. Econ.*, May 1969, pp. 344-46.

251. Lipsey, R.G., and Lancaster, K. "The General Theory of the Second Best." *Review of Economic Studies* 24, 1 (1956-57): 11-32.

252. Llewelyn-Davies, Lord. "Facilities and Equipment for Health Services: Needed Research." *M.M.F.Q.*, July 1966, Part 2, pp. 249-72.

253. Lombroso, C.T. et al. "Two-Dimensional Ultrasonography: A Method to Study Normal and Abnormal Ventricles." *Pediatrics*, July 1968, pp. 157-74.

254. London, M., and Sigmond, R.M. "How Weekends and Holidays Affect Occupancy." *The Modern Hosp.*, Aug. 1961, p. 80.

255. Long, M.F. "Collective-Consumption Services of Individual-Consumption Good: Comment." *Quarterly Jour. of Econ.*, May 1967, pp. 351-53.

256. ______"Efficient Use of Hospitals." In *The Economics of Health and Medical Care*. Ann Arbor: The University of Michigan 1964, pp. 211-26.

257. Long, M.F., and Feldstein, P.J. "Economics of Hospital Systems: Peak Loads and Regional Coordination." *A.E.R.*, May 1967, pp. 119-29.

258. Lorber, J., and Zachary, R.B., "Primary Congenital Hydrocephalus." *Arch. Dis. Childh.* 43 (1968): 516-27.

259. Luck, E. "The Problem of Duplicate Coverage and Overinsurance." *Inquiry*, Aug. 1963, p. 28.

260. Lytton, H.D. "Recent Productivity Trends in the Federal Government, An Exploratory Study." *Review of Econ. and Stat.*, Nov. 1959, p. 341.

261. Mabry, John H. "International Studies of Health Care." *Medical Care* 9, (May-June 1971): 193-202.

262. MacEachern, M.T. *Hospital Organization and Management*. Chicago: Physicians Record Co. 1935.

263. Mack, R.W. "Theoretical and Substantive Biases in Sociological Research." In M. Sherif and C.W. Sherif (eds.) *Interdisciplinary Relationships in the Social Sciences*. Chicago: Aldine 1969, pp. 52-64.

264. Mack, R.P. "Comments." In S.B. Chase (ed.) *Problems in Public Expenditure Analysis*. Washington, D.C.: Brookings Institution 1968, pp. 213-22.

265. Mann, J.K., and Yett, D.E. "The Analysis of Hospital Costs: A Review Article." *Jour. of Business*, Apr. 1968, pp. 191-202.

266. Manning, H.E. "The Future Governance of Public Hospitals." *Bull. N.Y. Acad. of Medicine*, July 1967, p. 707-12.

266a. March, J.G., and Simon, H.A. *Organizations*. New York: Wiley 1958.

267. Martin, Nancy. "Already There's Something Better Than Peer Review." *Medical Economics*, November 23, 1970, pp. 35-46.

268. May, J. Joel. "Physician Productivity and the Hospital: An Introduction." *Inquiry*, 5 (September 1969): 57-58.

269. *Measurement of Personnel Health Expenditures*. N.C.H.S. Series 2, No. 2. Washington, D.C.: U.S. Dept. of H.E.W., P.H.S., 1963.

270. *Medical Care for Low Income Families*. Special Issue. *Inquiry*, March 1968.

271. *Medical Care Prices*. A Report to the President. By the Department of H.E.W. (Washington, D.C., Feb. 1967.) (The "Gorham Report")

272. *Medicare and Medicaid: Problems, Issues, and Alternatives*. Staff Report, Committee on Finance, U.S. Senate, Washington, D.C., Feb. 9, 1970.

273. Metzner, C.A., and Winter, K. *Institutional Care for the Long Term Patient*. Ann Arbor: Bureau of Public Health Economics 1958.

274. Mishan, E.J. "Reflections on Recent Developments in the Concept of External Effects." *Canadian Jour. of Econ. and Pol. Science*, Feb. 1965. Reprinted in E.J. Mishan, *Welfare Economics*. New York: Random House, 1964, pp. 98-154.

275. ______ "A Survey of Welfare Economics, 1939-1959." *Econ. Jour.*, June 1960, pp. 197-265.

276. Miller, J.P. *Pricing of Military Procurements*. New Haven: Yale University Press, 1949.

277. Mohring, H. "Urban Highway Investment." In R. Dorfman (ed.) *Measuring the Benefits of Government Investment*. Washington, D.C.: Brookings Institution, 1965, pp. 231-91.

278. Monsma, George N., Jr. "Marginal Revenue and the Demand for Physicians' Services." In Herbert E. Klarman (ed.) *Empirical Studies in Health Economics*, Proceedings of the Second Conference on the Economics of Health. Baltimore, Md.: The Johns Hopkins Press, 1970, pp. 145-60.

279. Montias, J.M. "Socialist Operational Price Systems: Comment." *A.E.R.*, Dec. 1963, pp. 1085-93.

280. Montias, J.M. *Central Planning in Poland*. New Haven: Yale University Press, 1962.

281. "More Hospital Centered Practice Ahead." A Panel Discussion, *Medical Economics*, Feb. 19, 1968, pp. 75-82.

282. Morrill, R.L., and Earickson, R. "Variation in the Character and Use of Chicago Area Hospitals," *H.S.R.*, Fall 1968, pp. 224-38.

283. Muller, C.E. "Outpatient Drug Prescribing Related to Clinic Utilization in Four New York City Hospitals." *H.S.R.*, Summer 1968, pp. 142-54.

284. Muller, C.E. "Complexity of Surgery as a Factor in Patients' Hospital Bills." *Medical Care*, Mar.-Apr. 1967, pp. 100-16.

285. Muller, Charlotte E., and Worthington, Paul. "Factors Entering into Capital Decisions of Hospitals." Paper delivered at the Second Conference on the Economics of Health. Published in Herbert E. Klarman (ed.) with assistance of Helen H. Jaszi. *Empirical Studies in Health Economics*. Proceedings of the Second Conference on the Economics of Health. Baltimore, Md.: The Johns Hopkins Press, 1970, pp. 399-415.

286. Muller, C.E. and Worthington, P. "The Time Structure of Capital Formation: Design and Construction of Municipal Hospital Projects." *Inquiry*, June 1969, pp. 42-52.

287. Muller, C.E.; Herbst, M.; and Westheimer, R. "Use and Cost of Drugs for Inpatients in Four New York City Hospitals." *Medical Care*, Sept.-Oct. 1967, pp. 294-312.

288. Musgrave, R.A. *The Theory of Public Finance*. New York: McGraw-Hill, 1959.

289. Mushkin, S.J. "Why Health Economics?" In *The Economics of Health and Medical Care*. Ann Arbor: The University of Michigan, 1964, pp. 3-13.

290. Mushkin, S.J., and Collings, F. d'A. "Economic Costs of Disease and Injury." *Public Health Reports*, Sept. 1959, pp. 795-809.

291. Myers, Beverlee A. "Health Maintenance Organizations: Issues for Neighborhood Health Centers." Paper presented at the Workshop for Directors, Staff, and Board of Neighborhood Health Centers sponsored by the Group Health Association of America and National Association of Neighborhood Health Centers, Washington, D.C., April 13, 1971.

292. McCall, J.J. "The Simple Economics of Incentive Contracting." *A.E.R.* 60, 5 (December 1970): 837-46.

293. McKean, R.N. "The Use of Shadow Prices." In S.B. Chase (ed.) *Problems in Public Expenditure Analysis*. Washington, D.C.: Brookings Institution, 1968, pp. 33-64.

294. McKinney, S. "Hospital Statistics–Are We Asking the Right Questions?" *Inquiry*, Dec. 1966, pp. 28-34.

295. McNerney, W.J. "M.D.'s Need Incentives for Medical Efficiency," an interview. *Medical Economics*, Nov. 10, 1969, p. 25 ff.

296. McNerney, W.J. "Does America Need a New Health System?" Paper delivered to the Detroit Economic Club, Feb. 3, 1969. (Reproduced.)

297. Nash, R.M., and Gregg, R.D. "Discrimination and Its Effects on Hospital Effectiveness." *Medical Care Review*, November 1968, pp. 853-88.

298. Navarro, Vicente; Parker, Rodger; and White, Kerr L. "A Stochastic and Deterministic Model of Medical Care Utilization." *H.S.R.* 5, 4 (Winter 1970): 342-57.

299. Nelson, Phillip. "Information and Consumer Behavior." *Journal of Political Economy* 78, 2 (March/April 1970): 311-29.

300. Neuhauser, Duncan. "Evidence of Change." In George Bugbee (ed.) *Urban Community Hospital in Transition*. Proceedings of the Twelfth Annual Symposium on Hospital Affairs, April 1970. Conducted by the Graduate Program in Hospital Administration and Center for Health Administration Studies, Graduate School of Business, University of Chicago.

301. Newhouse, Joseph P. "The Economics of Group Practice." P. 4478-1, Santa Monica: The RAND Corporation, February 1971.

302. ______ "Toward a Theory of Nonprofit Institutions: An Economic Model of a Hospital." *A.E.R.* 60, 1 (May 1970): 64-74.

303. ______ "A Model of Physician Pricing." *The Southern Journal of Economics* 37, 2 (October 1970): 174-83. Reprinted in *RAND Paper* P-4011-2, Feb. 1971.

304. ______ *Toward a Rational Allocation of Resources in Medical Care.* Ph.D. dissertation, Harvard University, 1968.

305. Newhouse, Joseph, and Taylor, Vincent. "The Subsidy Problem in Hospital Insurance." *The Journal of Business* (University of Chicago), 43, 4 (October 1970).

306. ______ "A New Type of Hospital Insurance: A Proposal for an Ex-

periment." October 1970, P-4485. Santa Monica, California: The RAND Corporation.

307. ——"The Economics of Moral Hazard: Further Comment." P-4080-1, August 1969. Santa Monica: The RAND Corporation.

308. Newell, D.J. "Problems in Estimating the Demand for Hospital Beds." *J. Chronic. Dis.*, Sept. 1964, p. 749.

309. Newman, P. *An Analysis of the Factors Involved in the Costs of Health Services and Commodities from 1929 Through 1963 And a Projection of These Costs Through 1975.* Ph.D. dissertation, New York University, 1967.

310. *New York City and Its Hospitals: A Study of the Roles of Municipal and Voluntary Hospitals Serving New York City.* Report of the Commission on Health Services, Hospital Council of Greater New York. New York, July 20, 1960.

311. Norman, John C. "Medicine in the Ghetto." *New England Journal of Medicine* 281, 23 (Dec. 4, 1969): 1271-75.

312. Nulsen, F.E., and Becker, D.P. "Control of Hydrocephalus by Valve Regulated Shunt." *Jour. of Neurosurgery* 26 (1967): 362-74.

313. Ohlen, R.B. "Seven-Day Versus a Five-Day Week–A Comparative Utilization Analysis." *Hospital Topics* 47 (December 1969): 26-32.

314. Packer, Arnold H., and Shellard, Gordon D. "Measures of Health-System Effectiveness." *Operations Research* 18, 6 (Nov.-Dec. 1970): 1067-70.

315. Palmiere, D. "The General Hospital as a Community Institution." Unpublished paper, January, 1969 (Ann Arbor).

316. Patierno, R.T. "Progressive Patient Care–The Practical Answer to Rising Hospital Costs." *Phys. Ther.*, Mar. 1968, pp. 234-36.

317. Pauly, M.V. "Efficiency, Incentives and Reimbursement for Health Care." *Inquiry* 7, 1 (March 1970): 114-31.

318. Pauly, M.V. "The Economics of Moral Hazard: Comment." *A.E.R.*, June 1968, pp. 531-37.

319. Pauly, M.V. "Efficiency in Public Provision of Medical Care." Ph.D. dissertation, University of Virginia, 1967. Published in revised version as *Medical Care at Public Expense.* New York: Praeger, 1971.

320. Pauly, M.V., and Drake, D.F. "Effects of Third Party Methods of Reimbursement on Hospital Performance." Paper delivered at the Second Conference on the Economics of Health. In Herbert E. Klarman (ed.) with assistance of Helen H. Jaszi. *Empirical Studies in Health Economics.* Proceedings of the Second Conference on the Economics of Health. Baltimore, Md.: The Johns Hopkins Press, 1970, pp. 297-314.

321. Payne, B.C. *Hospital Utilization Review Manual.* Michigan State Medical Society, June, 1966 (Reproduced).

322. ——"Use of the Criteria Approach to Measurement of Hospital Utilization." *A Handbook for the Medical Staff.* Chicago: American Medical Association, 1965.

323. Peck, M.J., and Scherer, F.M. *The Weapons Acquisition Process.* Boston: 1962.

324. Pellegrind, E.D. "Regionalization–An Integrated Effort of Medical School, Community, and Practicing Physician." *Bull. N.Y. Acad. Med.,* Dec. 1966, pp. 1193-1200.

325. Penchansky, R. and Rosenthal, G. "Productivity, Price, and Income in the Physicians' Services Market–A Tentative Hypothesis." *Medical Care*, Oct.-Dec. 1965, pp. 240-44.

326. (Piel, G.) *Community Health Services for New York City*, Report and Staff Studies of the Commission on the Delivery of Personal Health Services. New York: Praeger, 1969.

327. ______"Public Authority and Voluntary Initiative in New York City's Health Services, I and II." *New York Medicine*, August 1969, pp. 346-49, and Sept. 1969, pp. 381-84.

328. *Pilot Study on Patient Charge Statistics.* N.C.H.S. Series 2, No. 28. Washington, D.C.: Dept. of H.E.W., P.H.S., 1968.

329. Piore, N. "Metropolitan Areas and Public Medical Care." In *The Economics of Health and Medical Care.* Ann Arbor: The University of Michigan, 1964, p, 60-71.

330. Platt, R.D. "Utilization of Facilities for Heart Surgery." *N. Engl. J. Med.* 284 (June 17, 1971): 1386-87.

331. Pollack, Jerome. "The Voice of the Consumer: Cost, Quality, and Organization of Medical Services." In John H. Knowles (ed.) *Hospitals, Doctors, and the Public Interest.* Cambridge, Mass.: Harvard University Press, 1965, pp. 167-86.

332. Pryor, F.L. *Public Expenditures in Communist and Capitalist Nations.* Illinois: Irwin, 1968.

333. Rafferty, John A. "Patterns of Hospital Use: An Analysis of Short-Run Variations." *Journal of Political Economy* 79, 1 (January/February 1971): 154-65.

334. Ravitch, M.M. "The Anachronistic City Hospital." *Med. Times*, Mar. 1968, pp. 328-31.

335. Rayack, E. *Professional Power and American Medicine.* Cleveland: The World Publishing Co., 1967.

336. Reder, Melvin W. "Economies of Scale in Medical Practice: Comment." In Herbert E. Klarman (ed.) with assistance of Helen H. Jaszi. *Empirical Studies in Health Economics.* Proceedings of the Second Conference on the Economics of Health. Baltimore and London: The Johns Hopkins Press, 1970, pp. 274-77.

337. ______"Some Problems in the Measurement of Productivity in the Medical Care Industry." In V.R. Fuchs (ed.) *Production and Productivity in the Service Industries.* New York: N.B.E.R., 1969, pp. 95-131.

338. ______"Reply." In V.R. Fuchs (ed.) *Production and Productivity in the Service Industries.* New York: N.B.E.R., 1969), pp. 148-53.

339. ______"Some Problems in the Economics of Hospitals." *A.E.R.*, May 1965, pp. 472-80.

340. *Report of the National Advisory Commission on Health Manpower*, Volume I, Washington, D.C., 1967.

341. *Report of the National Conference on Medical Costs.* Washington, D.C.: U.S. Dept. of H.E.W., 1967.

342. Revans, R.W. "Research into Hospital Management and Organization." *M.M.F.Q.*, July 1966, Part 2, pp. 207-48.

343. Rice, D.P. "Estimating the Cost of Illness." *A.J.P.H.*, Mar. 1967, p. 424-40.

344. ______*Estimating the Cost of Illness.* P.H.S. Publication No. 947-63. Washington, D.C., 1966.

345. ______*Economic Costs of Cardiovascular Diseases and Cancer, 1962.* H.E.S. Series 5, P.H.S. Publication No. 947-5. Washington, D.C., 1965.

346. Rice, R.S. "Analysis of the Hospital as an Economic Organism." *The Modern Hospital*, April 1966, pp. 87-91.

347. Riedel, D.C., and Fitzpatrick, T.B. *Patterns of Patient Care.* Ann Arbor: The University of Michigan, 1964.

348. Ro, K.-k. "Incremental Pricing Would Increase Efficiency in Hospitals." *Inquiry*, Mar. 1969, pp. 28-36.

349. ______"Patient Characteristics, Hospital Characteristics and Hospital Use." *Medical Care*, July-Aug. 1969, pp. 295-312.

350. ______"Determinants of Hospital Costs." *Yale Economic Essays*, 1968, pp. 185-257.

351. Ro, K-k. and Auster, R. "An Output Approach to Incentive Reimbursement for Hospitals." *H.S.R.*, Fall 1969, pp. 177-87.

352. Robertson, R.L. "Issues in Measuring the Economic Effects of Personal Health Services." *Medical Care*, Nov.-Dec. 1967, pp. 362-68.

353. Roemer, M.I. "Bed Supply and Hospitalization: Natural Experiment." *Hospitals*, Nov. 1, 1961, pp. 35-42.

354. ______"Hospital Utilization and the Supply of Physicians." *J.A.M.A.*, Dec. 9, 1961, pp. 989-93.

355. ______"How Medical Judgment Affects Hospital Admissions." *Modern Hospital*, April 1960, p. 142.

356. Roemer, M.I., and DuBois, D.M. "Medical Costs in Relation to the Organization of Ambulatory Care." *New Eng. J. Med.*, May 1, 1969, pp. 988-93.

357. Roemer, M.I.; Moustafa, A.T.; and Hopkins, C.E. "A Proposed Hospital Quality Index: Hospital Death Rates Adjusted for Case Severity." *H.S.R.*, Summer 1968, pp. 96-118.

358. Rorem, C.R. "Capital Financing for Hospitals." Health and Hospital Planning Council of Southern New York, Inc. New York, 1968.

359. Rosenthal, Gerald. "Price Elasticity of Demand for Short-Term General Hospital Services." Paper delivered at the Second Conference on the Economics

of Health. Published in Herbert E. Klarman (ed.) *Empirical Studies in Health Economics*. Proceedings of the Second Conference on the Economics of Health. Baltimore, Md.: The Johns Hopkins Press, 1970, pp. 101-117.

360. Rosenthal, G.D. *The Demand for General Hospital Facilities.* Hospital Monograph Series No. 14 Chicago: American Hospital Association, 1964.

361. Rothenberg, Jerome. "Comment." In Herbert E. Klarman (ed.) with assistance of Helen H. Jaszi. *Empirical Studies in Health Economics*. Proceedings of the Second Conference on the Economics of Health. Baltimore, Md.: The Johns Hopkins Press, 1970, pp. 222-28.

362. Rottenberg, S. "The Allocation of Biomedical Research." *A.E.R.*, May 1967, pp. 109-118.

363. Rourke, A.J.J. "Utilization Review May be More Effective Than Believed." *Modern Hospital* 117, 2 (August 1971): 137.

364. Ruggles, N. "Recent Developments in the Theory of Marginal Cost Pricing." *Review of Economic Studies* 17 (1949-50): 107-26, reprinted in R. Turvey. *Public Enterprise.* New York: Penguin Books, 1968.

365. Ruffin, Roy J., and Leigh, Duane E. "Charity, Competition, and the Pricing of Doctors' Services." The University of Iowa and Washington State University, 1971.

366. Runyan, J.W. Jr.; Phillips, W.E.; Herring, O.; et al. "A Program for the Care of Patients with Chronic Diseases." *Jour. of the American Medical Association* 211 (January 19, 1970): 476-79.

367. Russell, Louise B., and Davis, Karen. "The Demand for Outpatient Care: Time Series Evidence." Social Security Administration, April 1971.

368. Saathoff, Donald D., and Kurtz, Richard A. "Cost per Day Comparisons Don't do the Job." *The Modern Hospital* 99, 4 (October 1962): 14-16.

369. Sanazaro, P.J., and Williamson, J. "End-Results of Patient Care." *Medical Care*, March-April 1968, p. 128.

370. Schneider, J.B. "Measuring the Locational Efficiency of the Urban Hospital." *H.S.R.*, Summer 1967, pp. 154-69.

371. ______ *Planning the Growth of a Metropolitan System of Public Service Facilities: The Case of Short Term General Hospitals.* Ph.D. dissertation, University of Pennsylvania, 1966.

372. Schonfeld, H.K. "The Development of Standards for the Audit and Planning of Medical Care: Audit of Hospital Outpatient Care." Paper delivered at the Conference on Auditing Outpatient Care, University Hospitals, Minneapolis, Minn., March 29, 1968.

373. Schonfeld, H.K.; Falk, I.S.; et al. "The Development of Standards for the Audit and Planning of Medical Care: Good Pediatric Care–Program Content and Methods of Estimating Needed Personnel." *A.J.P.H.*, Nov. 1968, pp. 2097-2110.

374. Schultze, C.L. *The Politics and Economics of Public Spending.* Washington, D.C.: Brookings Institution, 1968.

375. Schwartz, Jerome L. "Early Histories of Selected Neighborhood Health Centers." *Inquiry* 7, 4 (December 1970): 3-16.

376. Schwartzman, D. "Uncertainty and the Size of the Firm." *Economica*, N.S., Aug. 1963, pp. 287-96.

377. Scitovsky, A.A. "Changes in the Costs of Selected Illnesses." *A.E.R.*, Dec. 1967, pp. 1182-95.

378. *Secretary's Advisory Committee on Hospital Effectiveness, Report*. Washington, D.C.: U.S. Dept. of H.E.W., 1968.

379. Seeman, M., and Evans, J.W. "Stratification and Hospital Care: II. The Objective Criteria of Performance." *American Sociological Review*, April 1961, pp. 193-204. Reprinted in W.R. Scott, and E.H. Volkart, *Medical Care*. New York: Wiley, 1966, pp. 488-501.

380. Shain, M., and Roemer, M.I. "Hospitals and the Public Interest." *Pub. Health Rep.*, May 1961, pp. 401-10.

381. ______ "Hospital Costs Relate to the Supply of Beds." *Modern Hospital*, April 1959.

382. Shapiro, S. "The Outcomes of Care Provided Through Prepayment Organized Practice." Paper delivered at the 97th Annual Meeting of APHA, Nov. 9, 1969.

383. ______ "Group Practice Plans in Governmental Medical Care Programs: III. Serving Medicaid Eligibles." *A.J.P.H.* 59, 4 (April 1969): 635-41.

384. Schelton, D.S.; Schesinger, R.H.; and Fibiger, H.W. "Bed Utilization." *Phys. Ther.* 48 (March 1968): pp. 228-30.

385. Sheps, Cecil G. "Trends in Hospital Care." *Inquiry* 8, 1 (March 1971): 27-31.

386. Shortell, Stephen M., and Anderson, Odin W. "The Physician Referral Process: A Theoretical Perspective." *H.S.R.* 6, 1 (Spring 1971): 39-48.

387. Shubik, Martin. "A Curmedgeon's Guide to Microeconomics." *Journal of Economic Literature* 8, 2 (June 1970): 405-34.

388. Silver, Morris. "An Economic Analysis of Variations in Medical Expenses and Work-Loss Rates." In Herbert E. Klarman (ed.) with assistance of Helen H. Jaszi. *Empirical Studies in Health Economics*. Proceedings of the Second Conference on the Economics of Health. Baltimore and London: The Johns Hopkins Press, 1970, pp. 121-40.

389. Sigmond, R.M. "Sources of Capital Investment in Health Care Facilities." In *Costs of Health Care Facilities*. Report of a Conference Convened by the National Academy of Engineering, National Academy of Sciences. Washington, D.C., 1968, pp. 66-80.

390. ______ "Capitation as a Method of Reimbursement to Hospitals in a Multihospital Area." In *Reimbursement Incentives for Hospital and Medical Care* Washington, D.C.: U.S. Dept. of H.E.W., S.S.A. Research Report No. 26, 1968, pp. 49-60.

391. Skinner, C.G. "Hospitals and Allied Institutions." In W.J. McNerney

Hospital and Medical Economics, Vol. II. Chicago: Hospital Research and Educational Trust, 1962.

392. Sloan, R.P. *This Hospital Business of Ours.* New York: Putnam, 1952.

393. Smith, C.A. "Survey of the Empirical Evidence on Economies of Scale." In *Business Concentration and Price Policy*. Princeton: Princeton University Press, 1955, pp. 213-30.

394. Smith, H.L. "Two Lines of Authority: The Hospital's Dilemma." *The Modern Hospital*, March 1955. Reprinted in E.G. Jaco (ed.) *Patients, Physicians, and Illness*. New York: Free Press, 1958, pp. 468-77.

395. Somers, Anne R. "The Rationalization of Health Services: A Universal Priority." *Inquiry* 8, 1 (March 1971): 48-60.

396. ——— *Hospital Regulation: The Dilemma of Public Policy*. Princeton, N.J.: Industrial Relations Section, Princeton University, 1969.

397. ——— "Hospital Costs and Payment: Suggestions for Stabilizing the Uneasy Balance." *Medical Care* 7, 5 (September-October 1969): 348-60.

398. ———"Some Basic Determinants of Medical Care and Health Policy: An Overview of Trends and Issues." *H.S.R.*, Fall 1966, pp. 193-209.

399. Somers, Herman M. "Delivery of Health Care: Do We Know Where We Are Going?" In George F. Rohrlich (ed.) *Social Economics for the 1970's*. Cambridge: University Press of Cambridge, Mass. and New York: The Dunellen Company, Inc., 1970, pp. 99-113.

400. ———"Financing of Medical Care in the United States." *New Eng. J. Med.*, Sept. 29, 1966, pp. 702-09.

401. Somers, H.M., and Somers, A.R. *Medicare and the Hospitals*. Washington, D.C.: Brookings Institution, 1967.

402. ——— *Doctors, Patients, and Health Insurance*. Washington, D.C.: Brookings Institution, 1962.

403. Stambaugh, J.L. "A Study of the Sources of Capital Funds for Hospital Construction in the United States." *Inquiry*, June 1967, pp. 3-22.

404. Steep, M.A., and Tilley, T.J. "Outpatient Diagnostic Benefits and the Effects on Inpatient Experience: A Three Part Study." *Inquiry*, June 1965, pp. 3-12.

405. Steinberg, M.R. "Hospital Charges Are Much Too Low." An interview. *Medical Economics*, March 17, 1969, pp. 218-35.

406. Stenn, F. "Seven-Day Utilization of the Hospital." *Illinois Med. Jour.*, July, 1968, p. 51.

407. Stevens, C.N. "Hospital Market Efficiency: The Anatomy of the Supply Response." Paper delivered at the Second Conference on the Economics of Health. Published in Herbert E. Klarman (ed.) with assistance of Helen H. Jaszi. *Empirical Studies in Health Economics*. Proceedings of the Second Conference on the Economics of Health. Baltimore, Md.: The Johns Hopkins Press, 1970, pp. 229-48.

408. Stewart, Charles T., Jr. "Allocation of Resources to Health." *The Journal of Human Resources* 6, 1 (Winter 1971): 104-22.

409. Stiefel, J.B. "Use and Costs of AHS Coordinated Home Care Programs." *Inquiry*, Oct. 1967, pp. 61-68.

410. Stigler, George J. "The Theory of Economic Regulation." *The Bell Journal of Economics and Management Science* 2, 1 (Spring 1971): 3-21.

411. Strauss, A.L. "Medical Organization, Medical Care and Lower Income Groups." *Soc. Sci. & Med.* 3 (1969): 143-77.

412. Swartzman, Gordon. "The Patient Arrival Process in Hospitals: Statistical Analysis." *H.S.R.* 5, 4 (Winter 1970): 320-29.

413. Taylor, Vincent. "How Much is Good Health Worth?" Santa Monica: the RAND Corporation, P-3945, July 1969.

414. ______"The Price of Hospital Care." P-4090, Santa Monica: The RAND Corporation, May 1969.

415. (Teamster Reports, 1.) *The Quantity, Quality and Costs of Medical and Hospital Care Secured by a Sample of Teamster Families in the New York Area.* New York: Columbia University School of Public Health and Administrative Medicine, 1962.

416. (Teamster Reports, 2.) *A Study of the Quality of Hospital Care Secured by a Sample of Teamster Family Members in New York City.* New York: Columbia University School of Public Health and Administrative Medicine, 1964.

417. Teng, Clarence. "The New York City Health Budget in Program Terms." RM-5774-NYC, Santa Monica: The RAND Corporation, May 1969.

418. Terenzio, Joseph V., and Manning, Henry E. "New York City." *Hospitals* 44, 13 (July 1, 1970): 65-69, 72-75.

419. Torrens, Paul R., and Yedvab, Donna G. "Variations Among Emergency Room Populations: A Comparison of Four Hospitals in New York City." *Medical Care* 8, 1 (January-February 1970): 60-75.

420. Trussel, R.E. et al. *Family Medical Care Under Three Types of Health Insurance.* New York: Foundation on Employee Health, Medical Care and Welfare, Inc., 1962.

421. Turvey, R. "On Divergences Between Social Cost and Private Cost." *Economica*, N.S., Aug. 1963, pp. 309-13.

422. Tyroler, H.A. "The Classification of Disease." In Merwyn R. Greenlick (ed.) *Conceptual Issues in the Analysis of Medical Care Utilization Behavior.* Dept. of H.E.W., Public Health Service, Hlth. Svcs. & Ment. Hlth. Admin., October 1969, pp. 33-57.

423. Vickrey, W. "Some Implications of Marginal Cost Pricing for Public Utilities." *A.E.R.* 45 (May 1955): 605.

424. Wakar, A., and Zielinski, J. "Socialist Operational Price Systems." *A.E.R.*, Mar. 1963, pp. 109-27.

425. Waldman, S., " 'Average Increase in Costs'—An Incentive Reimbursement Formula for Hospitals." In *Reimbursement Incentives for Hospital and Medical Care.* U.S. Dept. of H.E.W., S.S.A., Research Report No. 26, Washington, D.C., 1968, pp. 39-48.

426. Warren, R.L. *Patient Profiles*. Buffalo: Hospital Review and Planning Council of Western New York, 1965.

427. Weinerman, E. Richard. "Research on Comparative Health Service Systems." *Medical Care*, 9, 3 (May-June 1971): 272-90.

428. Weinerman, E.R. "Changing Patterns of Medical Care: Their Implications for Ambulatory Services." *Hospitals, J.A.H.A.*, Dec. 16, 1965, p. 67.

429. Weinerman, E.R. et al. "Yale Studies in Ambulatory Medical Care V. Determinants of Use of Hospital Emergency Services." *A.J.P.H.*, 1966. Reprinted in *Medical Care in Transition, Reprints from the American Journal of Public Health*, Vol. III. Washington, D.C.: U.S. Dept. of H.E.W., P.H.S., 1967, pp. 397-416.

430. Weisbrod, B.A., "Income Redistribution Effects and Cost-Benefit Analysis." In S.B. Chase (ed.) *Problems in Public Expenditure Analysis*. Washington, D.C.: Brookings Institution, 1968, pp. 177-208.

431. ______"Some Problems of Pricing and Resource Allocation in a Non-Profit Industry–The Hospitals." *Jour. of Business*, Jan. 1965, pp. 18-28.

432. ______"Collective-Consumption Services of Individual-Consumption Goods." *Quarterly Jour. of Econ.*, Aug. 1964, pp. 471-77.

433. Wessen, A.F. "Hospital Ideology and Communication Between Ward Personnel." In E.G. Jaco (ed.) *Patients, Physicians and Illness*. New York: Free Press, 1958, pp. 448-68.

434. Williamson, O.E. "A Dynamic Stochastic Theory of Managerial Behavior." In A. Phillips, and O.E. Williamson, (eds.) *Prices: Issues in Theory, Practice, and Public Policy*. Philadelphia: University of Pennsylvania Press, 1967, pp. 11-31.

435. ______"Peak-Load Pricing and Optimal Capacity Under Indivisibility Constraints." *A.E.R.*, September 1966, pp. 810-27.

436. Willis, J.T. "The Community Hospital Concept for the Charity Hospital System in Louisiana and the Impact of 'Medicare and Medicaid' on its Implementation." *J. Louisiana, Med. Soc.*, May 1967, pp. 187-92.

437. Wilson, Glenn. "The Organizational Structure of a Comprehensive Medical Care Program in a University Medical Center." *A.J.P.H.* 61, 5 (May 1971): 957-61.

438. Wilson, R.N. "The Physician's Changing Hospital Role." *Human Organization.* Winter, 1959-60, pp. 177-83. Reprinted in W.R. Scott and E.H. Volkart. *Medical Care.* New York: Wiley, 1966, pp. 406-20.

439. Wing, Paul, and Blumberg, Mark S. "Operating Expenditures and Sponsored Research at U.S. Medical Schools: An Empirical Study of Cost Patterns." *The Journal of Human Resources* 6, 1 (Winter 1971); 75-102.

440. Wirick, G., Jr. *Health Care Facility and Personnel Needs: An Annotated Bibliography*. Bureau of Hospital Administration. Ann Arbor: University of Michigan, 1966.

441. Wolkstein, I. "Incentive Reimbursement Plans Offer a Variety of Approaches to Cost Control." *Hospitals* 43 (June 16, 1969): 63-67.

442. Wolkstein, I. "The Legislative History of Hospital Reimbursement." In *Reimbursement Incentives for Hospital and Medical Care.* U.S. Dept. of H.E.W., S.S.A., Research Report No. 26 Washington, D.C., 1968, pp. 1-16.

443. Yett, Donald E. "Causes and Consequences of Salary Differentials in Nursing." *Inquiry* 7, 1 (March 1970): 78-99.

444. Yett, D.E. "An Evaluation of Alternative Methods of Estimating Physicians' Expenses Relative to Output." *Inquiry* (March 1967); 3-27.

445. Young, J.P. "A Conceptual Framework for Hospital Administrative Decision System." *H.S.R.*, Summer 1968, pp. 79-95.

446. Zemach, Rita. "A Model of Health-Service Utilization and Resource Allocation." *Operations Research*, 18, 6 (Nov.-Dec. 1970): 1071-86.

Index

About the Author

Born in Budapest, Hungary, in 1930, **Sylvester E. Berki** came to the United States in 1946. After six years as a professional soldier he entered Columbia University from which he received the B.S. *(magna cum laude)*. He did his graduate work in Economics at Yale where he was a Ford Fellow in 1960-61. During 1963-67 he was Assistant Professor in the Economics Department and the Sloan Institute of Hospital Administration at Cornell University. Since 1967 he has been in the Department of Medical Care Organization in the School of Public Health at the University of Michigan, where he is currently Associate Professor.

Professor Berki has been a consultant to the Urban Institute and the Institute of Medicine of the National Academy of Sciences. His publications on national health insurance have appeared in *Inquiry* and the *Annals* of the American Academy of Political and Social Science.